T0143237

# A Plague of Paradoxes

Worlds of Desire
The Chicago Series on Sexuality, Gender, and Culture
Edited by Gilbert Herdt

# A
# Plague
# of
# **Paradoxes**

## AIDS, Culture, and Demography
## in Northern Tanzania

## Philip W. Setel

THE UNIVERSITY OF CHICAGO PRESS

*Chicago & London*

Philip W. Setel is senior research associate at the University of Newcastle upon Tyne School of Medicine and project director of the Adult Morbidity and Mortality Project.

The University of Chicago Press, Chicago 60637
The University of Chicago Press, Ltd., London
© 1999 by The University of Chicago
All rights reserved. Published 1999
08 07 06 05 04 03 02 01 00 99      5 4 3 2 1

ISBN (cloth): 0-226-74885-5
ISBN (paper): 0-226-74886-3

Library of Congress Cataloging-in-Publication Data

Setel, Philip.
    A plague of paradoxes : AIDS, culture, and demography in northern
Tanzania / Philip W. Setel.
        p.      cm. — (Worlds of desire)
    Includes bibliographical references and index.
    ISBN 0-226-74885-5. — ISBN 0-226-74886-3 (pbk.)
    1. AIDS (Disease)—Tanzania.   2. Chaga (African people)
I. Title.   II. Series.
RA644.A25S378   1999
362.1′969792′00967826—dc21                                        99-16509
                                                                                                     CIP

# Contents

# List of Illustrations

**Figures**

**Tables**

# Preface and Acknowledgments

This book was completed as the United Nations AIDS organization, UNAIDS, increased its estimate of the number of people around the globe living with HIV/AIDS from over 20 million to more than 30 million (UNAIDS 1997, 1998). Most of the affected were living in Africa. The message was clear: after more than a decade and a half of combat against the AIDS epidemic, it is growing worse. More than ever before there is a need to reassess what we know about this disease and how to mitigate its impact. If this study of AIDS in Northern Tanzania provides such an opportunity for reflection and prompts constructive action and dialogue, it will have accomplished its aims.

Elsewhere (Setel 1995a) I have thanked those whose help was crucial to this book. Some of those people have continued to be a source of guidance, support, and inspiration. In particular, I must thank the women of KIWAKKUKI—stronger than ever after nearly a decade of community-based action on AIDS—and the Lefroy, Machui, and Mrema families in Kilimanjaro. I also wish to thank again Professor M. T. Leshabari, Professor Eustace Muhondwa, and Dr. George Lwihula, of Muhimbili University College of Health Sciences, and to add thanks to Dr. Sylvia Kaaya, also of Muhimbili.

Fieldwork was made possible with the kind permission of the Tanzanian Ministry of Health, the National AIDS Control Programme (headed at the time by Dr. Klinton Nyamuryekungé), the Tanzanian Commission for Science and Technology (COSTECH), and with the support of my local counterpart in Kilimanjaro, Dr. Watoki Nkya, and his colleague Dr. William Howlett. Thanks are also due to the Urio and Mndasha families for more homes away from home than one could wish for. I was also very fortunate that Aud Talle and Donna Kerner were in the vicinity to throw a rope to an occasionally floundering neophyte fieldworker in Tanzania.

In the United States I was extremely fortunate to have the guidance of Jane Guyer, Donald Pollock, and Allan Hoben. Stephanie Spencer, Halldora Gunnarsdóttir, Nancy Abelmann, Glorian Sorensen, and Hank Bonney have also provided support from the beginning. Stacie Canning Colwell gave invaluable comments throughout the revising of the manuscript, as did Päivi Hasu, from the University of Helsinki. My mother, Susan Setel, resurrected the English teacher in her and was a punctilious proofreader. Donald Pollock, Dorothy Broom, and colleagues in the "embodiment" reading group at the Australian National University helped frame many of the theoretical issues. I have done my best not to garble their clearheaded insights. Knut-Inge Klepp gave important help on many of the sections dealing with HIV/AIDS epidemiology. Basia Zaba provided many valuable comments on the entire book, and particularly on the historical and demographic aspects of HIV/AIDS and fertility. I am particularly grateful to Gil Herdt for his enthusiasm and advice in the transformation of a disjointed doctoral thesis into the monograph that you have before you. I am also very grateful to John C. and Pat Caldwell and colleagues at the Health Transition Centre, National Centre for Epidemiology and Population Health, at the Australian National University, where much of the final manuscript was prepared. Peggy Daroesman, Bob Hefner, Dorothy Broom, Julia Byford, Ann-Maree Bortoli, Stacie Colwell, and Don Pollock provided great moral support. Thank you.

The research for this book was conducted with grants from the Social Science Research Council and American Council of Learned Societies Joint Committee on African Studies, with funds provided by the Rockefeller Foundation and by a junior fellowship grant from Health in Housing, a WHO Collaborating Center at the State University of New York at Buffalo. Much of the revision was done under a postdoctoral research fellowship for demographic anthropology funded by the Andrew W. Mellon Foundation through the Australian National University.

Finally, I must thank, as a group, the people I am so fortunate to have in my families and, in particular, my life partner and inspirer of healthy *tamaa*, Suzy. I close these prefacing remarks with words that are a constant reminder to me of the fight against AIDS and are as true today as when they were first taught to me by the women of KIWAKKUKI in 1991:

*Kwa Pamoja Tuukabili UKIMWI*

Together We Confront AIDS

# CHAPTER 1

## "Hey, Listen!"

### Starting with a Song

This is a book about an epidemic and the cultural and demographic circumstances out of which it emerged. The HIV/AIDS epidemic emerged into global consciousness in the early and mid-1980s. By 1998, more than two-thirds of the people living with HIV (Human Immuno-deficiency Virus) resided in sub-Saharan Africa (Table 1.1). Nearly 40 percent of Africa's burden of HIV/AIDS was borne by nine countries in East and Central Africa, where five and a half million people were estimated to have died. Over 11 percent of all the adults in the region—over eight million—were believed to be HIV infected. Tanzania has been among the hardest hit in the epidemic. In 1983, Tanzania recorded its first case of AIDS. In the ensuing twelve years, the country reported significantly more cases of AIDS than any other country in Africa (over 100,000) to the World Health Organization (WHO). By 1995, AIDS had become the leading cause of death among adults in at least three Tanzanian districts (Ministry of Health and AMMP 1997). At the end of 1997 the country ranked second, compared with its eight immediate neighbors, in the estimated number of infected people and estimated deaths, and seventh in estimated adult prevalence (UNAIDS 1998). As the epidemic began to take hold in the 1980s, the northern Tanzanian region of Kilimanjaro (Figure 1.1) had among the highest case rates in the country of what came to be known simply as *ugonjwa huo*, "that disease."

As the epidemic continues to exact its toll, research on its nature, origins, and meaning multiplies. New volumes on nearly every aspect of AIDS—clinical, molecular-biological, epidemiologic, and social scientific—appear daily, and still the epidemic grows (UNAIDS 1997, 1998). From a public health and social policy standpoint, the enormity

Table 1.1 Global and East and Central African AIDS Pandemics, December 1997

| | Number of People Living with HIV (est.) | Adult Prevalence (% est.) | AIDS Deaths Cumulative to 1997 (est.) |
|---|---|---|---|
| Global | | | |
| Australia and New Zealand | 12,000 | 0.11 | 7,000 |
| Eastern Europe | 190,000 | 0.09 | 5,400 |
| North Africa and Middle East | 210,000 | 0.13 | 42,000 |
| Carribean | 310,000 | 1.82 | 110,000 |
| East Asia and Pacific | 420,000 | 0.05 | 11,000 |
| Western Europe | 480,000 | 0.23 | 190,000 |
| North America | 860,000 | 0.55 | 420,000 |
| Latin America | 1,300,000 | 0.52 | 470,000 |
| South and Southeast Asia | 5,800,000 | 0.61 | 730,000 |
| Sub-Saharan Africa | 21,000,000 | 7.41 | 9,600,000 |
| TOTAL | 30,600,000 | 0.97 | 11,700,000 |
| East and Central Africa | | | |
| Burundi | 260,000 | 8.30 | 200,000 |
| Rwanda | 370,000 | 12.75 | 170,000 |
| Malawi | 710,000 | 14.92 | 450,000 |
| Zambia | 770,000 | 19.07 | 590,000 |
| Uganda | 930,000 | 9.51 | 1,800,000 |
| Democratic Republic of Congo | 950,000 | 4.35 | 470,000 |
| Mozambique | 1,200,000 | 14.17 | 250,000 |
| Tanzania | 1,400,000 | 9.42 | 940,000 |
| Kenya | 1,600,000 | 11.46 | 600,000 |
| TOTAL | 8,190,000 | 11.55 | 5,470,000 |

Source: UNAIDS 1998.

of AIDS stems from its infectiousness, incurability, and the physical, emotional, and economic hardship that it causes. From the perspective of anthropological understanding, the epidemic gains added significance because it moves along pathways that lie at the very heart of biological and social reproduction. By "social reproduction," I mean the processes, institutions, and values by which populations perpetuate themselves and their identities from generation to generation. These processes and institutions are always in flux.

Our ability to comprehend and respond to AIDS will ultimately depend on how we understand the dynamics of transmission in social and cultural context. This account focuses on how AIDS emerged at the intersection of culture, demography, and the regional political economy of Kilimanjaro. For the residents of Kilimanjaro, AIDS has been a plague of paradoxes. Paradox and irony are at the core of the social experience of the epidemic and at the center of modern life more

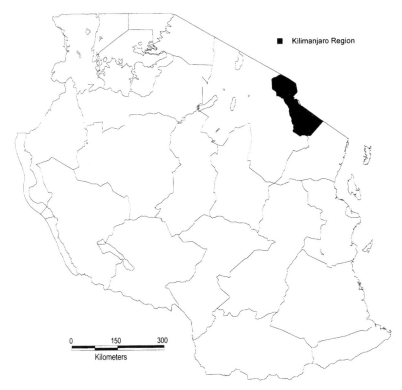

Figure 1.1. Map of Tanzania showing Kilimanjaro Region. (Philip Setel and Don de Savigny)

generally. Indeed, modernity itself contains an internal contradiction for Chagga.[1] On one hand, colonial and postcolonial institutions (such as the church and Western education) were seen as escape routes from increasingly crowded mountain slopes where, over time, fewer and fewer households could be successfully sustained by agriculture. On the other hand, these same "escape routes" came to be associated with vulnerability to AIDS.

Contemporary sexual ideologies in Kilimanjaro are tied to these contradictions: for example, so-called traditional mores are in reality based upon "imagined" values inherited from an equally imagined idea of the past. Despite clearly discernible patterns of behavior, present-day sexual culture is spoken of in terms of chaos; confusion hides the principles of the system's own internal organization. Other ironies emerge within the context of the epidemic itself. Perhaps the most dramatic example is the way in which vulnerability to HIV has been attributed to the excesses of "bad moral character" and "desire" among the young; yet vulnerability and risk are as much born out of demographic and economic necessity as individual behavior. Local concepts of "moral character" and "desire" among young people, we shall see, are profoundly contradictory aspects of the experience of AIDS in Kilimanjaro.

In addition to these cultural ironies are epidemiological and demographic ones. The tensions between sexual risk and reproductive ambitions in the age of HIV have too seldom been made explicit in AIDS research. There has been practically no research on the overlapping concerns of family planning programs and HIV/Sexually Transmitted Disease (STD) prevention (Zaba, Boerma, and Marchant 1998:3). Mitigating the effects of the HIV epidemic depends largely on finding ways of influencing both sexual *and* reproductive behavior. The link is straightforward: infection with HIV is a necessary precondition for the subsequent development of the clinical condition of AIDS.[2] HIV can be spread by any practice that brings infected body fluids from one individual into contact with the blood and/or the mucous membranes of another. In Africa sexual intercourse is by far the commonest mode of transmission (see Mann, Tarantola, and Netter 1992).[3] Clearly, patterns of sexual action and risk must be at the center of an account of AIDS in Africa. Yet the social and cultural circumstances that bring people together in the first place in most of Africa are inextricably linked to individual and group expression of reproductive agendas among very poor and economically insecure men and women, people who have extremely limited access to quality health care, culturally appropriate health education, and the technical means to protect themselves. In its fullest sense, the paradox of AIDS is that this *new* disease is enmeshed in *historically shaped* social environments. The epidemic is not a discrete event. The transformation of sex and reproduction over time, through many kinds of human agency and in many formal and informal settings, has shaped both the epidemiology of AIDS and the terms in which it is comprehended.

My objective, then, is to unravel the contradictions in contemporary sexual and reproductive life in Kilimanjaro and to demonstrate how AIDS has been experienced in this context. Cultural process and demographic change form the foundation of the analysis. In Kilimanjaro, epidemiologic and demographic accounts—both professional and popular—constitute much of the conceptual ground on which the epidemic has been played out.

The analysis of cultural experience and paradox in the age of AIDS is based upon a number of postulates. These are: that cultural practices pertaining to sexuality, social reproduction, and shifting life courses have given the epidemic substance and meaning; that the epidemic's epidemiologies are inextricably linked to demographic contexts; and that, owing in large part to the syndrome's enduring ambiguities, knowledge and experience about AIDS (again, both popular and professional) constitute essential and often competing social realities of the epidemic.

An epidemic may be seen as a social process of disorder structured in terms of person, place, and time. These concepts have cultural and scientific definitions that often overlap only partially. Following Farmer, Schoepf, and others who have used a history, political economy, and culture approach to the study of AIDS in developing countries (e.g., Kaijage 1989; Schoepf 1991b, 1992; Farmer 1992; Weiss 1993), I place the issues of "person, place, and time" in a broadly historical framework. The book moves from a model of productive and sexual/reproductive values in the past to an analysis of how AIDS related to sexual action and the predicament of productive life for young adults in the 1980s and 1990s.

In charting these changes, anthropology and demography go together. AIDS in Africa could offer no better case for the admonishment made in 1968 that "unless basic demographic variables [are] taken into account, even basic ethnography would be misleading and inadequate" (Yengoyan, paraphrased in Kertzer and Fricke 1997b:10). While epidemiologists studying AIDS often focused on a concept of risk configured in terms of individual dichotomous variables, demographers have taken a population perspective.[4] The structure of risk for AIDS in Africa, they argue, is intimately connected to forces such as mobility and fertility regimes, and the cultural forces that shape them (see, e.g., Caldwell, Caldwell, and Quiggin 1989; Larson 1989).[5]

The following song lyric foreshadows many of the issues that the rest of this book will examine. "Hey, Listen!" is a popular epidemiology that situates AIDS (or UKIMWI, in Swahili) in culturally defined terms of person, place and time.[6] It is a parable, a poem about a new disease, a warning to Tanzania's young urban lovers—especially the youth of Moshi, the city in which the song is set, and the regional capital of Kilimanjaro. The song evokes many of the components of the AIDS paradox: blame, ambiguity, confusion, vilification of young people, desire, moral character, the conundrum of older generations, and a mixture of ineptness and helplessness among medical professionals.

Above all, the song demonstrates that local ideas about AIDS and its causes were deceptively straightforward when reduced to matters of individual behavior. These ideas were based upon demonstrably inconsistent "moral discourses" about risk.[7] As Farmer (1992) has shown in Haiti, the way in which culture shapes the expression of suffering and illness has been deeply affected by colonialism and local population dynamics. And yet in Haiti, as in Kilimanjaro, "accusation—*the assertion that human agency had a role in the aetiology of AIDS*—is the dominant leitmotif" (Farmer 1992:192; emphasis added).

The song "Hey, Listen!" is an allegory of human agency—of intentions and misdeeds—in the age of AIDS. The song, largely a spoken narrative, is a story of a "Beautiful Girl." This young woman is seduced and infected with HIV by a "Young Man." In this story, symbols of wealthy urban life and modernity (such as cell phones and Volvos) stand alongside a list of modes of HIV transmission and clinical symptoms of AIDS. "Hey, Listen!" is a tale of dissembling and denial, of a hidden give-and-take. It tells of a relationship that might have seemed rather ordinary to many young Tanzanians in the early 1990s were it not for a "disease that has just been announced called UKIMWI."[8]

> Hey, Listen!
> Lovers in the streets, you!
> Lovers in the clubs, you!
> They are dangerous, I'm telling you.
> There's a disease that's just been announced called UKIMWI.
>
> Lovers in the places that serve beer, you!
> Lovers of roasted meat, you!
> Lovers in the markets, you!
> They are dangerous, I'm telling you, young man
> don't play with fire.
> Look as the waters rise, let them wash by, and then you may pass
>     in peace.
>
> The other day I was in this bar. I was just sitting there and this very good-looking guy came in the door. He was wearing this really fancy suit. He sidled up to the bar and ordered, "Hey! You have beer? Bring one fast!" It came to the table. While he was sitting there, he started to think. What he was thinking about we will never know, but just at that moment, the door of the bar opened and in walked a beautiful girl.
>
> She had on a gorgeous dress, her hair was done, she had on makeup, and her shoes cried as she walked: "kwa, kwa, kwa, kwa . . ."
>
> Young man: Ho! Today I'll be feeling better! Hey! Halloo, dahling! Dahling! I think I've seen you somewhere before . . .

Girl: Hardly. Where would that have been?

Young man: Come on, now. What will you drink? Beer, *mbege,* or soda?[9]

Girl: If I drink *mbege* it makes me cough; soda gives me gas. All I drink is the hard stuff.

Young man: Oh! Hey! Bartender! Bring two bottles of beer and some gin!

The drinks came, and while they were drinking, the young man began to boast, "Welcome! No problem with me! All the taxis here in town are my wealth; the red ones, the blue ones, the green ones, the yellow ones. Look at all the nice houses here in town. All of them are mine. Oh boy, today you are really lucky. I don't usually talk with little folks like you—only the Big Shots. So just take it easy." And he thought, "The sweetness of booze and words will get this girl asking for a ride."

Girl: Hey, brother, hey! What time am I going to get home, anyway?

Young man: No sweat. There's one of my cars—a Volvo—that always comes to pick me up and take me wherever I want to go. Today it's at your disposal, so just relax until later.

The time passed: seven, eight, nine, ten, eleven . . . and finally they heard on the radio, "This is the midnight news bulletin announced by . . ." The girl turned and said, "Hey brother, who am I going to go with tonight?"

Young man: Oh, sorry, Charlie! I forgot to tell you. Us Big Shots move around with phones in our pockets, and my phone just told me that that Volvo of mine got a puncture, so you'll have to cool it at a guest house near here; one of mine.

When they left, we do not know; where they went, we do not know; what took place, we do not know . . .

Three years passed. The girl was telling her father, "Father I feel very sick. Sometimes I cough, sometimes I vomit, sometimes I have diarrhea, or dizziness, or a fever from time to time, and my mouth is so dry. I don't even feel like eating."

Father: Go to the hospital to Mzee Kimbeleza. He'll give you medicine.

Girl: Hello? Mzee?

Mzee: Yes? What is your problem?

Girl: I'm terribly ill, but I want you to examine me to find out for yourself.

Mzee: Aha! You are pregnant.

Girl: Doctor, are you nuts? I tell you I'm sick. Give me some medicine.

Mzee: Aha! Take these. Use them for three days and come back and tell me how you're doing.

Three days pass and she returns.

Girl: Doctor, those pills were useless. So come on, give me an injection, OK?

Mzee: I have nothing else for you here, except to give you a letter to Mawenzi Hospital, where they have many experts, many tests, many medicines.

The girl left, and she prayed, "But won't I get better? God, help me!" When she left and went to Mawenzi, the doctor received her, and after examining her, he said, "We have no help for you here. I'm writing you a letter to go to KCMC where they have many experts, many tests, many medicines."[10]

She left right away for KCMC, but on the way she became confused. She entered a restaurant and was told, "Here we serve *ugali* [maize porridge]; we don't sell medicine."

Finally, she arrived, and the doctors took her letter and examined her and told her, "Sister, I'm very sad. The cure for this disease of yours is not yet available in this world. You must go and stay on Ward Sixteen for dangerous patients until you pass from this world."

Girl: But doctor! What disease do I have?

Dr.: You have the disease called UKIMWI.

Girl: Doctor, are you crazy? How could I have been infected by UKIMWI? Just look at me! What are you afraid to tell me?

Dr.: I have no problem with you. If you plant a cabbage, you will harvest a cabbage; if you plant greens, you will harvest greens; if you sow promiscuity and worldly desires . . . we have no other help for you here.

Girl: There's nothing I can give you to get rid of this?

Dr.: We don't take UKIMWI bribes here. Now get out of here, quick!

Girl: My friends! All of my jewelry and my clothing—who will wear them? My friends! Fear UKIMWI! He swore to me that we would have a proper wedding and seal the marriage, and look! He is killing me! My friends, fear UKIMWI! My friends, I am dying. Am I speaking the truth or am I deceiving you? Fear UKIMWI! UKIMWI is very dangerous. Even Kemron doesn't cure it.[11] Don't be deceived. UKIMWI has no cure! Haiyooo! . . .

Let us briefly consider the narrative content of the song, beginning with the villain: the *kijana*, the young man, the carrier of AIDS, who possesses the power to conjure beautiful women through the sheer magical force of his "bar ruminations." This *kijana*'s cynical pursuit and satisfaction of desire, his seductive and fanciful excess, his empty promise of access to icons of modern urban wealth (cars, houses, and phones), and his duplicity in failing to honor his alleged commitment of marriage all point to the invisible pathology of HIV, which brings about the death of the beautiful girl. Who is our villain? A young man from Kilimanjaro. In the song he comes and he goes like his flesh-and-blood counterparts are said to; rootless and mobile, slipping into a bar alone, then into a guest house with a woman, and then out of the narrative, alone once again, leaving the woman, her family, and the hospital helpless to remove the lethal stain of his fugitive desire.

What about the beautiful girl? Summoned by the unspoken wishes of a man, she nevertheless negotiates for what she herself desires, a desire that seems tentative and contingent despite her dress and make-up, and the clacking shoes that draw attention to her body. She personifies the way in which AIDS in Kilimanjaro was experienced as both medically ambiguous and existentially absolute. Confusion and ambiguity shadow her path toward what listeners know is a foregone conclusion. First there is the mystery of what passed between the young man and his vulnerable partner in the guest house. Then, as she struggles to learn the cause of her illness, she is told in an ironic and careless blunder that she is pregnant. Later, as her condition becomes clearer to the listener, she grows confused, and in her denial she desperately attempts to seek a cure in maize porridge and to bribe the doctors, as if changing the signs of HIV from positive to negative could work a sympathetic magic of the blood.

And who is to cope with this tragedy? The voices of authority in handling this illness are all male: the father, the physicians. It is the older, educated (and apparently more morally upstanding) generation who must manage the descent into death of its wayward daughters and its absent, errant sons. Indeed, we hear nothing of the fate of the young man, who has also presumably become ill and died; the song conveys no sympathy for his plight. It should also be pointed out that this part of the lyric neglects to identify a major aspect of the lived experience of HIV disease: the care of AIDS patients falls mostly to women. The moralistic response of the song's second doctor to the beautiful girl's plight is also significant. Upon hearing her entreaties, the only solace he offers is a preachy "wages of sin" prognosis about cabbages, greens, and desire.

The remainder of the book will account for many of the themes of this song. It will consider not only the cultural logic of the story but also the contradictory experiences and perspectives of young people like the men who wrote it, and the role of national and international AIDS organizations in the representation of the epidemic (both to Tanzanians and to other scientists). After reading this book, glance over these lyrics once again; I hope that you will understand how, for people in Kilimanjaro, just a few words about failing to honor a commitment to marry could, when experienced in context, evoke a tragic "folk demography" of youth and an epidemiology of AIDS. The themes of "Hey, Listen!" are at the heart of this account: the dubious social and demographic position of young people; gender, ambiguity, and experience; the visible invisibility of sexual relations; the paradoxes in the medical involvement with the epidemic; the cultural coming to grips with AIDS; and desire and moral character.

## Bodies and Discourse in a Study of AIDS

This subsection addresses primarily an anthropological audience. It moves temporarily away from the theme of paradox and toward a consideration of theory and method in an anthropology of AIDS. While I have attempted to use general terms and to explain ideas in detail, it has been necessary to employ some technical terms and concepts, and to assume some familiarity with contemporary trends and questions in social theory. In order to address these anthropological concerns, we need to explore the relationship between discourses, texts, bodies, and action. Nonanthropological readers may wish to skim this section, or move directly to the summary of epidemiologic issues in the section "Announcing a Disease." The main point to carry forward is this: my central concern with the biological aspects of the epidemic is *not* with deriving precise epidemiologic estimates of HIV prevalence or assessing the demographic impact of AIDS.[12] Rather, I am primarily concerned with how epidemiology and demography tell stories about AIDS, reproduction, and sexuality that encode cultural meanings.

Among researchers who have discussed how AIDS in Africa has been represented in television reports, newspaper articles, policy statements of religious organizations and governments, and epidemiologic studies (e.g., Chirimuuta and Chirimuuta 1989; Treichler 1989; Bledsoe 1990; Patton 1990:77–97; Packard and Epstein 1991; Seidel 1993), few have done fieldwork directly on the topic. Those who have not, have been unable to observe *in context* the cultural dynamics surrounding the creation of the representations they interpret, to scrutinize the social and political conditions under which they are produced.

In her consideration of AIDS, gender, and medical discourse, Treichler posed the question, "What is the nature of the bodies most at risk for AIDS? What is their discursive history?" (1988:244). This

account of AIDS in Kilimanjaro seeks to answer the first of these questions, and expands upon the second. Cultural context informs the
meaning of AIDS in ways not exclusively tied to discourse; a focus on
the *discursive* history of bodies often has too much discourse, too little
history, and too few bodies. By definition, cultures and societies order
human existence for both individuals and groups. In doing so, they
undergo constant, internal self-correction. They also encounter forces
such as colonialism, warfare, epidemics, or demographic and techno-
logical change that transform them, changing the conditions in which
they perform the work of organizing meaning and experience.

Epidemic diseases such as AIDS, indeed all diseases, may be seen
as a disruption of society's organizing processes. Thus, cultures order
and give some structure and meaning to the experience of disorder
when it occurs as a physical disease or illness. These disruptions take
place through the medium of human bodies on discrete, yet interdependent, levels (see Turner 1984:85ff.). Since the late 1980s it has been
increasingly common to read of "the Body" in social and anthropological theory (e.g., Scheper-Hughes and Lock 1987; Martin 1992; Lock
1993). Unpacking the layers of meaning and experience surrounding
AIDS in Tanzania, however, does not fit well into a paradigm of the
Body. By this I mean that it does not justify the use of the singular term
"Body" as a master trope—whether in anthropological, sociological,
or biomedical terms.[13] Seen in cultural context, bodies and illness are
connected in a dynamic flow of the generation of meaning, or signification, that entails a cultural and corporeal hermeneutic of disordered
*persons,* of disruptions to the proper performance of agency and meaningful action (see Pollock 1996:320ff.). Rather than employing a discursive idiom of the Body as an externally inscribed and structured object,
I shall emphasize an idiom of process, of living and dying *bodies* as
dynamically unfolding and directed *processes* that are organized and
changed in time and space by culture.

These issues require further explanation as they apply to AIDS and
sexuality. For the moment, however, I wish to elaborate on the relationship between "bodies" and "persons." For the purposes of this inquiry,
the bodies of young people in Tanzania are treated as material and
action-oriented aspects of personhood; bodies are both vehicles and
processes through which meaningful action is manifest and in which
powerful capacities of production, reproduction, and representation
are located. Persons are thus corporeal agents of meaningful action,
located at an ever-unfolding juncture of biological existence and socio-
cultural experience. Sexual relationships are expressions of meaningful

action; they are more than forays into desire, evidence of long-term love and commitment, the outcome of prescriptive relations, or the results of economic necessity.

Although it is necessary to be as precise as possible about epidemiologic and demographic issues, the most central issue about the *biological* aspects of AIDS in this study pertains to the way in which biology (i.e., epidemiology and demography) has contributed to the cultural experience of the epidemic. The task is to describe what bodies *do,* and not to enter into the intractable debate over what the Body *is.* The "cultural semantics of action" (Pollock 1996:321) necessary for this task can only be derived from an interpretive ethnographic project grounded in fieldwork. Furthermore, any model of cultural semantics of action must contend with a range of local perspectives on the relevance of bodies (biological and social), minds, persons, personalities, selves, sexes, sexualities, and genders to AIDS.

These multiple perspectives are represented through both discursive and nondiscursive means. This makes fieldwork essential to a thorough account. Much of the meaning of AIDS is generated at the level of action itself, unmediated by communicative speech acts or linguistic expression of any kind (see, e.g., Clifford 1988). In the absence of fieldwork, analysis of cultural materials by outsiders too easily becomes disconnected from the contexts in which these materials have emerged. The case for linking analysis done without fieldwork to the perspectives of Africans themselves and to their experiences of AIDS is consequently weakened. Once a text has been stripped from the context of its production, the specific historical, cultural, and political locations of its producers become nearly invisible, as do the immediate responses of its local audiences. Thus, it is not merely the tightly knit symbolism of texts such as "Hey, Listen!" that leads us into a study of AIDS, culture, and demography. It is also the appreciation that this song is a product of specific actors in specific circumstances, and that these actors are themselves a key to the story.

Although fieldwork is essential to an understanding of cultural aspects of AIDS, it is not sufficient to such an understanding in and of itself. Anthropologists who have conducted fieldwork often overstep the limitations of their data. These include qualitative and quasi-qualitative studies on AIDS in Africa that rely primarily upon texts and narratives generated through fieldwork (e.g., interviews, semi-structured questionnaires, and focus groups; see Irwin et al. 1991; World Health Organization 1992; Caprara et al. 1993; Konde-Lule, Musagara, and Musgrave 1993; McGrath et al. 1993; Huygens et al.

1996; Nnko and Pool 1995, 1997; Mogensen 1997). Many of these studies explicitly claim to address the *experience* of sexuality, risk, and AIDS. However well personal or focus-group-generated narrative may *represent* experience, clearly there is a conceptual confusion in suggesting that one can stand for the other. This is not to discount the importance of narratives and discourse, but to place them in a wider frame that examines "experience" in both narrative/linguistic and non-narrative/nonlinguistic manifestations. Examples of the latter are assessed, and often quantified in demographic and epidemiologic studies.

The first line of the narrative in "Hey, Listen!" draws attention to the social context of its composers—to their demographic predicament and the representational strategies they use communicate it. The song begins, "The other day I was in this bar. . . ." Immediately, we know that this story is being filtered through a narrator. The use of the first person draws attention to the total phenomenon of this song; it becomes more than a stylistic hook with which to catch the listener's ear. The artists are well known by their clan names, which identify them as Chagga, and the song contains numerous references to specific locations in Kilimanjaro, notably hospitals. The narrator goes on to offer a particular vision of the moral character of other members of his own society, of the dangerous new disease his peers are facing. In part of the song (not translated), the singer exhorts young people to "leave promiscuity and adultery, leave a profligate lifestyle [*uhuni*]."

In the 1990s, the young men who composed this song lived in a section of Moshi dominated by Kiboriloni, the largest regional market and one of the locations singled out as "dangerous to lovers" in the lyric. The lyricist is the son of a Lutheran pastor, and in 1992 many of his social activities were connected with a nearby church. Like many other young Chagga men, he had a strong sense of attachment to the mountain, but no productive opportunities on the slopes, where his grandfathers inherited lands, farmed, married, reproduced, and, in turn, divided their ever-shrinking land holdings among their own sons. Also, like many of his peers, he relied on a combination of activities for income, little of which derived from agricultural labor. Much of his income came from selling pirated and prerecorded cassettes from a tiny kiosk in Kiboriloni market and traveling to Dar es Salaam and Arusha to market tapes of the music he played with his partner.

These young adults and the characters they create in "Hey, Listen!" were living an urban-oriented existence and telling us about disease and social process. What was so "telling" was not their "discourse" in song or speech, but their *physical presence* in certain spaces at once real and representational (Tanzanian towns) and their absence in other locations (rural villages) at a certain moment in time: an era of economic decline and epidemic disease.

Significantly, the band's message had relevance to many people beyond this American anthropologist. In 1992, educators from a large, internationally funded AIDS research and intervention project hired the bands to play for the public at the opening ceremony of a drop-in AIDS education center in the middle of Moshi town. Yet even before the publicity generated by this appearance, "Hey Listen!" was well known in Kilimanjaro. During my daily activities I often heard the song's bouncy, rhythm-machine beat, keyboard bass progressions, and accordion chord changes. Clearly this performance appealed to many local actors and to the representatives of the international health community in Kilimanjaro whose purpose was to combat the spread of AIDS in the region. In the way that all successful art does, the song somehow rang true to the way in which many people in Kilimanjaro experienced AIDS.

## Sexuality, Personhood, and AIDS

In Kilimanjaro, all of the issues mentioned above were connected to the local experience of sexuality. Before we proceed, then, a few words are also necessary about the use of the concept of sexuality in this book.[14] Many constructionist agendas for the study of sexuality are based upon an a priori rejection of connections between sexuality and reproduction, social or biological (e.g., Vance 1991). This separation is not supported by the ethnographic case presented here. In Kilimanjaro, sexuality, gender, and reproduction have remained implicitly connected in many, if not most, contexts. Proponents of the view that sex and reproduction are inherently separate domains of experience have maintained that accounts that fail to "de-link" them fall into a "cultural influence" model that is mired in outdated essentialist views about the very nature of sex (Vance 1991). Yet constructionism itself is by no means immune from essentialism (Setel 1994). To suppose it so leads directly to the implication that only *other* theoretical perspectives (such as those of physicians, epidemiologists, and cultural influence anthropologists) bring hidden agendas to the topic.

Other analysts of illness, sexuality, and social power in Africa have addressed the question of how a radical constructionism can be applied to African case materials (see Vaughan 1991:7–10; Jeater 1993:18, 37).

They argue, as do I, that a constructionism that is predicated upon poststructuralist Euro-American models of "fractured subjectivities" and of separable sex, gender, and reproductive domains does not necessarily fit African contexts. Demanding that African cases fit into the strictures of postmodern theory is little short of a new version of intellectual colonialism (Vaughan 1991:17). A truly constructionist perspective would deny the possibility of disinterested deconstruction. It would frankly acknowledge that those of us who write about, study, and attempt to fight AIDS all bring outside agendas to our projects, that we are all involved in creating the very processes we seek to address. Any analysis of AIDS, constructionist or otherwise, ultimately contributes to the play of power and knowledge in the epidemic.

When it comes to HIV and sexuality, one can certainly agree with Vance that a great deal is at stake. One merely has to glance at the age and sex distribution of HIV and the age-specific fertility rates for young Tanzanians to appreciate why sex, gender, reproduction, and risk are seen as critical and linked problems facing young people. Thus, the task of this account is to explain the cultural ontogeny of the connections and/or disconnection of sex and reproduction over time, not to assume they are inherently separable.

The concept of sexuality employed here is framed as a historically, demographically, and culturally circumscribed aspect of human experience ideologically and experientially linked to social reproduction.[15] For local actors, AIDS and sexuality have "revealed" deep contradictions in social reproduction and development. Demonstrating this requires not only an analysis of the epidemic in the present, but a historical study linking contemporary forms of reproductive power and sexuality to transformations in long-standing hierarchies of generation and gender. If the words of "Hey, Listen!" reverberate behind discussions of nineteenth-century reproductive regimes and the scientific epidemiology of HIV, then readers will understand how for residents of Kilimanjaro, AIDS has been simultaneously immediate and shocking on one hand, and all too familiar on the other.

For Tanzania and for Africa more generally, AIDS, sex, and reproduction are bound together and surrounded by forceful cultural ideologies about relations of production and reproduction. After all, there is no social reproduction without biological reproduction, and (for all but those with access to modern reproductive technologies) there is no biological reproduction without sexual relations. However one chooses to draw one's analytical boxes, these processes are self-evident for people in Kilimanjaro and so form the starting point for this study.

This does not mean, however, that local exegesis can be substituted for anthropological analysis. Because they are given the task of perpetuating cultural worlds, local actors both articulate and embody ideologies and values that have shaped the taken-for-granted character of sexuality and reproduction. These ideologies form a conduit "through which particular relations of domination become inscribed in the taken-for-granted shape of the world—in definitions of the body, personhood, productivity, space and time" (Comaroff 1985:5). As such, they must be discerned not only in "discursive" or "signifying" practices, but also in "power relations [that] materially penetrate the body in depth, without depending even on the mediation of the subject's own representations. If power takes hold on the body, this isn't through its first having to be interiorised in people's own consciousnesses. There is a network or circuit of bio-power, or somato-power that acts as the formative matrix of sexuality itself" (Foucault 1980b: 186). The demographic history of Kilimanjaro and the numerous ways in which sexuality has been channeled, authorized, and prohibited over the past century make up such a formative matrix. Although subjective and personal, sexuality remains beyond the capacity of individuals to define at will in terms of identity and consciousness or, in the absence of technological intervention, epidemiologic and demographic consequence.[16]

Thus, sexuality is about much more than what takes place on an interpersonal level between sexual partners; it is embedded in a whole array of contextual forces that are antecedent to any particular encounter. The significance of sexual action encompasses not only individual desire and interpersonal power dynamics but also the patterned relationships among persons, their bodies, and social process for a population as a whole. Through the extended discussion of AIDS in Kilimanjaro that follows, I am concerned with demonstrating how the disordering effects of the epidemic are simultaneously creative of new meanings and revealing of long-standing values which surround social reproduction.

The account of AIDS offered here should sound a warning note to anyone who is comfortable with a notion of "traditional African sexuality." As Vance has noted, it is now a commonplace to acknowledge that sexuality in Europe and America has a complex history and has been shaped by numerous social forces (e.g., Katz 1976; Foucault 1980a; Laquer 1990). Although there is now over twenty years' worth of studies on contemporary cross-cultural issues of gender and sexuality, histories of sexuality in African contexts remain scanty. While some (e.g.,

Schoepf 1992:357–59) explore regional diversity in precolonial sexual life, most tend to revolve around the adaptation of sexual values to urban life and the emergence of new kinds of sexual relationships in cities, or in connection with industrial capitalism and missionization (e.g., Epstein 1981; van Onselen 1982a, 1982b; White 1990; Bauni 1992; Ahlberg 1994).

The tools and materials for accounts of change in precolonial African sexualities are limited, but they are not absent. Where historical considerations have been addressed, as in the case of emergent sexual arrangements among Yoruba, the problem has been framed as one of "destabilization" of traditional systems (Caldwell, Orubuloye, and Caldwell 1991). With the exception of studies such as Jeater's, much of the debate about "African sexualities" versus "sexuality in Africa" has been strikingly ahistorical beyond the colonial era. It focuses on cross-cultural diversity and context to the exclusion of internal heterogeneity and change.[17] Epstein's study of domesticity in the Zambian Copper Belt in the 1950s, for example, shows how customs from village life that related to sexuality and domesticity (customs that were historically antecedent to the conurbations of the mining industry) were by turns reinvented, reasserted, and improvised upon in the urban sphere. Yet his study does not entertain the notion that these traditional values may themselves have been undergoing long processes of change. Instead, they were like a force of conservatism in the new contexts of the town. Thus, innovative erotic acts, as when husbands began to suck their wives' breasts during sex, were interpreted by some women as witchcraft attacks. We do not hear about the women and men who may have enjoyed this or other inventive practices or whether such activities were emerging in rural areas as well. Nor do we know whether these practices were, indeed, novel. Perhaps they were merely uncommon, or began to receive a different kind of cultural attention.

When it comes to understanding AIDS, this feature of the literature is very important. Looked at uncritically, it has tended to reinforce the empirically unsubstantiated proposition that sex in rural Africa is steeped in tradition-bound routine that only began to change under the forces of modernity and the encounter with colonialism. Far too many analyses of AIDS have employed such false assumptions, pathologizing sexuality in Africa when it crosses the world-changing urban-rural divide (see, e.g., Pela and Platt 1989; Rushing 1995). It is quite ironic that a hundred years ago Europeans denigrated Africans as immoral for engaging in precisely the imagined sexual regimes (mistakenly) thought in the 1990s to be protecting rural Africans from AIDS.

In Tanzania, these naive assumptions of stable traditional village sexuality versus the comparative sexual looseness of modern urban life are contradicted by at least one large-scale study (Rutenberg, Blanc, and Kapiga 1994). In short, the history of sexuality and AIDS in Kilimanjaro should temper glib characterizations of change in patterns of sexuality and nuptiality in Africa as indicative of increasing entropy, of social decline, and of AIDS as the taken-for-granted outcome of urbanization and consequent cultural loss.

In Kilimanjaro, sexuality, sexual morality, and the links among gender and productive and reproductive life have always undergone change. In the 1980s and 1990s, an appearance of increasing randomness in sexual life was not a revolutionary break from the past, but represented a kind of structured indeterminacy that informed many self-representations of sexuality. Without this indeterminacy, actors could not have operated as they did. This cultural need for ambiguity in sexual relationships is often misrepresented as "indiscriminate." Even when self-representations of sexual life seem to emphasize pleasure or numerous contexts for sexual expression, it is not valid to assume that there is an absence of concepts and practices of sexual discipline (Ahlberg 1994:226).

## Announcing a Disease: The Early Epidemiology of AIDS in Tanzania

The first three cases of AIDS in Tanzania were diagnosed in 1983 in the northwestern region of Kagera. The following year, three regions reported cases of AIDS: Kagera (106 cases), Tabora (2 cases), and Kilimanjaro (1 case). After the establishment of the National AIDS Task Force in 1985, all 20 regions in mainland Tanzania began reporting cases, and by the end of 1995, the country as a whole had reported 53,247 cases of AIDS to the World Health Organization—more than any other country in Africa at the time (World Health Organization 1995). The age and sex structure of cumulative case rates through 1997 (Figure 1.2) shows how the burden of AIDS cases was just beginning in 1992, when the bulk of the fieldwork for this book was carried out, and increased into the late 1990s, when additional fieldwork was carried out.[18] It also indicates a common pattern in the African epidemic, with peak prevalence among women between twenty and thirty-five years old, and men between twenty-five and forty-five.

In 1992, the government estimated that only one in three or four cases of AIDS was being diagnosed and reported (NACP 1992), an esti-

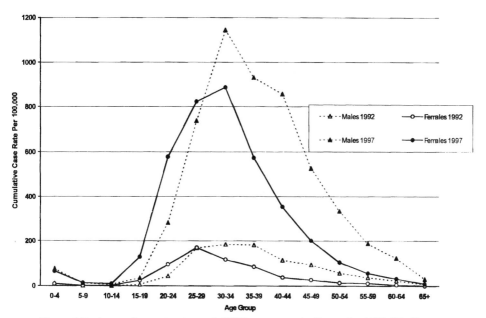

Figure 1.2. Age and sex structure of AIDS case rates in Tanzania, 1983–97. (Source: NACP 1992, 1997)

mation which has assumed huge importance in the social experience of coping with the disease at interpersonal, family, and community levels. If, despite reporting difficulties, the age structure of these cases is an accurate representation of the distribution of infections in the national population (and most sources concur that it is), the need to understand the context of young people's sexuality and how they have been perceiving and responding to AIDS becomes clear. Given a mean latency period between infection and onset of symptomatic HIV infection of five to ten years (Killewo et al. 1993; Ainsworth and Over 1994; Boerma, Nunn, and Whitworth 1998), the bulk of infections in both men and women must begin occurring from the late teens into the early twenties.

There are no meaningful estimates of HIV seroprevalence for the entire Tanzanian population. Attempting to cite a single rate for the nation would be a dubious task, and one of limited utility. A "national AIDS rate" would hide important factors relating to risk (e.g., age, sex, and location within the national context). The Ministry of Health and National AIDS Control Programme (NACP) have attempted to chart the progress of the AIDS epidemic in the population as a whole through "sentinel surveillance." Blood donors and pregnant woman attending antenatal clinics were designated by the NACP as "sentinel" groups. The rates of HIV infection among these subgroups were taken to provide a rough marker of the state of the epidemic in the general population. Sentinel figures must be viewed with a great deal of caution, and serious questions have been raised both about the reliability of the data and about using sentinel results to represent the HIV prevalence in the adult population as a whole (Borgdorff et al. 1993; Mnyika 1996:5–8; Zaba and Gregson 1998).[19] Although the NACP was aware of these concerns, HIV seroprevalence figures from blood screening activities were still "the most reliable estimates available for seroprevalence in the population at large" (NACP 1992:7).[20]

In 1992, 4.3 percent of all blood donors in Tanzania were HIV-positive (age- and sex-adjusted rate). By 1997 this had climbed to 7.6 percent for males and 11.6 percent for females (NACP 1992, 1997). This translated into an estimated 1.5 million HIV-infected adults. In most of Africa the ratio of male to female cases of HIV/AIDS was low compared with America and Europe. In 1997 the male to female rate ratio was 1.05, and the case ratio was 0.99. This indicates that the burden of the epidemic was falling on men and women in roughly equal proportions. Population-based seroprevalence surveys (which are the most reliable way to assess the prevalence of disease in a community) were conducted in several locations (Barongo et al. 1992; Killewo et al. 1990; Mnyika et al. 1994). They indicated a slightly higher female to male ratio of infection and peak prevalence among young adults from twenty-five to twenty-nine years of age.

While the epidemic began to spread, Tanzanians produced stories, rumors, songs, and parables about it. During the late 1980s and early 1990s they were also inundated with news stories about the growing scourge. At times stories about AIDS in Tanzania's English-language press outnumbered articles on other health issues by more than three to one (Setel 1989). Many of these articles focused on the looming specter of a massive epidemic, drawing upon alarmist facts and figures from the rapidly growing epidemiological literature on AIDS in Africa. Like popular representations of AIDS, the professional epidemiology of the epidemic has had its own set of motifs, symbols, and subtexts. These issues, and epidemiological assumptions about the "who, when, and where" of AIDS, will be analyzed later at length. At present, it will suffice to review what was known about the state of the epidemic in Tanzania the early 1990s. It is important to note that popular perceptions of risk and contagion contained in cultural texts such as "Hey,

Listen!" coincided demonstrably with an increasingly heavy burden of AIDS in Tanzanian society.

In Kilimanjaro, medicine and epidemiology contributed greatly to the social experience of the epidemic; medical practice and international health interventions were part and parcel of the local cultural context of AIDS. Medical practice contributed some core terms through which local actors themselves—doctors, farmers, and townspeople—came to comprehend the arrival of AIDS. Medicine became engaged with local narratives of population history and the changing moral character of adulthood expressed through sexuality and mobility. Over against "folk epidemiologies" (Muhondwa 1991) of AIDS, the cultural values ascribed to biomedicine in Kilimanjaro made a substantial contribution to the social experience of AIDS in the region.

In the West, the metaphorical life of AIDS in the 1980s flowed directly from the way it emerged and spread through communities of persons who used their bodies in ways that stereotyped and stigmatized them as noneconomically productive and nonreproductive members of society (Setel 1991b). These include intravenous drug users in the former case, and prostitutes and men who have sex with men in the latter. In Africa, the situation is practically the reverse. The metaphorical life of the epidemic is rooted in its emergence among those whose bodily praxis is simultaneously connected to productive and reproductive life, and to radical (and often culturally devalued) shifts in the organization of social reproduction. These include urban elites with money, truck drivers, and mobile men and women between twenty and forty years old. People in these categories are often thought to engage in risky sex and then "carry the disease home" to a rural agricultural population. Of course this is an oversimplification of AIDS epidemiology over time. Nevertheless, these perceptions set the tone for much of the first decade of the epidemic.

It should also be borne in mind that the epidemiologic knowledge base of the first ten to fifteen years of the AIDS epidemic in Africa has been a hodgepodge of figures from different kinds of studies among numerous population subgroups in scattered locations (de Zalduondo, Msamanga, and Chen 1989; Barnett and Blaikie 1992:15–17; Gould 1993:76–77). To an extent, as de Zalduondo et al. pointed out, this "mosaic" represents the diversity of the epidemic itself. When we look to the future, Tanzania will continue to be one of the world's most severely AIDS-affected countries (United Nations 1994). In the ten years from 1995 to 2005 declining national mortality rates will likely be reversed, and the life expectancy at birth may be up to seven years shorter than it would have been in the absence of AIDS. Because of the epidemic, population growth will probably be marginally slower, and mortality among twenty-five to forty-nine year olds (as a percentage of total deaths) will have risen about 10 percent between 1980 and 2005, solely because of AIDS (United Nations 1994:63). In the hardest-hit areas, AIDS is certain to bring about fundamental transformations in the structure and daily existence of communities (Ainsworth and Over 1994).

Despite the bleakness of these projections, recent research has shown that HIV prevalence rates in severely affected parts of Uganda and western Tanzania have begun to drop (Konde-Lule 1995; Pool et al. 1996; NACP 1997:24). People, it appears, are responding to their experience and understanding of the epidemic in such as way as to protect themselves from HIV. One of this book's main arguments is that the impact of AIDS education may be seriously limited by circumstances far beyond the control of educators or program implementers. Nevertheless, this study may contribute to these positive signs of decline in the disease through a better understanding of how AIDS has been experienced in its cultural and demographic context.

### Ending with a Rumor: The Social Life of My Social Life

It is well and good to problematize the location of the subjects of one's research, to note that epidemiologists, educators, and young people occupied particular positions of interest with relation to the AIDS epidemic, and that these positions affected their experience of it. It is equally important, however, to expose oneself, as the arbiter of this account, to such scrutiny. Here I shall briefly reflect upon how my "embodied vantage point" as a young, white, American male influenced my research.

In his study on Tamil personhood, E. Valentine Daniel states that the elements of culture revealed through anthropological endeavor are essentially cultural products in and of themselves. To some extent, culture emerges out of a synthesis of viewpoints. It is "spun in the communicative act engaged in by the anthropologist and his or her informants, in which the anthropologist strives to defer to [their] creativity" and reflects self-consciously upon the differed meanings that arise out of this engagement (Daniel 1984:13). Yet a reciprocal act may clearly take place. Indeed, as an anthropologist, I was, myself, spun into the account—forced from behind the aloof protection of my black notebook and made a subject of rumor and conjecture by dint of my mere presence as a white researcher and my "professional" interest in the sexuality of African men and women roughly my own age.

The nature of anthropological fieldwork, of immersing oneself to as great a degree as possible in the worlds of those one seeks to comprehend, entails at some point becoming subject to the frames of reference of cultural "others." Not only do fieldworkers negotiate life and work in unfamiliar settings, but those we encounter slot us into their ways of understanding persons and action in a manner that removes control of some of the conditions of research from the researcher. In Kilimanjaro, this process had less to do with whatever dialogue passed between me and my friends and informants and more to do with my eighteen months' presence in Moshi and surrounding areas between 1991 and 1993; with my sex; with my skin color and nationality; with my car; with my presence at Saturday night discos; and with the company I was seen to keep.

This point was brought embarrassingly home to me one day when, on the way to an interview, I dropped a flat tire off to be patched at a sidewalk workshop. As I heaved the spare out of the back of my car, the craftsman, or *fundi*, a man called Habib, gave me a sly smile. There on the street, for all passersby to hear, he loudly asked (in quite basic terms) about the state of my sex life.[21] As I investigated the reasons behind this humiliating ambush, it emerged that a rumor about me had begun to circulate in Habib's neighborhood, where I had a network of young adult informants. The word seemed to be that my "research project" on young people was nothing more than an elaborate ruse for me to screen desirable sex partners. I was said to have recruited a cadre of young men to go on scouting missions in search of suitable candidates, whom I would then "interview" for my "study."

Fortunately, I have no reason to believe that the rumors about me had any significant negative effect on my research, although I took steps to counteract the rumor and began using female research assistants more frequently to conduct interviews with young women.[22] The rumors were not intended as a serious allegation but more as a ribald joke made at my expense. The critique embedded in the teasing, however, brought into focus how tenuous are the boundaries between fieldwork and field life in long-term ethnographic research. These ambiguous boundaries centered on the facts that I was a single young man with (comparatively) considerable financial resources, and that I was not engaged in "work" in the sense that most people used the term—a routine, recognizable, paying occupation or activity in a specific location such as a shop, an office, or a hospital.

Thus, I was being teased according to local perspectives on manhood, sex, work, and race. Within this framework, I was seen as a sexual time bomb. The combination of my youth, money, and mobility and an apparent surfeit of free time (all I seemed to do was move around the social landscape, talking to people and writing in a book) signified a lighted fuse connected to a powder keg of unrestrained desire. This purported lack of self-restraint was assumed to be bidirectional, as most people took for granted the willingness of my female "informants" to respond to the overtures of a lover from the wealthy white world—a gendered dynamic of cross-cultural fieldwork that has been uncomfortably evident to other anthropologists, but seldom candidly discussed among us (Hammar 1993; Setel 1995d; see also Ratliffe 1996; Yelvington 1996; and Hooper 1990:62–76, for a journalist's personal narrative).

My supposed sexual conquests were seen in light of my particular purpose for being in Tanzania in the first place. Not only was I portrayed as a young man with an inflated sexual desire who exploited those he met to satisfy his sexual wants, but I was supposedly doing so under the ostensibly munificent guise of helping to combat AIDS in Tanzania. Research such as my own was often associated with the development sector. It was frequently assumed that I had a great deal of influence with the "donors" *(wafadhili)* who sent me, and could channel loans or donations to those who assisted me. In essence, I fit into at least four kinds of narrative formulas associated with AIDS and sex. The first was simply the application of the notion that "turnabout is fair play." If I felt it was my right to ask them embarrassing personal questions, shouldn't I be prepared to answer the same? The second played on cultural configurations of youth and the moral value of work. The third was about race and easier access to partners, and the fourth had to do with the suspicions, tensions, and contradictions built into structurally unequal social relations in the international health sector's response to the epidemic (Setel 1997). Thus, the particular way in which I was being ridiculed was part of the very process I had come to regard as central to an understanding of how AIDS had emerged, was understood, and was responded to by people in Kilimanjaro.

Despite my young Tanzanian friends' frequent denigration of Moshi and environs as an unexciting cultural backwater (often as measured by the diminishing quality and number of discos), there were many rich and parallel cultural worlds operating there. During the course of my stay, I moved among several of them. Some I merely visited while conducting a household survey, looking for a traditional healer (*mganga*) who was reputed to treat people with HIV/AIDS, attending a wedding, or visiting someone who was ill. But others, such as the Moshi neighborhood where Habib's workshop was located and a village in the rural ward of Mbokomu, were places in which I was rarely permitted the luxury of drawing clear distinctions between my work identity and the rest of my life. What is evident from Habib's surprise question is that the social conditions under which anthropological fieldwork takes place are ultimately subject to precisely the cultural outlooks that the anthropologist seeks to decode and interpret.

The immediacy of the fear of AIDS, the complexities of adult sexuality, the difficulties in negotiating gender relations, and the frightening ambiguities in encountering those with long-term illnesses were all part of my daily life for a year and a half (albeit in a fundamentally different way than for those among whom I worked and lived). All of these experiences were, by necessity, bracketed by certain characteristics about me as human being which were immutable in this setting. This said and acknowledged, I will try to convey the quality of these experiences in hopes that it will add to the reader's appreciation that all research, not just everybody else's, is "situated."

The interdisciplinary objectives of this account pose a number of theoretical and representational challenges. To give just one (admittedly oversimplified) example: How does one handle contradictions between popular ideas about AIDS and the scientific epidemiology of the disease without reducing "culture" simply to misinformation (from a biomedical standpoint) or "epidemiology" to a purely epistemological phantasm of Western concepts of body, person, and disease (from a constructionist standpoint)? My solution to the representational dilemma is not to demand of this account that it tell *the* story of AIDS in Kilimanjaro. There is no single story of AIDS in Kilimanjaro. Rather there are competing, overlapping narratives—cultural, historical, demographic, epidemiologic, and political economic.

Thus I present more than a chronicle of the cultural paradoxes of AIDS and the social contexts out of which they emerged; local forms of knowledge and practice are but two privileged sources of data. For while scientific epidemiologies of AIDS may be eminently "deconstructable" as cultural products, the disease processes measured by these social artifacts are all too material. The cultural representations offered by Tanzanians with whom I lived and spoke are in turn balanced against available analysis of demographic data and the scientific epidemiology of AIDS in the region. There is no single, paradigmatic analysis offered here, but an acknowledgment that, like the syndrome itself, the cultural experience of AIDS in Kilimanjaro is perpetually ambiguous and irreducibly plural. An account of this disease is thus best left open-ended, reflecting a recognition that all disciplinary perspectives are inherently partial. This is only partly an acknowledgment of the "antiparadigmatic moment" in anthropology identified by Marcus and Fischer (1986). It also speaks to the intellectual honesty in Merton's much older call for "theories of the Middle Range," which do not aspire to the status of paradigm to begin with: "It would seem reasonable to suppose that sociology will advance in the degree that its major concern is with developing theories of the middle range and will be frustrated if attention centers on theory in the large. I believe our major task *today* is to develop special theories applicable to limited ranges of data—theories, for example, of class dynamics, of conflicting group pressures, of the flow of power and the exercise of interpersonal influence—rather than to seek at once the 'integrated' conceptual structure adequate to derive all these and other theories" (1949:9).

However much failing to insist upon narrative flow and a "final analysis" may be regarded as a shortcoming, I believe that doing so reflects an honest appraisal that AIDS, as it has been lived and experienced in Kilimanjaro, is a far too nebulous, multidimensional, and internally inconsistent entity to pin down and fix with a single story line or a single disciplinary paradigm.

# CHAPTER 2

## Not a Promised Land: Historical Instabilities in Social Reproduction

> What the young generation wants nowadays is not a plenitude of children, but only full stomachs.
>
> Gutmann (1926:58)

> A Chagga without a *kihamba* is not a social being.
>
> Clemm (cited in Iliffe 1979:460)

> Every step in Chagga history seems to be characterized by paradox.
>
> Howard (1980:75)

### Social Reproduction in the Precolonial Era

The idea that "once upon a time" there were clear and rigidly obeyed cultural rules and social institutions governing sexuality is no truer for Africa than it is for Europe. In Africa, as in Europe, histories of sexualities and the mechanisms of social reproduction to which they have been linked (or from which they have become decoupled) have undergone constant transformation, though without completely losing continuity with the past. Schoepf has cautioned that in Africa, "if historical reconstruction of social relations is a difficult intellectual enterprise, an archaeology of sexuality is virtually impossible to establish for the periods without written records and beyond the reach of memory. The absence of such records does not justify constructing either a methodologically indefensible 'ethnographic present' or a timeless ethnographic past of tradition" (1992:357). In this chapter, I attempt precisely this type of archaeology. The stories it reveals lie at the heart of the paradox of contemporary sexuality for the Chagga. Again, this paradox derives from the fact that the success of Chagga "demographic tradition" was a major source of its own undoing.

Indeed, much of the literature on AIDS in Africa is based on the presumption that sexual values have only become "destabilized" in the encounter with external forces such as colonialism, capitalism, and modernity.[1] When anthropologists and demographers have debated this topic, it has been almost exclusively in connection with the ripple effects of colonialism (Caldwell, Caldwell, and Quiggin 1989; Ahlberg 1994), and rarely as part of a theoretical vision of longer-standing "traditions of invention" in African cultures (Guyer 1996). While Chagga sexual histories are unique in Kilimanjaro, they should not be thought of as unique *to* Kilimanjaro. The kinds of transformations evident in northern Tanzania in the mid-to-late twentieth century were experienced elsewhere in Africa. At a time when Chagga were beginning to explore alternative marriage strategies, Shona speakers in Southern Rhodesia, for example, were developing an explicit and historically unprecedented "moral discourse" about sexuality in the colonial context (Jeater 1993). Among Yoruba, urbanization and modernity have also transformed sexual life and the operation of sexual networks (Caldwell, Orubuloye, and Caldwell 1991; Renne 1993). It is time to put to rest the notion of a historical "sexual norm" in any regional or continent-wide sense.

In Kilimanjaro, various local authorities staked their claim to knowledge of what traditional sexual mores were supposed to have been. Naturally, a great deal of local discourse about AIDS has been configured around these imagined mores, how they have been abandoned and have replaced modern desires, and how this "loss of culture" has been explicitly connected to a crisis in sanctioned modes of reproduction. This kind of folk model has been echoed in a great deal of scholarship on AIDS in Africa, but has too seldom been examined critically; the dominant voices that put forth this narrative have too seldom been challenged. The parties who make this case are often major stakeholders in the political uses of particular forms of historical consciousness about sexuality and social reproduction. Thus their standpoints and the local histories upon which they base their claims must be critically examined.

The past one hundred years have been radically different from previous times in the rate and qualitative scope of social and cultural change. Nevertheless, this does not mean that the precolonial era was devoid of a dynamic history in sexuality. Sexuality, as a culturally shaped aspect of life, has always undergone adjustments in response to internal or regional dynamics in Africa—as have religion, agriculture, and political organization. Despite the existence of a set of core reproductive values, an array of sanctioned sexual relationships appears always to have existed in the mountain system. The dominant ideologies and sexual values against which the AIDS epidemic have been compre-

NOT A PROMISED LAND     29

hended flowed out of a dynamic *kihamba*-based system of social reproduction, which reached ascendancy during the nineteenth century. The
*kihamba* (plural, *vihamba*) is the family-farmed garden plot on which
Chagga reside on the slopes of Kilimanjaro. Fields under seasonal cultivation that were not the sites of permanent households were called
*shamba* (plural, *mashamba*).

Tensions have long existed between ideal modes of cultural reproduction associated with the *kihamba* and the dynamic demography of
the mountain. These links transcend time and generation to connect
the *kihamba*-based life of the 1890s to AIDS and social instability in the
1990s. We can appreciate how AIDS has played upon age-old themes
for residents of northern Kilimanjaro only through a consideration of
these historical linkages. Although these connections are often erased
in collective memory, they are plain to see in what contemporary
Chagga believe about the development of a person's moral character
and the sexual conduct of adults in the age of AIDS.

It must be acknowledged at the outset, however, that it is extremely
difficult to find evidence for a formal model of demographic and sexual
regimes before the very recent past. Nevertheless, the available material does enable us to sketch the contours of the system. In Kilimanjaro,
a cultural-demographic regime rooted in the perpetuation of the *kihamba* served to inculcate in individuals a core set of reproductive and
sexual values. The entire system, however, existed on unstable demographic ground, and at the edges a set of cultural practices and institutions existed that circumvented or subverted ideal sexual process and
values. The reasons that sexual values and reproductive practices developed in the way they did are not always clear. The general direction
followed by the path of culture change in these domains of experience,
however, can be discerned.

The cultural and demographic analysis in this chapter is often based
upon traveler and missionary accounts, the extensive ethnography of
Bruno Gutmann and Otto Raum, and oral histories of population dynamics taken with older Chagga men and women in the early 1990s.
These sources paint a rough picture of ideology and experience in sexual life in the mid-to-late nineteenth century. They also illuminate the
gaps between local theory and practice in sexual life. The palette, however, is limited. The cultural materials consist of words of songs taught
to children and recollections of initiation rituals that were all but extinct
by the time Gutmann recorded them. Gutmann was a German missionary and ethnographer who lived in Kilimanjaro earlier this century,
and much of his material was based upon the collective memory of

just a handful of informants (Winter 1979:65). Much of Raum's (1940) account, meanwhile, is merely a recapitulation of Gutmann's.

In addition to the limitations the data place on a local history of sexuality, only the merest of sketches of precolonial demographic conditions is possible. Fertility, migration, morbidity, or mortality cannot be quantified or even sharply delineated. Nevertheless, the early ethnographic literature on Chagga culture does reveal certain key facts. Most significant, it appears certain that the core institutions that guided young people into reproductive life had already been in flux for at least one or two generations by the time large-scale forces such as population pressures and the European presence in East Africa began to affect the mountain system.

## The *Kihamba* Regime

For the residents of the chiefdoms on Mount Kilimanjaro, who came to be known collectively as the Chagga (Figure 2.1), production and reproduction were based on the perpetuation of the clan and the *kihamba*.[2] The *kihamba*, then, can serve as a trope for modeling the demographic regime operating on Kilimanjaro into the early part of this century. The *kihamba* existed on many levels at once—material and metaphorical. The *kihamba* was the lineage reproducer, agricultural producer, and the provider of material for shelter. It was a unit of political capital and the living manifestation of key cosmological processes. Yet, first and foremost, it was none of these, but in its varied cultural topography, and with shifting emphases over time, it has simultaneously been all of them.

Following Lesthaeghe, I employ the concept of the *kihamba* demographic "regime" to imply both continuity and change: "The links between the organizing principles of a society and the specific features of its reproductive regime . . . are not only of importance for gaining insight into demographic variations at a particular point in time, but they are of even greater value for the understanding of the various paths followed in the course of social change. More specifically, as changes in the spheres of political organization, division of labor, social stratification, economic exchange, cultural differentiation, and demographic regulation are not likely to proceed in a synchronized fashion, a clearer view of the relations between 'production and reproduction' is essential to understanding individual and group strategies" (Lesthaeghe 1989:13). Social change in Kilimanjaro reflected the asynchrony inherent in this concept of regime. This asynchrony had drastic consequences for gender relations. Jeater has noted that in nineteenth-

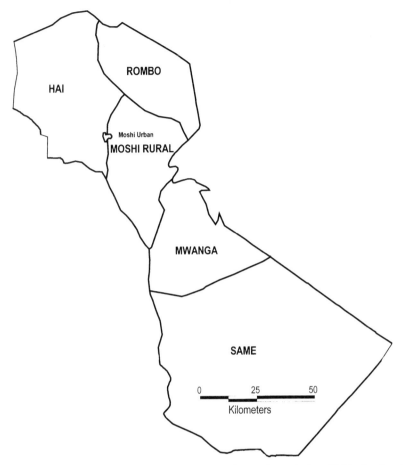

Figure 2.1. Map of Kilimanjaro Region showing district boundaries. (Philip Setel and Don de Savigny)

century southern Rhodesia "the ways in which people experienced themselves as men and women were inextricably linked to the production process" (1993:23). The same may be true of all systems in which there are more or less culturally rigid sexual divisions of labor. For Chagga, ruptures in the cultural dynamics of sexuality and gender relations accompanied changes in the production process of the past century. These ruptures are well hidden in today's imagined oral demographic histories, in the stories of sexual discipline in an era when men and women knew their places in the regime.

For Chagga, the *kihamba* approached "a total social fact" in the sense that Mauss (1967) used the term. The gardens structured the expenditure of human energy within households and symbolized hierarchies of generation, gender, and clan. The heterosexuality and procreation enacted there were, in terms of local cosmology, the basic "model of the most powerful forces of the universe" (Moore 1976:367). The *kihamba* anchored social and cultural life. The cosmos was enacted beneath the cover of the banana plants, mapped onto familiar objects of *kihamba* life, and lived out within the *kihamba* boundaries. Reproductive ideology was built upon the bedrock of this worldview, and hierarchical concepts of masculinity and femininity were anchored in it (Moore 1977). Sexual first principles governed the conditions under which male and female entities (human or symbolic) were meant to come into contact. The proper combination of these entities was the key to ordered reproduction; their improper mixture evoked destruction and death. The *kihamba* was the stage upon which these dramas were played; it was the only location in which the combination of male and female was authorized.[3] The formal organization of each *kihamba* not only provided a cultural map of linked productive and reproductive relations, but it also charted a model of the ideal gendered and generational life course. The unborn, the living, and the dead were all co-resident there. In the fertile soil beneath the banana plants lay buried the bones of the ancestors and the umbilical cords of their male issue. The *kihamba* represented prosperity, proliferation, and the supremacy of an ordered succession of generations beneath the umbrella of the patriclan.

The *kihamba* linked together the maintenance of daily life within households, the perpetuation of patrilineages, and adult procreative and productive life. Social reproduction was inextricable from Chagga kinship both to agnates and affines. One served the former group (generally speaking, one's "blood relations") through the maintenance of the *kihamba* and through fertility. One assisted the latter group (one's relations through marriage) through exchanges in bridewealth transactions and the lending of child labor to a wife's natal clan. Thus, the social efficacy of individuals was linked not only to a process of reproduction in and for one's own lineage but also to a world in which interlineage relations after marriage were ideally mediated by important acts of exchange.[4]

*Vihamba* gardens were also the source of subsistence and of agricultural surplus.[5] Ecologically, the *kihamba* zone on Mount Kilimanjaro comprises the land between three and seven thousand feet in elevation, mainly on the southern and eastern sides of the mountain. Land below this altitude has been seasonally cultivated with maize during the twentieth century and less intensively with millet in the nineteenth century. Land above seven thousand feet has largely remained forested. Before the introduction of coffee as a cash crop, the produce of the *kihamba* sustained people in many ways. It was consumed and stored by Chagga families and used in cultural and ritual transactions, and surpluses were sold at market to other Chagga and to outsiders.

Over the course of a few generations in the late nineteenth and early twentieth centuries, two aspects of the *kihamba* regime (the importance of maintaining good relations with patrilineal kin, and the customs of *kihamba* inheritance) contributed to increasing pressures and tensions on young people entering reproductive life. Within the *kihamba* regime, one maintained one's social identity in a context of clear-cut interdependencies under the overall control of elder men and lineage heads (though with crosscutting allegiances to one's age mates and the chief). Ingratiating oneself to male patrikin was critical to gaining access to resources necessary to marry and to progress through the life course. Fathers provided cattle, and patrikin provided beer for bridewealth payments. Fathers controlled access to land for first and last sons. Displeasing a parent could lead to a diminished or forfeited inherited share of herds, a curse upon one's health or fertility, or, worst, expulsion from the lineage. Thus, securing one's status was not merely a matter of performing mundane and ritual tasks but entailed living within kin-based hierarchies of generation and gender in which one's position was subject to constant evaluation and sanction. Even after a man's death, his surviving kin could exercise a great deal of discretion in the disposal of his property to potential heirs.[6]

Perhaps more profoundly, the customs of primo- and ultimogeniture in *kihamba* inheritance contributed to social and familial strife as population growth and land scarcity increased in the *kihamba* zone.[7] Before a land crisis in the twentieth century made the expansion of ideal settlement patterns impossible for most Chagga clans, the households of adult male descendants of male ancestors usually occupied clusters of contiguous *kihamba* gardens. Although there are no population estimates, even early travel accounts describe the area as densely populated. First and last sons inherited *kihamba* lands, and men had to establish a *kihamba* before marrying. Middle sons had to fend for themselves, though in practice siblings and grandfathers often looked after them. Barring such assistance, middle sons cleared new lands and established *vihamba* of their own on previously unused tracts. When new *kihamba* land was required, it was added, if possible, in such a way as to maintain the contiguity of land holdings of a lineage. Through the social organization of reproduction, the *kihamba* regime ensured the maximal use of limited *kihamba*-zone land.[8] Yet, by virtue of being culturally and ecologically anchored to the limited resource of fertile mountain land, the *kihamba* regime contained an inherent paradox: it was based upon unstable and unsustainable relationships among altitude-dependent agricultural production, regional trade, population growth, and particular forms of inheritance (Moore 1986).

The earliest European impressions of Kilimanjaro (from the mid-to-late 1800s) indicate that by the nineteenth century, the *kihamba* regime was in full swing. The accounts of settlement patterns and the natural setting of Chagga society were sometimes naively idyllic. They employed biblical hyperbole and likened Kilimanjaro to the Garden of Eden (New 1873:392) or declared it a Promised Land.[9] To Chagga of the time, however, the *kihamba* was not a timeless bucolic idyll; it represented a social order on the verge of drastic change.

The *kihamba* regime, it must also be noted, supported the political and economic interests of men over those of women, but did so within relations of carefully delineated interdependencies within marriage, among siblings, and between fathers and daughters. Despite an ideology in which men stood in a categorically superior position to women, women nevertheless exerted substantial control over productive and reproductive resources (see Moore 1986:121). Men and women relied on one another on the *kihamba,* as did younger men upon their elders, or brothers of different birth order upon their siblings.[10] Hence, the "domestic compound [was the] spatial archetype of ideal domesticity." For sexually active men and women, the *kihamba* and its attendant penumbra of ideal domesticity were an "*achieved* state of maturity and productivity which is crucially linked to marital status" (Moore 1996: 114; emphasis added). Sex was work.

The group strategies of the *kihamba* regime were maintained by the participation of individual men and women. The work of reproducing these men and women—not just biologically, but culturally—made the *kihamba* central to their lives. Ritual and child-rearing practices created the actors who drove the regime forward and, in turn, changed it. These men and women pioneered new approaches to sexual and reproductive partnerships. In the past, as today, clear-cut ideologies of sexual discipline stood against the murkier realities of daily life.

## The Production of Reproductive Agency
### Imitation and "Empersonation"

The reproductive and sexual values of the *kihamba* regime were passed on through a socialization process that focused on the development of proper conduct. Proper conduct, in turn, was inculcated through imitation and a process I shall term "empersonation." The intentional acts of individuals had huge consequences throughout the life course, and this message was reinforced from an early age. Here it is worth stressing the obvious: a cultural focus on one's action was a focus on the use of one's body. Chagga have had an explicit tradition of making cultural interpretations about persons through assessments of the day to day use of bodies. Bodies were the medium through which Chagga learned about proper personal development on a daily basis. The cultural symbolism of the human body was not reserved only for life-crisis events such as birth, initiation, marriage, and death.

The mundane task of socializing children was frequently the responsibility of grandparents. From birth, grandparents and other adults immersed children in a repertoire of songs, stories, rituals, and lessons that were part of a training for adulthood. These lessons, which once "saturated" the Chagga world (Gutmann 1932:1), were frequently based upon a practice which has remained essential to the cultural production of persons in this part of Tanzania: imitation.[11]

On one level, imitation was merely part of the way Chagga children grew up. On another level, it points to a more complex set of relations between bodies, action, persons, and meaning. This set of relations made up a process that might be called the empersonation of bodies. "Empersonation" intentionally evokes the word "impersonate," with its connotation of social relations of conscious and unconscious mimesis in the mediation of the somatic and the cultural (Lock 1993:144; Taussig 1993). Empersonation was effected through exercise of what Taussig (1993) has termed the "mimetic faculty." Taussig's concept of mimesis is very close to the concept of imitation *(-iga)* employed by people in northern Tanzania. What mattered in learning to become adult was the *correct performance of imitative action.* Children learned that to imitate one's elders of the same sex was the central, ordained technique for becoming a person, the way to acquire the knowledge and skills appropriate to being a man or woman.[12] "Imitate!" commanded the lessons of elders, "Look, my grandchild! You must imitate. If you did not want to imitate (at your present age), you would not be a human being" (Gutmann 1932:230). "A child that never imitates," young people were warned, "never becomes human" (231). Thus each child had to use his or her body to actualize the values the child had learned. Raum (1940:255ff.) considered that the point of the imitative play of Chagga children was not "mere imitation" in the sense of rote reproduction of modeled action, but the representation of patterns of social relations. Thus parents looked with favor upon children's games that imitated marriage and the chief's court.

In the twentieth century, there was a cultural emphasis on the role of imitation in socializing children that verged on preoccupation. A hundred years after most of the childhood rituals and songs had fallen into disuse, a loss of parental control over the objects and role models children imitated was considered one of the central problems of modern life in multi-ethnic Moshi Town. This was ironic, considering that Chagga themselves were a group defined by diversity of language, heritage, and local variation of "tradition." Because imitation has been so central to the acquisition of character, a great deal was at stake in the early exposure to good and bad role models. Worries about the "imitating bad moral character" *(-iga tabia mbaya)* emphasize that for Chagga, cultural reproduction has been acknowledged as an inherently moral undertaking, the product of the proper use of bodies to acquire personhood in a relational world. For Chagga, as for Kaguru to the south in Tanzania, the corporeal axes of sex and age were "inextricably connected and both in turn convey[ed] order and flux in time and the pathos of their effects upon the social person" (Beidelman 1987:141).

For Chagga, human bodies appear never to have been conceived of as separable from their role in mediating social relationships. There appears never to have been a highly articulated model of "the Chagga Body" in a biological sense.[13] Even the fear and malevolence associated with infants born with deformities were cultural anxieties about their somatic incapacity to become effective agents of social reproduction, or evidence of poor relations with parents or parents-in-law. As persons developed, their bodies became more salient to the agency of meaningful action. Organs, tissues, and bodily products attained unique powers to mediate personal and group relations. For example, saliva (particularly that of the mother's brother), when combined with leaves of *masale* (the dracaena hedgerows that marked the boundaries of the *vihamba*), was a powerful healing agent; the exchange of blood created bonds between men. Chagga ethno-anatomical notions also displayed how physiology could be socially relational.[14] The torso and chest possessed a unique cultural ontology as *mrima,* the seat of "all tendencies and desires," and the belly churned with emotions. The head, neck, eyes, the right side of the body (which belonged to the patriclan), and the genitals were beacons of "emanation" for one's wishes and feelings (Winter 1979:146–48). Rituals involving the piercing of earlobes, the extraction of teeth, circumcision, and clitoridectomy (discussed below) incised cosmological principles into flesh.[15]

As one grew older and culture validated one's sexual capacity, bodies became sources of immense power. The sex organs and the secretions of sex and reproduction could be creative when combined in the proper ways and at the proper time, and destructive when improperly mixed or used. Menstrual blood and semen, together with the cooperation of the propitiated ancestors, could produce human life—but only after initiation. On the other hand, male and female figurines and pots in human form with exaggerated genitalia were especially powerful devices used in calling down curses upon malefactors (Moore 1986: 334–35).

Thus empersonation, or mimesis, made actual the metaphorical connections among individuals and social institutions such as clans and chiefdoms; among social groupings of men and women, elders and juniors; and between individuals and the specific groups to which they belonged, such as age grades *(rika)*.[16] Chagga children were simultaneously cultural products and (re)producers: "The mimetic faculty carries out its honest labor suturing nature to artifice and bringing sensuousness to sense . . . granting the copy the character of the original, the representation the power of the represented" (Taussig 1993:xviii).

### *Initiation,* **Mregho,** *and* **Shiga**

The rituals associated with becoming an adult are particularly revealing of Chagga sexual ideologies. Specifically, they conferred the culturally defined states of being "closed" and "opened." These states were critical to fertility. Chagga initiation symbolically sealed men and opened women.[17] Both of these states were then publicly *concealed* in such a way as to emphasize the former and downplay the latter. Initiation also legitimated the imminent achievement of domestic life and sanctioned sexuality: "Circumcision not only confers the legal status of an adult, but his [sic] sexual rights, too. These consist in the permission to found a homestead, to marry . . . and to procreate" (Raum 1940: 312).

Initiation was the clearest example of how reproductive ideology in the *kihamba* regime was inculcated into the bodies of successive generations.[18] Initiation relied upon cooperation between superiors and inferiors across generations. The ritual closure of men's bodies at initiation (discussed below) required an elder age set voluntarily to relinquish the symbolic power to reproduce. In a related way, adult men shared in the responsibility for preserving a woman's fertility, her "openness," which commenced at menarche and was confirmed with her own initiation and circumcision.[19] The treatment men accorded their wives could also affect their openness; an improperly or poorly built house might "close" a woman, making her infertile.

Men acquired their power to reproduce through the grove initiation ceremonies. The most elaborate of these ceremonies for which there is any record were conducted in the mid–nineteenth century and required boys to stay for periods of up to five months in sacred forest groves high on the mountain. The key moment of the grove initiation was the symbolic closure of men's anuses through the figurative setting of the *ngoso,* or anal plug. The *ngoso* was the essence of men's sanctioned sexual and reproductive potential; without it they were little better than children.

The *ngoso* contained a number of contradictions. First, men were symbolically, not literally "closed" by the anal plug. Second, the supposed transformation of male physiology was meant to be a secret known only to men. Women and children were meant only to know that after initiation, men completely digested their food and no longer defecated or farted. Yet women's initiation made explicit reference to the *ngoso,* thereby subverting its secrecy. Third, in spite of this common knowledge, both men and women pretended that the *ngoso* was a secret; open discussion of the topic drew heavy penalties, such as confiscation of cattle, for transgressors. The ramifications of the *ngoso* are discussed in more detail below.

Given the apparent centrality of the *ngoso,* it is surprising to note that over time the important step in coming of age for boys shifted from the grove initiation to the single act of circumcision.[20] Nevertheless, this was the case; by the late 1920s male group initiation had all but ceased in most parts of the mountain (Gutmann 1926:288).[21] Circumcision for men, however, was not imbued with anything like the same power and drama as the *ngoso* and was not configured symbolically to perform the same cultural work as anal closure (i.e., to "close" men and so activate their fertility). Although the ethnographic record does not offer an explanation for their demise, there is evidence that *ngoso* initiations were in decline well before there could have been any substantial external influence from missionization or colonial suppression.[22]

Even if we are unable to discern the reasons for their decline, the initiation rituals nevertheless illuminate the cultural construction of sexual values. Their decline demonstrates the larger point that "traditional" cultural institutions central to the production of social identities and sexual values were in flux in the precolonial era. Circumcision, which was to become the most enduring aspect of initiation, was but the first step in the ritual cycle. Boys were eager to take it, and sometimes banded together to demand it. On the morning of the circumcision the boys, the circumciser, and his assistants retreated to the *kihamba* where the surgery took place. The removed foreskins were buried and guarded for a two-month period, after which they were disinterred, mixed together with manure, and scattered over *kihamba* land. Thus circumcision itself was one of the most potent reminders to boys that their sexuality and their fertility were physically intertwined with the maintenance of the *kihamba*.

The grove procession followed circumcision and took place high in the mountain forest, outside the *kihamba* zone and nearer the mountain peaks.[23] Once at the grove, the elder charged with instructing the incipient *rika* made a welcoming speech likening the bodies of the initiates to the *vihamba*: "The *vihamba* are the creation of former days and have been tested by former generations, so the elder will start with your body as he starts the cultivation of a field" (Gutmann 1932:319).[24]

The height of the grove ceremonials involved the concentration of male waste, its consecration, and the setting of the *ngoso*, the anal closure.[25] The grove ceremony leader was lowered into the pit and blessed the fertility of the initiates. After this, the grove leader symbolically set the *ngoso* by touching a live grasshopper to the tongue of each initiate. The leader then released the grasshopper, which became the sign of the blood bond among the *rika* mates and the pact of secrecy among the men. Henceforth these grasshoppers were forbidden food to men.

What circumcision literally carved in flesh, grove initiation figuratively carved into identity. The closing and stitching of the anus was graphically, though not literally, inscribed into the body of each man. The setting of the *ngoso* was supposedly effected by plugging and stitching shut the anus; this caused complete digestion of food and was the "very foundation of . . . manhood" (Gutmann 1932:291).[26] Upon returning as a "closed" and united *rika*, men were no longer to speak to women of the need to defecate or to fart.[27] Under no circumstances were they to reveal to younger women or children the physical fiction of their state of cultural closure. Thus, the signal event of male initiation in the nineteenth century was not the removal of a boy's foreskin, but the symbolic closure of his anus. The cultural associations between the attainment of fertility, masculinity, and entering a state of closure were recurrent themes during the whole initiation process.[28]

Chagga ideas about biological reproduction placed a great emphasis on the man's contribution to the process. Again, the *ngoso* was a charter for male primacy in a reproductive regime based on complementarity between unequal elements (i.e., men and women). Cultural ideas of male power were also evident in the *mregho*, or tally stick. Initiation and *mregho* not only placed men at the center of social reproduction but positioned them as the agents of successful biological reproduction as well. *Mregho* was yet another cultural technique for emphasizing the metaphorical links between reproduction, individual bodies, and the *kihamba* world of intra- and interlineage power relations. In the song cycle accompanying *mregho*, familiar objects became metaphors for the dependence between unequal relational parts. These included the relations of mother to fetus, ancestor to unborn, male to female, chief to clan, and elder to junior (Gutmann 1932:17).[29]

The agency of male ancestors in fetal growth within the female body was striking; each organ and limb that developed was said to sprout in response to a pinch or a pull from the grandfathers (Raum 1940: 561).[30] To abuse a pregnant woman was to assail the sacred and invisible work of male ancestors. The strong association of pregnancy with patrilineality was emphasized by the notion, still common in the 1990s, that gestation varied according to patrilineage. Chagga held, as have many Bantu-speaking groups, that women supplied the fleshy substances of blood, milk, and fat but that an adequate supply of semen through frequent sexual intercourse early in pregnancy was required for full fetal development and the development of the skeleton. Men, however, could be carried away with their own sense of reproductive power and had to be reminded bluntly that women played any role in the development of the fetus at all: "Once you have spat your 'cream' into her, you shall go off and leave the rest of the work to her and God . . . you may not brag as if the child were solely yours. Know rather that woman has her laborious part in it" (Gutmann 1932:26).

The significance of male initiation in relation to women's roles in reproduction becomes clearer when viewed in the context of female initiation teachings. For young women, clitoridectomy and initiation teachings *(shiga)* were analogous in many ways to the male initiation. Although much less has been written of women's rites, what has been recorded indicates that they bore close parallels to those of the men.[31] Women's rites, however, did little to confer women's rights. As Raum noted of *shiga*, "The same ideology . . . which justifies the social gradation according to sex is used to bolster up the authority of old age" (1939:564). Women's initiation did not merely bolster *kihamba* power relations, however. It also challenged them by asserting that women were in fact the original owners of the *ngoso* and that the men had stolen procreative power from them.[32] Later, we shall see other ways in which Chagga women's institutions challenged the ideology and practice of male superiority.

As we have seen, imitation in daily life and the ritual cycle culminating in initiation were the major techniques used to inculcate reproductive values into young people during the nineteenth century. Children were taught early in their lives to imitate in order to internalize an ideology of hierarchical relations. Through imitation, they rehearsed activities associated with male and female gender. The songs and lessons of the grandparents and the initiation teachings bolstered participation in the *kihamba* regime and emphasized a model of moral character that included a sense of accountability of the socially more powerful to the less empowered.

Chagga ritual focused on the bodies of young people as the mechanism for activating their reproductive potentialities. All of these techniques entailed the symbolic use of the *kihamba* as both a fertile metonym and productive metaphor for Chagga society, culture, and cosmology. All of these practices, however, were enacted in an unstable and unsustainable material and demographic environment. The internal coherence of the *kihamba* regime and its dominant reproductive ideologies were under internal pressures and tensions before the arrival of major external influences. Initiation was already undergoing change at the turn of the century. Similarly, the cultural ideal of the proper bridewealth marriage was also becoming transformed. Pressures and tensions in reproductive life can be seen not only in the way young people entered adulthood but also in the emergence of alternative sexual and reproductive unions to bridewealth marriage. This alternative array of male-female relationships emanated from accelerating processes of social and political differentiation and the demographic stresses that emerged shortly before the colonial era.

## Demographic Dissonance and Sexual Polyphony
### Precolonial Population Dynamics and Population Growth

Chagga began to face demographic pressures at a time when colonialism was also becoming a serious presence in the mountain system. These pressures undoubtedly prompted some degree of change in sexual and reproductive life. It would be tempting to offer a brand of demographic determinism in modeling the impetus for change. The story might run along the following lines: Population growth led to agricultural intensification and ultimately to land shortage, which, in turn, led to out-migration; the Chagga successfully exploited, then overpopulated the mountain and were forced into new ways of viewing sex and social reproduction. Colonialism, Christianity, and the commodification of *kihamba*-zone land gave an added push. The existence of alternative reproductive unions at the time might be seen as further evidence of a cultural need to adapt to these circumstances.

This reductionist story takes us only so far. The strains that emerged in Kilimanjaro are best seen as a product of more complex interactions. These primarily concerned practices that favored politically empowered agents (especially men and lineage elders) and the rapidly shifting material and demographic constraints in which they strove to push their advantage. While population growth, stratification, land shortage, and colonialism did require a cultural response, the particular character of local responses was neither predetermined by these phenomena nor open to entirely novel moves. Rather, these forces were confronted as new, if unprecedented, challenges to the cultural ordering of social life. The contradictions in sexual life and social reproduction in the *kihamba* regime before the turn of the century stemmed in part from the paradoxes of demography and ecology. They also derived from the malleability in sexual life rooted in local cultural process, a malleability that in later years was responsive to (not dictated by) a move from rural to urban spaces, conversion to world religions, and enrollment in capitalist modes of production.

Despite a regional picture that suggests the contrary, demographic pressures appear to have been at work on Kilimanjaro during the precolonial era. Again, precolonial population dynamics, particularly with regard to movements in levels of fertility, morbidity, and mortality, are extremely difficult to reconstruct. The problems are compounded when one tries to model, even notionally, for a relatively small area such as Kilimanjaro.

The interpretation of nineteenth-century population dynamics within the mountain system offered here, however, departs from the received wisdom. Koponen (1996) paints the general picture for the region, and Moore (1981) does so for Kilimanjaro. It is one of cataclysmic mortality and low-to-moderate fertility in the late nineteenth century followed by a decline in mortality and a fertility boom beginning sometime after 1925. Koponen's account paints precolonial demography with too broad a brush; it is too unproblematic in applying regional dynamics to diverse human and disease ecologies at a subregional level, and inconsistently applies the idea that colonialism prompted shifts in fertility and mortality in some cases but not others. In her discussion of demographic change in Kilimanjaro Moore concurs with Koponen's assessment and argues that high mortality and low fertility persisted into the colonial era and that infant mortality dropped rapidly and fertility increased dramatically only after the arrival of Europeans (1988:236ff.).

There are a number of facts that point toward a different model of population dynamics on the mountain. With regard to infant and child mortality, for example, Gutmann believed that death rates escalated, rather than declined, in the colonial era (Koponen 1996:29). Furthermore, data about low child death rates recorded among Christian converts in the 1930s cited by Moore are dubious. Her figures (about one death per thousand) in an era long before the wide availability of Western health-curative services, antibiotics, or primary health care are implausible. They contrast too strongly with an under-five mortality rate in Kilimanjaro between 1992 and 1996 of sixteen per thousand (Ministry of Health and AMMP Team 1997), and contemporary European rates of between five and eight per thousand.

While there may have been no generalized shortage of land, even the sketchy account of precolonial population dynamics made possible by available sources and interviews with older Chagga gives a sense that a land crisis was looming for at least some of the population before the arrival of Europeans. Early colonial observations also contradict the idea that population density on Kilimanjaro had been low into the 1920s and 1930s (TNA 5.449).

By custom only first and last sons directly inherited *kihamba* lands. Middle sons had to rely upon brothers, elder male kin, or their own ingenuity to obtain a *kihamba*. Moore has argued that the structural vulnerability of middle sons to landlessness in inheritance was more a potentiality than a reality before the lowering of mortality and the raising of fertility. The problem of middle sons would not have been a concern for many Chagga, she argues, until surviving children totaled about five or six per woman (an event she places in the late 1920s or 1930s). The child mortality question aside, this model assumes an equation of *female* fertility with *marital* fertility. In the last century, Chagga marriages were preferably polygynous. Thus, Moore's model would only work if the number of monogamous marriages, male death rates, and child/infant mortality combined to yield only slightly over two surviving sons per marriage.

If we think of the situation in terms of marital fertility as represented by male fertility and polygyny, the picture changes. Any polygynous man (the preferred situation) whose surviving sons exceeded the total number of his wives plus himself stood an even chance of having one or more middle sons who could not be accounted for in a "break-even" model of precolonial primo- and ultimogeniture. If Chagga women

were surviving to about age fifty and if they had seven births on average under moderate mortality conditions, we could expect that each
wife would have an average of three surviving adult sons. Thus a polygynous family with two co-wives and three surviving sons each had
a good chance of producing a middle son. Having any more than one
other co-wife required about two surviving sons per woman in order
to create a need for an adult man to use other means than direct inheritance to acquire a *kihamba*.

It may also be pointed out that there is no evidence that there were
demographic limitations (other than delaying male age at marriage)
on achieving a polygynous marriage. This may suggest a condition of
sustained population growth, since polygyny can only be perpetuated
in a bounded community if the population is growing, there is a steep
slope in age distribution, and / or some men never marry. There are no
reports of a crisis in the availability of wives in precolonial Kilimanjaro,
nor of efforts to acquire wives from groups off or away from the mountain. To be sure, the evidence often points in contradictory directions.
Nevertheless, there is reason to question the depth of the nineteenth-
century mortality crisis on the mountain, the timing of land shortage,
and the abruptness in onset of the twentieth-century population boom
as they have been previously portrayed.

In previous centuries, in-migration was the most obvious source of
population increase in Kilimanjaro. From its beginnings some four to
five hundred years ago, it appears that Chagga society was born out
of regional ferment, of people of diverse origins seeking political autonomy, fleeing violence and cattle raiding, escaping drought and famine,
forced to move because of the decimation of cattle herds due to disease,
and questing for fertile land (Dundas 1924; Lemenye 1953; Stahl 1964;
Makundi 1969; Odner 1971). By the nineteenth century, when Swahili
traders, European missionaries, and early colonialists began to arrive
from the coast, Chagga had formed a number of discrete chiefdoms,
each of which possessed distinct variants of core ritual complexes and
a distinct dialect of the Chagga language. From the mid-nineteenth century onward, the picture is cloudy; some sources suggest a population
increase, while others point to either a decline or little to no growth.
There are no numerical estimates that can be regarded as reliable base-
lines; those that do exist must be discounted as pure speculation.[33]

By the turn of the century, much of the land in the *kihamba* zone
appears to have been occupied. When viewed from afar by explorers,
the mountainside revealed the presence of an easily discernible pattern

of heavy and uniform *kihamba* habitation, with little forest remaining at lower altitudes and no concentration of people in villages (Rebmann, cited in Krapf 1860:197; Johnston 1886:91).

Yet population growth was certainly not without its checks. As in all societies, cultural institutions affected the starting and timing of fertility among Chagga. There appear to have been severe punishments for sexual activity among uninitiated youth that resulted in a birth. These included the threat of death for the young parents and the infant. While fertility was a virtuous necessity, there was also a sense of proportion; families that were too prolific were tauntingly said to be like wild animals (Gutmann 1926:37). For adults, among whom marriage in one form or another appears to have been nearly universal, postpartum abstinence (or at least fertility avoidance) was the most common technique of fertility limitation. Chagga also had a specific term (*ititsha mweri*) for techniques used to work out a woman's ovulatory cycle and maximize (or minimize) chances for conception. There is evidence that the prescribed three-year birth interval was among the longest in late precolonial Tanzania (Koponen 1988:325).[34] Abortion and various techniques of contraception were also practiced in order to avoid mistimed births.[35] Chagga, along with a few other groups in Tanzania, practiced "terminal" fertility avoidance; according to the cultural logic of male initiation, when a new age grade was initiated, the officiating age grade was meant to cease reproducing. This practice may have functioned to keep family sizes smaller than they might otherwise have been (assuming a late age at marriage for men, and assuming that young wives did not typically have extramarital reproductive partners).

There were other checks on population growth, including disease, disruption, and famine. Warfare over access to trade routes displaced some of the local population westward to Mount Meru (Le Roy 1889: 345) and caused hunger through the destruction of crops and looting of livestock (Iliffe 1979:70; Koponen 1988:171). There was also an undetermined amount of intra- and interchiefdom slave trading.[36] The precolonial epidemiology of the area, however, is nearly as unknowable as the precolonial demography; no figures exist to provide any prevalence or incidence data for disease. Infectious diseases associated with fairly high mortality, such as smallpox and plague, were reported from the area from the mid-1800s onward. Direct references to sexually transmitted diseases are found in initiation lessons recorded in the early twentieth century, and syphilis may have been a specific element of certain Chagga curses earlier than that (Gutmann 1926:563).[37] Malaria was well known to Chagga, and descending the mountain during the rainy season was avoided for this reason.[38] Other prevalent diseases included yaws and leprosy.

The unequal distribution of power and resources within chiefdoms, clans, and families meant that in addition to the emerging land pressures at the turn of the century, dislocation, morbidity, and mortality were also unequally distributed. The health effects of increasing differentiation were exacerbated by frequent periods of localized food scarcity (Howard 1980:39–40). In the late nineteenth century, a "political ecology" (Turshen 1984) of morbidity and mortality was beginning to emerge in the increasingly differentiated social world of Kilimanjaro. Wealthier Chagga, for example, commented that famine was preferable to smallpox, for, while the former struck only the poor, the latter took rich and poor alike (Schanz 1913:33). Tuberculosis, which has experienced a great resurgence as a companion scourge to AIDS, made its entry into Chagga disease ecology shortly after the turn of the century. This disease has been a significant cause of morbidity in Kilimanjaro, where the British established the territory's tuberculosis hospital in the 1920s.

Although there is evidence for a period of heightened mortality in the early colonial era due to such causes (Gutmann 1926:66; Koponen 1988:178), the indications are that growth has been the dominant feature of population dynamics in Kilimanjaro for the past 150 years.[39] This claim is supported by the existence of a lengthy birth interval, the apparent ease with which polygyny was sustained, and the frequently overlooked (though unquantifiable) role of in-migration from surrounding areas. Local oral demographic histories collected from older men and women in the former chiefdom of Mbokomu indicate a degree of displacement between chiefdoms in the late nineteenth century. A scarcity of land forced people to move from crowded high altitude locations to uninhabited tracts on the lower margins of the *kihamba* zone. All of these issues, however, require more research.

## The Array of Precolonial Male-Female Relations

Given this constant demographic change, it is not surprising to find that accounts of "traditional" Chagga marriage and sexual expression exist side by side with narrations of subversive trends and tendencies. The numerous recognized forms of sexual and reproductive unions mentioned in the literature suggest that there were divergent pathways for accommodating growing numbers of adults—many of whom did not have equal access to the material wealth necessary for establishing a "proper" bridewealth *(ngosa)* marriage after initiation.[40] Men could not enter into *ngosa* negotiations without access to land and cattle through their fathers (or the benevolence of brothers or grandfathers) and other patrikin.[41] They also needed the assistance of these relations for the preparation of several large prestations of beer. Once negotiations commenced, couples often began to have sexual relations.[42] The payment of bridewealth was often gradual; a woman's clan occasionally demanded final installments upon her death in old age. In addition to *ngosa* marriages, leviratical unions and sanctioned bride capture (which often involved more limited exchange than *ngosa* marriages) were also within the realm of sanctioned reproductive unions.

Toward the end of the nineteenth century, however, a wider array of non-*ngosa* unions developed that subverted or circumvented the strictures of bridewealth. Some of these appeared to have been oriented more toward sexual gratification than ordered social reproduction. Whether or not these relationships emerged as a result of a demographic bottleneck in access to cattle and land is impossible to say.[43] They may have also been prompted, for example, by a shifting age structure brought about by increasing numbers of young people (due to higher fertility, better survival, and in-migration) and changes in mortality patterns.[44]

In Kilimanjaro men and women began to assert an increasing measure of innovation and self-determination in sexual matters. References to at least twelve different types of sexual and reproductive relationships are scattered throughout early ethnographies and cultural accounts, primarily in the work of Gutmann. In addition, women often took the initiative in establishing liaisons with men they desired. As among many Tanzanian groups, sex before marriage (but after initiation) appears to have been permitted in the precolonial era as long as it did not lead to pregnancy (Raum 1940:68). Childbirth outside marriage was not sanctioned; the offspring of nonmarital unions faced denial of paternity or infanticide (Gutmann 1926). Sexual activity that resulted in pregnancy before initiation was especially aberrant. More than any other form of illicit sex, fertility among the uninitiated contradicted the most central tenets of the cultural authorization of fertility: initiation and the *ngoso*.[45]

It seems that women asserted themselves most strongly in the flirtations of youth. They arranged trysts at marketplaces, dances, or at the houses in which marriage-aged women sometimes co-resided. Although girls were often betrothed to men from childhood, many seemed simply to bide their time until they decided on their own course of action, whereupon they might cancel a betrothal or engagement arranged by a parent or guardian.[46] Young women were said to have the power to entrance men through ingesting a small amount of blood from an incision on the arm. Lovers could also conclude a more binding and (presumably) more erotic "blood pact" by sucking a small amount of each other's blood from cuts made near the genitals (Gutmann 1926:129). Women had specific techniques of assertive action in pursuit of marriage, not just sex. "Bringing oneself to the husband" (*Ikusitsa ko mi*) was one such strategy; "By using this form, a woman determines her fate with complete independence" (28). Women who selected their own husbands in this manner were often pregnant upon their arrival at their intended's homestead and were said to be as eager to conceal this fact as they were to establish a legitimate marriage.

Nonmarital liaisons were well known and scripted, although the negative consequences for beginning an affair that was not meant to lead to marriage were emphasized. In initiation lessons, men were surreptitiously instructed on how to arrange an affair with a married woman while at the same time being warned that they would fall ill from doing so.[47] "Opening a hut" was a more regularized form of extramarital sexuality. For polygynous men, this may well have been a prelude to obtaining an additional wife. While infidelity on a woman's part was normally grounds for a beating, separation, or termination of marriage, there were specific circumstances in which a woman was encouraged to seek a relationship outside her marriage.[48]

By the early twentieth century initiated men began to exert a larger degree of autonomy in the selection of spouses. Bride capture (as likely to imply elopement as abduction and rape) was the clearest example of contradicting the established order represented by an *ngosa* marriage.[49] It seems reasonable to speculate that the increase in bride capture observed by Gutmann may have been brought about by a demographic bottleneck for initiated men who did not possess any of the increasingly scarce *vihamba* land but nevertheless wanted to marry.[50]

Sexual responses to social change in Kilimanjaro were as much the province of personal initiative as they were the outcome of processes of proletarianization, conversion to Christianity, or adherence to "custom." In colonial Zimbabwe, as in precolonial Kilimanjaro, new cohorts of young men and women entering into adulthood sought ways of asserting autonomy. Gradually, they established new and culturally acknowledged forms of relationships, relationships that fit better with their own desires and the dictates of their changing productive lives.

The particular shape that sexual strategies took depended a great deal on the creative application by individuals of culturally constructed conventions of gender roles.

The core sexual ideologies of the Chagga past were never connected to a stable system of social reproduction. Given this situation, it seems that the way in which young people established themselves in marriage and sexual life merely entered a new, albeit qualitatively different, phase in the colonial era. The later codification of "traditional" sexuality in local discourse was part of a process of dislocation that will be examined in more detail in the next chapter. Despite the existence of clearly defined ritual traditions that expressed enshrined marital values, innovation characterized the *kihamba* regime at the turn of the century. The *kihamba* regime appears never to have reached any sort of static state in cultural or demographic terms. Rapid population growth, catalysts such as colonialism, the introduction of coffee cultivation, and an increasingly stratified social world compelled further change in the twentieth century.

The *kihamba* regime was the demographic story of nineteenth-century Chagga culture, with population growth as its leitmotif and land crisis its denouement. Dissonance in the system came from tensions between the ideals of initiation, marriage, and *kihamba* maintenance and the realities faced by younger generations. In the early colonial era, an expanding population and internal struggles over resources produced strains within Chagga culture. An increasing reliance on productive activities ancillary to *kihamba* cultivation, and a range of culturally acknowledged alternative sexual and marital arrangements, reflected this state of affairs. Gender, sexual values, and social and biological reproduction nevertheless remained linked to cultural models of male and female life courses that appear to have been in flux.

Within a matter of a few decades, many Chagga vigorously adopted new institutions such as the church, the school, and the clinic and a new source of wealth in coffee farming. While the rate of growth and change in Kilimanjaro may be a subject of debate, the magnitude of its impact upon Chagga culture and society is not in dispute. Many people in Kilimanjaro, as in southern Rhodesia, were able to "think about themselves as men and women in ways which had no place in the lives of their grandparents" (Jeater 1993:227). Yet Chagga brought several cultural values forward into their encounter with colonialism and modernity, values of key relevance to the moral demography of contemporary Kilimanjaro. Chief among these was a valorized concept of ordered social reproduction grounded in a *kihamba*-based life course.

For men, this entailed accountability toward siblings, spouses, and patrikin. For women, it meant participation in a reproductive regime that gave them precisely delineated spheres of control in social and domestic life. Over time, the challenges posed to the moral order of the *kihamba* regime coalesced into a moral demographic narrative of cultural dislocation and disordered social reproduction, a narrative which became central to the cultural life of AIDS in the 1990s.

Ethnographers have long drawn attention to the artifice of Chagga nostalgia over the decline of "culture" and "tradition" (Raum 1940: 289–90). Indeed, for most of this century, Chagga have been discussing their demographic predicament and the contradictions it has posed. They have been aware that the rapidity of social change has left them increasingly unable to regenerate an ideally ordered cultural world according to older, *kihamba*-based models of kinship duties, marital obligations, and family formation.

These nostalgic dialogues have taken the form of a set of oral demographies with moralistic themes and of local discourses about population dynamics, the waning cultural integrity of reproductive life courses, and economic decline. The moral aspects of these discourses stem from the fact that they have involved explicit judgments of personhood and character. The connections between morality and demography are made possible by the fact that, for Chagga, "character" is embodied in issues closely related to local population dynamics. These include gender roles in reproduction, adult sexuality, fertility, mobility, morbidity, and even mortality. In particular, cultural critiques of men's behavior and changing concepts of desire have been central to these moral demographies and, later, to cultural explanations about the origins of AIDS. It must be borne in mind, however, that near universal knowledge of AIDS influenced the way in which individual men and women recounted local population histories in the 1990s. Regardless of whether the epidemic is vanquished, there will never again be an oral demography in Kilimanjaro that is not conceived in the shadow of the epidemic.

# CHAPTER 3

## Population, Men, and Movement: (M)oral Demographies of Desire and Risk

> A have-not dishonors his manhood.
> > Moral from an *mregho* lesson (Raum 1940:331)

### Disease, Mobility, and Risk

If one considers the relationship between disease patterns (including STDs) and mobility in Africa during the twentieth century, it is easy to see why local ideas about AIDS in Kilimanjaro were often related to cultural stories about population dynamics. In Kilimanjaro, as in South Africa, much about AIDS could be summed up as a case of "old crisis, new virus" (Jochelson, Mothibeli, and Leger 1991:158). To begin with, the colonial era certainly represented a sea change in young men's (and hence young women's) access to the means of self-replacement according to the models prescribed under the *kihamba* regime. These changes, examined below, emerged out of a growing population competing for increasingly scarce *kihamba* lands. This was the result of the paradox of the success of the *kihamba* regime, combined with specific external forces. The roots of this scarcity and the competition it provoked were in the rapidly differentiating rural society and the introduction of coffee, which made *kihamba* lands valuable possessions and productive of wealth in an entirely new way. The result of this demographic and economic squeeze was an out-migration of men from the *kihamba* zone that started in the first decades of the century and increased through at least the 1980s.

Overall, it is difficult to know what "health" in a community sense may have looked like to those living through this era of population change. On one hand, the calamitous regional rates of morbidity and mortality of the end of the nineteenth century had subsided. On the other, colonialism was causing rapid shifts in the disease ecology of large sections of the African population. Many of these changes depended upon discrete kinds of dislocation and movement. These in-

cluded participation in expanding trade networks in rural areas, a
move to a mine or a town, seasonal plantation work, or military con-
scription. Some of these were voluntary and some directly or indirectly
coercive. All of them, however, had a potential effect on disease patterns.

There were shifts both in the epidemiology and the overall burden
of prevalent diseases, and new pathogens were introduced.[1] Men and
women were displaced from familiar modes of social reproduction,
enrolled in industrialized labor forces, and encountered poor living
conditions in the towns and cities to which they moved (Packard
1989:3). Across Africa, sharp rises in mortality and morbidity due to
conditions such as tuberculosis, malnutrition, and diseases associated
with poor sanitation were seen among labor migrants during the early
part of the century.

Colonial responses to African diseases like malaria and tuberculosis
equated race and vulnerability in ways not unfamiliar in the AIDS era.
Colonial authorities took measures to segregate migrants from Europeans on the grounds that the Africans themselves, rather than the conditions in which Africans were forced to live, were responsible for the
rise in morbidity (Curtin 1985; Packard 1989:52; Schoepf 1991b:94). Mobility also separated men and women for long periods of time, placing
them in different disease ecologies and thereby introducing or exag-
gerating differentials of risk among them (e.g., Turshen 1984; Cordell,
Gregory, and Piché 1992:49–61). In the postcolonial era these trends
have continued, and population movement and urbanization have remained important dynamics in epidemiologic change across the continent (Good 1991:4).

### Mobility and STDs

Lack of attention to the sociocultural bases of STDs in Africa has been
systematic in a vast literature that includes more than two thousand
references (Barton 1991; Caraël 1996:58). Yet even where these bases
are revealed, connections to fertility, infertility, and reproduction are
too rarely made. Ignoring how AIDS relates to fertility, as well as to
mobility, represents a failure to address dynamics at the very heart
of the epidemic. The previous chapter has shown how culture both
influenced and responded to demographic conditions. As men, in particular, became more mobile, their long-term outlooks on viable lifeways and reproductive careers changed along with their exposure to a

variety of illnesses, including STDs. As with other diseases, the spread of STDs in Africa has long been associated with the mobility of men and women for trade and labor (Setel 1999a).

The link between social and demographic change in Africa and the epidemic spread of STDs prompted debates among colonial medical personnel that foreshadowed later concerns about AIDS. These concerns coalesced into familiar discursive formulations that overwrote the subtler social dynamics of epidemiology and movement or, as in the case of malaria and tuberculosis, simply equated risk and race. Depending on the context, these epidemiologic "creation myths" could be applied to either sex. During the late nineteenth and early twentieth centuries in South Africa, for example, the notion of "migrant-as-vector" was applied to male miners in South Africa for both TB and STDs (Packard 1989; Jochelson 1991). During the 1940s and 1950s, a similar story was told about the movement of women from Haya areas of western Tanzania, many of whom engaged in commercial sex work (Kaijage 1993). In Uganda, another narrative formulation of disordered African sexuality and STDs predominated. Between the 1910s and 1930s, physicians, missionaries, and colonial officials generally blamed high rates of syphilis on the removal of social controls over female sexuality (Vaughan 1991:130ff.).[2]

Early epidemiologic studies of the spread of AIDS in Africa started with this conventional wisdom about mobility and risk and ignored fertility issues altogether. Researchers reasoned that the epidemiology of HIV would both mirror historical routes of STD transmission and expand along emerging networks of geographic mobility and urbanization (see Quinn 1994; Cohen and Trussell 1996:64–66). Although men dominated most of the migration networks studied, some were the province of women. In addition to the movement of Haya women in Tanzania to and from urban areas and neighboring countries, the circular migration of Ghanaians to Abidjan (Ivory Coast) was dominated by women (Anarfi 1992:243–44).[3] Among Sereer in rural Senegal, migration has also been circular and gendered (Garenne, Becker, and Cardenas 1992:272–73). Through the early 1990s, young Sereer women often moved to Dakar for several successive dry seasons to work and to prepare for marriage. By sixteen years of age, many took urban lovers. Sereer men have migrated for longer periods, but not to cities. They have tended to remain in rural areas and to establish long-term "fiancée" relationships or to purchase sex. This has led to somewhat different axes of risk and mobility for the sexes. In other parts of Senegal that experience similar seasonal migration most married couples have been regularly separated for seven months of each year (Enel and Pison 1992:251). During separations, the behavior of men and women has differed, with up to half of men taking extramarital partners in other rural areas where they travel to tap palm wine, and women (ostensibly) remaining abstinent at home villages.

The phenomenon of truck-stop communities and subcultures provides an extreme example of the relationship between geographical mobility, gender, and risk for STD and HIV infection (Forthal et al. 1986; Lwihula 1990; Nguma, Leshabari, and Mpangile 1991; O'Connor, Leshabari, and Lwihula 1992; Orubuloye, Caldwell, and Caldwell 1993). In these settings, well-paid male truck drivers who travel for long periods of time away from their homes meet female traders, bar maids, and hotel workers, who are economically marginalized. These situations have led to obvious risks for the rapid spread of the epidemic, but have also revealed unique adaptations of cultural principles related to polygyny. In northern Nigeria, men who cannot maintain a single permanent home establish a semipermanent one at each stop. In some cases they conclude marriages with women there, further developing a version of roadside domesticity. Many women, meanwhile, may fill this role for several men at once—sometimes with the tacit knowledge of their various husbands, sometimes without (Orubuloye, Caldwell, and Caldwell 1993:44–45).

These truck stops, where men may engage in polygyny on a chiefly scale and women carefully orchestrate their cryptopolyandrous existences, emphasize the social and epidemiologic consequences of mobility. In areas with high rates of geographic, economic, and social mobility, movement has been at the core of transformations in the forms, timing, and stability of marriage and has played a role in altering marital fertility (Timæus and Graham 1989:386). Because of such disruption to social reproduction, mobility has also been at the center of struggles over the (loss of) control of female and male sexual activity both in- and outside marriage (Jeater 1993; Weiss 1993).

These strands of gender, movement, and shifting economic lifeways came together forcefully in the early AIDS epidemic in Kilimanjaro. The local dialogue about AIDS focused so exclusively on sex and sexual behavior that reproduction was often ignored. Yet reproduction was really at the heart of the debate. Epidemic disease and population dynamics under demographic and economic pressures intersected in both local narratives about HIV and the local manifestations of the epidemic.

## Chagga Moral Demographies and the Birth of Desire
### The Concept of "Moral Demographies" and AIDS

While it is critical to demonstrate the empirical associations of historical patterns of mobility, urbanization, STDs, and nuptiality, it is equally important to document whether and how local populations themselves place AIDS in historical perspective.[4] Not only does this provide insight into how interveners might address local concepts of risk among population subgroups for short-term prevention education, but it can also illuminate deep elements of cultural debate about structural inequality and social instability relevant to broader development issues. In western Tanzania, for example, local perspectives on AIDS served to reactivate stigmas associated with female mobility and economic activity that were prevalent there since the 1930s. This can be viewed in the context of strains on cultural preferences of control over women in marriage and, ultimately, to controlling their access to land (Weiss 1993: 32–33). The historicized views of AIDS presented here and in chapters 5 and 6 reveal the more general need to comment upon the political and economic roots of the group experience of disease. As Farmer has shown in Haiti, decoding local understandings on the basis of what I have termed "moral demographies," helps "to explain *why* members of a particular community came to understand illnesses such as . . . AIDS in the manner in which they did" (Farmer 1992:256).

Understanding these local perspectives has a direct bearing on how we understand the position of those most vulnerable to infection. Failing to comprehend the links between demography, political economy, gender, marriage, mobility, and risk is to miscomprehend the issues of real relevance to perceptions of risk in Kilimanjaro. This point was brought home to me at an AIDS seminar run at a Lutheran church in western Kilimanjaro. The day was full of skits about the proper care of the AIDS ill and reducing shame, of presentations from regional officials about the state of the epidemic in the region, and of informational speeches about HIV transmission and the course of HIV infection. Afterward, one woman approached me and asked a very direct question: What good was all this education, she wanted to know, when none of it reached her husband? After all, she went on, he was the one who would infect her and for her to mention condoms (as a "good" wife) was simply inconceivable.[5] Thus the call for an interpretive anthropology that is "fully accountable to its historical and political-economy implications" (Marcus and Fischer 1986:86) in the AIDS epidemic is more than an appeal for generating richly contextualized accounts of sex. It is part of a project Farmer has termed a "responsible materialism" (1992:258).

In order to comprehend this woman's physical risk and her perception of it, we must examine the moral demographics of vulnerability in Kilimanjaro. Through "moral demography," various actors produce knowledge about the locations of bodies (migration), their status (morbidity and mortality), and the consequences of reproductive action (fertility). These demographic narratives told the story of AIDS and young people in Kilimanjaro. Furthermore, there was a gap between the formal demographics and the stories told about population dynamics on the local stage. The formal demographics of youth in the twentieth century might have led (and may in future lead) to a number of causal stories or explanatory models of the AIDS epidemic. Demography does not tell one *particular* story. The stories told are, at least in part, a function of the perspective of local actors making sense of a rapidly changing demographic regime. This knowledge inevitably becomes enlisted in the work of culture on a "discursive" level.[6] These moral demographies set the stage for the arrival of the epidemic, and they surrounded both the women left behind on the mountain slopes and those dislocated from the *kihamba* regime over the past century. These "ethnodemographies" also linked cultural concepts of "desire" and "moral character" to the wider structural conditions in which they emerged and became relevant ways of conceptualizing social and physical disorder.

It is important to bear in mind that changes in behavior related to risk of contracting new illnesses did not emerge solely from more individualizing modern institutions supplanting local, group-oriented ones. Rather, it arose out of the effects of new idioms on different subgroups of the population. Anthropologists have been warned about the facile application of ideas of "cultural logic" in accounts of emerging patterns of social organization. When explaining how local groups engage with external forces, the "problem with 'cultural logic,'" Guyer has noted, "is the primacy accorded to culture and the assumption of its 'logic'" (1981:126). Bearing in mind this caveat, it is nevertheless possible to see the moral aspect of Chagga oral demographies as deriving from the *kihamba* regime as it came to grips with change under colonialism.

Moral demographies are based upon a perceived link between concrete biological events, population processes, and cultural experience. The narratives raise questions about the relationship between biological bodies and social persons and how culture mediates this relationship. While bodies and actions do not in any way precede culture, they do precede certain forms of cultural work (such as the production of discursive or disciplinary knowledge). This notion builds upon insight latent in Africanist scholarship (see Riesman 1986; Jackson and Karp 1990).

This aspect of the idea of moral demography is not merely a way of recounting folk beliefs. It is intended to reproduce the palpable, but unexpressed, sense of an inchoate, embodied form of meaning. It is meant to challenge the subjugation of the somatic to the semantic, an "empirically untenable . . . tendency [within anthropology] to interpret embodied experience in terms of cognitive and linguistic models of meaning" (Jackson 1989:122). This linkage of bodies and meaning also related to what others, following Peirce, have called the "qualisign" or processes of "qualisignfication" (e.g., Munn 1986; Daniel 1994; Weiss 1996). The notion of bodies as qualisigns positions them as "signs that are mere qualitative possibilities in contradistinction to signs that are actualized and/or generalized . . . [a qualisign] is not a completed sign, but a sign of possibility . . . a sign that admits to the inexhaustibility of its representational mission; one never gets to the bottom of it" (Daniel 1994:229–30). Because this category of sign only exists in the context of systems of human action and meaning, it inherently, indeterminately, and unceasingly points to the *embodiment of values* produced by action (see Munn 1986:16–17).

The concept of moral demographies developed here incorporates this sense of an unfolding embodiment of values, values that are revealed over time through the qualities ascribed to actions associated with social reproduction.[7] The construction of persons through the significance associated with the uses and failures of their bodies in the moral demographies of Kilimanjaro is a process that remains open-ended. It has been and will remain subject to manipulation by actors with divergent interests in particular representations of action.

These demographic narratives place changes in the meaning of sexuality in the context of spatial and symbolic dislocation of younger cohorts off the mountain, and away from sexual values of social reproduction in the waning *kihamba* regime. Those who were dislocated experienced a cruel dilemma. On one hand the social conditions of sexual and reproductive life were changing rapidly. On the other, the cultural values and articulated codes of sexual ideology were increasingly based on a practice of Christianity (and occasionally Islam) that served mainly to bolster older, *kihamba*-regime ideals. So seamlessly

were world religions woven into Chagga cultural consciousness on this
score that a Lutheran pastor speaking at a World AIDS Day rally in
1991 called for the need to return to "our traditional Chagga culture
whether Christian or Muslim."[8]

In the late twentieth century, population growth and its consequences lay behind nearly all narratives of changing personal morali-
ties, behind familiar diatribes against young people and the erosion of
"customs and traditions" (mila na desturi). AIDS added sting to the
blame. People in northern Kilimanjaro took for granted that a combination of group experience and disordered individual action had brought
about the epidemic; for them, an awareness of one did not make sense
without the other. In their narratives external influences (such as colonialism) led to cultural loss, which, in turn, rendered men vulnerable
to seductive desires. This brought about family breakdown, and promiscuous sex. The result: AIDS. The moral demography of Kilimanjaro
reveals that the harmonies of individual aspiration and modes of social
reproduction under the kihamba regime were fading long before the
arrival of HIV. This was an attenuated calamity that foreshadowed the
epidemic.

What people thought about the relationship between individual versus group values was informed by local history and by local notions
of culture itself. The implication that culture has been locked in a losing
battle with the individual can surely be meaningful only if "culture"
is thought of in the most simplistic way as a set of norms, conventions,
or constraints that can be lost or jettisoned, rather than as something
intrinsic to human existence. When Chagga spoke of cultural loss, they
did so primarily in the simple sense of breakdowns in cultural rules
and convention. To accept this sentiment for the purposes of representing local ideas, however, requires anthropologists only to specify the
conditions under which this belief emerged, not to substitute it for our
own concept of cultural process and change.

It was common belief that broad social forces motivated particular
responses from individuals, and that the quality of these responses lent
insight into their moral character. These external forces included population growth and dislocation, extremes of wealth and want, and lack
of an ordered productive life. Conversely, individual attributes could
exacerbate the dissolution of group morality and foster the spread of
social dissolution or, in the case of AIDS, epidemic disease. In particular, these personal characteristics included a form of desire for both
persons and things called tamaa, and bad moral character, tabia mbaya
(or, in an extreme form, uhuni). While any of these topics could serve

as an entry point into the discussion of moral demographies in Kilimanjaro, the concept of desire is especially apt.

## The History of Desire

More than many other concerns, tales of cultural demise and AIDS
were united by the gravity attributed to disordered desire.[9] *Tamaa* was
commonly used to evoke the sense of a deeply felt urge, with negative
connotations. Excessive *tamaa* was synonymous with bad moral character, which in turn was revealed through the misallocation of one's
productive and reproductive resources and energies. This account of
*tamaa*, demographic narratives, and demographic conditions explains
why many people who moved away from the mountain were seen as
bad, morally vulnerable, and at risk of AIDS. Within the local stories
about people and population, Chagga culture engaged demography
in a selective and partial way. This engagement produced clichés of
disrupted reproductive sexuality and diminished social controls over
individual behavior long before the AIDS era—clichés which have continued to find their way with great regularity and questionable effectiveness into AIDS prevention and education.

The birth and growth of *tamaa,* an emotion with a history, contained
within it a layered set of implicit statements about personal disposition
and changes wrought by population dynamics and modernity.[10] Although a concept such as *tamaa* could be said to exist for individuals
in an extremely personal sense, to regard it as solely the product of
individual psyche, libidinous tendencies, or selfish longings stripped
of cultural constraint would be inaccurate.[11] Such a formulation does
not correspond to more considered local exegesis about *tamaa* or to the
range of contexts in which this type of desire could be said to apply
(discussed below). In its sexualized form, *tamaa* was a cultural carnality
of context, prompted at specific times in specific places by specific categories of objects and persons.

In 1991, at a training session for HIV/AIDS counselors at a Catholic
hospital outside Moshi, Esther Lema, a Chagga psychiatrist, articulated
a moral demography in which the dislocation of youth, and of men in
particular, was linked to the epidemic:

> What about our culture? What about Chagga culture? Is it intact?
> No. How was it in the old days? There was a big punishment for
> adultery and promiscuity—the Mangi could sentence you to
> death. They'd stake you down dead at the crossroads, even until
> 1968. This is all because Chagga culture has been polluted, and

mixed with European ways. . . . In the past, there was initiation and puberty training. Men learned their age sets and women were circumcised. . . . But it is true that today, Chagga culture has crumbled and is dead. The youth today are all tied up in the profligacy of the disco, bearing children out of marriage, and so on. Women are doing petty business, and men are all along the highways leaving home. The home is crumbling. Before, you never saw married women wandering around Arusha, or going to the border, or in the markets selling beer. Now it's totally different. There are even girls wandering all over the place. They go all the way to cities down south and their parents don't even know. AIDS comes from all of this. At Christmas the men come from outside, come home, and bring the gift of AIDS. They drink and make love, and try to get their women pregnant. . . . They come home and what do you do to stop this infection at Christmas? . . . We will end up having a funeral every day. We will be tired.[12]

Like the song "Hey, Listen!" this demographic denunciation was echoed in one form or another in countless settings in Kilimanjaro during the early 1990s. In this extract from her speech, Lema did not use the term "desire." Rather, she evoked it with references to the influence of external culture, to business life, and to itinerancy. For Lema's audience, the notion of *tamaa* was implicit in the conviction that the origins of AIDS were to be found in the demise of *kihamba*-based traditional culture. This, she indicated, was bound up with the seductive and character-destroying influence of mixing with "European ways," the long-term mobility of men coming home from "outside" at Christmas time, and the domestic delinquency of women engaged in the "wanderings of market life."

As Lema suggested, many people thought *tamaa* was inseparable from the development process, a product of the colonial encounter and the mixing of cultures in postcolonial society. As one friend, a thirty-six-year-old man living in Moshi, put it: "Life was very simple one to two hundred years ago. In the past, our grandfathers . . . had fruits, animals . . . they didn't have *tamaa*. *Tamaa* did not exist. *Tamaa* entered our society when foreigners came; when Europeans brought material goods that weren't known here—things like shoes, tables, cloth, plates, bowls, coats, boots, forks, knives, blankets, mattresses, beds, cars, lamps, metal sheeting, pressure lamps, flat irons. [So *tamaa* is always based on objects brought by Europeans?] It is always based on something you have seen. After all, you can't desire a 'Benz if you've never seen one."[13]

While some disputed whether or not *tamaa* itself existed before the colonial era, the arrival of Europeans certainly opened a Pandora's box of possibilities: "When foreign traditions and people migrated in, and education was introduced . . . we can say that it's not only the foreigners who contributed in the destruction of our tradition; even those who are educated have brought down their customs. That is why we can say *tamaa* was there from the beginning [but] that the chances of allowing it to overcome us were not there."[14] Objects for which one could feel *tamaa* were ones that were seen. The object of this desire had to be visualized. Thus, this particular type of desire was one of appearances, of surfaces, of representation. *Tamaa* fetishized specific types of objects from outside places. In particular, it fetishized money and the objects one could buy with it.[15] In doing so, it simultaneously drew attention to and hid the unequal power relations that were inherent in the production and distribution of these objects. The badness of money and the colonial conditions under which it was acquired nevertheless gave access to things that looked increasingly good. As the material conditions of life in Kilimanjaro changed during the century, so did ideas about what constituted good homes, families, and workable social relations of reproduction.

Again, Chagga felt that large-scale forces were responsible for the allure of the new. Some of these forces (such as population growth, land scarcity, and rural stratification) were inherently linked to the *kihamba* regime, while others (such as Christianity and European education) were colonial imports. Where *tamaa* pulled, these other factors pushed. Christianity and education were particularly important in the reorientation of ambitions and tastes.[16] In Kilimanjaro, "The Christian educated convert came to be regarded as an example of modern man" (Howard 1980:54). Particularly for elites, education offered new ways of establishing and maintaining personal and family prosperity (Lawuo 1980:85; Samoff 1974:39, 56); the expenditure of coffee money on education was "by far the most important cash investment" made in the development process (Moore 1986:129).[17]

Yet the appeal of education would later be regarded by some as having come at a high price. As one married woman stated, "In the 1960s many [men] started to move away. Now they only return once in a while. The difference, you see, is education. Now that they are educated, they marry women from other ethnic groups and pretend like they're strangers around here. They marry those women and learn things—some of which are good, maybe, but our customs and traditions are in pieces."[18] In the dominant moral demography of 1992, men's taking "outside" women had a doubly negative connotation: that of having sex outside marriage and of perpetuating a modern ethos of mixing customs by having partners from outside groups. Such actions, people asserted, were a like dagger in the heart of the promise of development, a mortal wound to the all-but-moribund reproductive program of the *kihamba* regime.

Chagga who were being displaced from the *kihamba* began to lose a sense of its day-to-day routines. Older patterns of relations between men and women across generations began to unravel. Many people began to take on an entirely new set of domestic tastes, values, and ambitions. A sense of being "modern" Africans and a firm belief in the benefits of development, most notably through education, quickly took hold: "With coffee cash . . . changes of style manifest themselves. The elite took up tea drinking. The taste for sugar spread. The Chagga purchased cooking oil, as well as soap, metal knives and spoons, china cups and plates. Each of these and many other new items peddled upcountry were trivial, but in aggregate they came to constitute a cultural commitment to an external economy" (Moore 1986:129). As my friend indicated, *tamaa* for things was thought to have been prompted by this dazzling array of what (from the vantage point of economic decline in the 1980s and AIDS in the 1990s) Chagga often viewed as the mixed blessing of modern life. As coffee money increased, even the most mundane technologies of living began to exhibit the influence of a modern aesthetic, and by the late 1920s several hundred privately owned shops in rural Kilimanjaro were selling products of Western manufacture (Lawuo 1980:39).[19] The play of Chagga children in the 1930s and 1940s was filled with caricatured colonial imagery divorced from the *kihamba* regime (Raum 1940:257–58). Children might imitate priests with pocket watches or schoolteachers with books.

Thus, the cultural commitment to an external economy was more than a reaction to demographic pressures. It entailed a new way of viewing the relationship between persons and the world of things, of growing desires in the context of an increasing displacement of persons from familiar reproductive and productive regimes. It is possible, therefore, to comprehend how Chagga could view desire for new things as part of a dubious realignment in the moral character of those at greatest remove from the *kihamba* way of life. These realignments were made visible through means and modes of production that had less and less to do with the household and kinship structures of the *kihamba* regime. It was all so simple and subtle, trivial even: men used coffee money to buy new dresses for their wives.

To understand *tamaa* is to understand that desire was not just lust, materialistic or sexual. It was an anxious predilection, born of the *ki-*

*hamba* and coffee cash, to acquire something better. It was produced in a specific and prosperous cultural and historical context, and, in recent years, it has been exacerbated by economic decline. This modernizing process does not imply a *loss* of culture—however much people in Kilimanjaro protested that it did—but rather its *transformation* and reconfiguration through aggregate application of cultural valuation to new and more diverse contexts.[20]

As Weiss noted with regard to the cultural significance of commoditization among Haya in the 1990s, "Far from being the predictable scourge of meaning in social relations, material forces and commodity forms . . . often *engender* . . . dense symbolic forms and practices" (1996: 177). The rapidity and apparent wholeheartedness with which Chagga were oriented toward modernity, commodities, and cash may at first seem puzzling. Why was such change not more incremental? Part of the answer, as Henrietta Moore has suggested, appears to be that such shifts may imply a wholesale reorientation of how cultural values are represented (Moore 1996:160–61). Among Marakwet in Kenya during the 1980s, for instance, changes of taste in housing styles and furnishings represented a fundamental and intentional alteration in the use of personal domestic space. The move away from traditional architectural forms and customary modes of furnishing and toward square houses and manufactured consumer items was not merely a matter of selecting from among a range of newly available forms.

*Tamaa* grew out of the conditions in which one formed one's most basic wants and hopes, one's *tabia* (moral character). This type of desire extended to a range of cultural settings—sexual, economic, domestic, political. When Chagga spoke of this broader set of ambitions, they generally framed the issue as one of "following," "pursuing," or "searching for" a good life *(kufuata* or *kutafuta maisha mazuri)*. By doing so, they drew attention to the idea that things worth having and ways worth living were inherently part of a quest that required movement and removal. As Maro, himself a Chagga, put it in his study of population and agriculture in Kilimanjaro, "The aspirations and ambitions of the people and their willingness and ability to accept new ideas and hard work, has been the prime mover towards 'modernization.' Nobody forced anybody to grow coffee or go to school, rather, *it was the desire to live 'a good life' . . . which motivated the people*" (1975:23; emphasis added).

True, no individual agents forced the sweeping changes taking place on the mountain. Yet force existed nonetheless in the groundswell of demographic change that pushed younger cohorts to invent or exploit new opportunities. As the material resources of the *kihamba* regime shrank, the productive horizons for young people had to expand—either locally or at a physical remove from the mountain community. The burgeoning population moved down and away from Kilimanjaro. They met with a corresponding movement of colonial institutions upward and into the *kihamba* world, penetrating Chagga lineages, households, and age grades, affecting the representational use of bodies and ambitions and desires of persons.

People in Kilimanjaro often felt that these population dynamics were driven first and foremost by individual motivations and choice—by the "desire to live a good life." *Tamaa* caused the dislocation and relocation of young people, and demographic and economic pressures were seen as secondary. Certainly this makes sense if one remembers that people only had the evidence of their immediate social networks upon which to form their perceptions. Thus many of the local population histories were suffused with a retrospective evaluation of the net effects for households and kinship of the life choices of young people and the desires which seem to have inspired them.[21] For those who moved, the sentimentalization of the mountain became enshrined in the well-known Chagga pilgrimages from elsewhere in Tanzania back to Kilimanjaro each year at Christmastime. In December each year, extra trains are scheduled from Dar es Salaam to Moshi, and buses are packed to capacity.

Desire, in the contemporary sense to which many Chagga refer to it, was born of demographic ferment and, as Lema indicated, out of the dislocation of young adults from a *kihamba*-based life. Behind the rush toward the new was the push of population growth and intensifying land pressures on the mountain. Given the growth of the population and the added pressures of the coffee-driven land squeeze, conditions for social reproduction on the mountain became untenable within a few decades. Many young men and women embraced alternative models for productive life and celebrated the material conditions in which to realize them.

The cohorts who were dislocated through this process, and the effects of their dislocation on those left behind, were at the center of the moral demographics of desire. When Ezra (a man with AIDS, whose story is discussed in chapter 6) told me about his life, he explained that after completing primary school, he was eager to get to town and break away from the strict upbringing of his father on the mountain. Ezra moved to Moshi in the mid-1960s and began earning wages there. He explained, "It was then I started to have *tamaa* for women. It was because of the surroundings. For me, life in the city was not very usual. There were people who drank beer, they went with women. . . . Little by little I started to look for a girlfriend. I didn't have to look very hard. There was one beer shop, and there was a woman there who liked me. She even came to my house looking for me."[22]

Clearly, the concept of desire, so central to the cultural life of AIDS, cannot be understood from a cultural insider's perspective without taking into account the social environment in which individuals were thought to have become so vulnerable to its predations. This environment emerged at the intersection of population growth, social stratification, land pressures, urbanization, and mobility.

### Dislocation: The Demographic Context of Desire

Given these local interpretations of population dynamics, we must also consider what was taking place at the time that did not find its way into local historical consciousness of population dynamics. The "formal" demography of Kilimanjaro and the social conditions in which it has been enmeshed demand a much more rigorous treatment than will be offered here. What follows is merely a sketch of the demographic contours of an integrated and attenuated crisis, a set of demographic themes that brought Chagga men and women to the brink of the epidemic and informed their understandings of it. AIDS fit into local demographic narratives through its links to desire. Desire, in turn, was seen to have motivated dislocation. Need, social disruption, geographic and economic mobility have thereby become tinged with an unprecedented virulence.

During the nineteenth century, the verdant mountain slopes drew new migrants, and, for the most part, those who settled there prospered. Kilimanjaro was fertile in more than an agricultural sense. Before the early 1900s and a coffee-inspired land grab, land shortages were already developing for some Chagga, and there were concerns in the colonial administration about population pressures building in parts of the kihamba zone.[23] Given the centrality of the kihamba to Chagga life, the fact that the total arable land between 3,500 and 6,000 feet on Kilimanjaro totals less than 500 square miles began to assume "staggering significance" in the face of this growth (Howard 1980:43). With many sons who required vihamba, the gardens underwent a relentless process of subdivision once all kihamba-zone land was taken, a cultural recipe for dislocation. Early on in the colonial period, the

seizure of land by Europeans hemmed in Chagga expansion, intensifying the pressures on the land.

Although most local narratives dealt with the post–World War II
era, several important conditions relating to this process were already
evident by the 1920s. Once coffee became established as a lucrative
cash crop, the land crisis became acute: "Coffee . . . made unoccupied
land valuable, and population growth made it scarce" (Moore 1986:
111).[24] The earliest response to the demand for suitable coffee-growing
land in the *kihamba* zone was to fill unoccupied plots with coffee trees.
On existing *vihamba,* land was diverted from food production to coffee
farming. By 1927, Chagga were commodifying and bureaucratizing the
anchoring symbol of their cultural worldview through the sale, purchase, and titling of *vihamba* lands. By the 1930s, "rural" Kilimanjaro
may have seemed something like an emergent, sprawling city, with
many areas approaching urban population densities and possessing a
concentration of churches, schools, clinics, and shops more typical of
towns.

Thus, the political economic roots and consequences of the land crisis
in Kilimanjaro, and the role of cash cropping in it, must not be overlooked. As land use changed, land value increased. This aspect of local
demography tinged the experience of dislocation with an economic
cast; stability and instability were intimately connected to unequal access to the means of social reproduction, access that was increasingly
favoring a privileged rural elite. More powerful clans were able to extend authority over remaining land on Kilimanjaro, and plots shrank
and fragmented. A widening gap emerged between land-rich and land-
poor.

In these circumstances, even the most structurally secure, such as
male members of powerful clans, or first- and last-born sons, faced
decreasing prospects for completing a *kihamba*-based circuit through
the life course. In the Usambara Mountains, about 150 miles to the
south of Kilimanjaro, Sambaa communities were contending with similar pressures (Feierman 1993). Privileged clans there exerted a similar
degree of control over available land, a move that ultimately affected
patterns of male out-migration. Nor were such dynamics limited to
northeastern Tanzania. In other East African locations with patrilineal
inheritance and where ecological conditions favored an intensification
and expansion of mixed banana and coffee cultivation, growing numbers of young people were being displaced (Kasfir 1993).

In Kilimanjaro, the ramifications of growth and accelerating dislocation were stark. *Mangis* (the Chagga chiefs) and settlers clashed over

access to rural labor (TNA 5.449), and more and more men were drawn inexorably into the plantation economy. Men worked on the farms during the week and only returned to home areas on weekends (Iliffe 1979: 154).[25] While significant numbers of people were accommodated locally through increased demands for food production for local consumption, movement, whether long- or short-term migration or daily or weekly commuting, became unavoidable for many young people.[26] By the 1960s and 1970s, Kilimanjaro was said to be the most overpopulated region in the country in terms of rural carrying capacity (Moore 1971). Nearly all the older men in one part of the mountain (Marangu) had been born on the land on which they were living, yet nearly two-thirds of them had two or more sons whom they expected to be landless (Maro 1975:13). Even though they were nominally resident in rural wards, half of these young men were either unemployed or working in the urban areas of Moshi or Arusha (17).

Although there are no quantitative data that specifically tie the rapid acquisition of remaining *vihamba* land in the mid-1990s to male out-migration, it is reasonable to suppose that there was indeed a close link between the two. It seems reasonable to suggest, further, that rural differentiation starting early in the coffee era may also have exerted demographic pressures. In Chagga moral demographic narratives it was not only the sheer volume of growth and the disrupting effects of migration that mattered but also the consequences of the change it produced in reproductive sexuality. Questing for alternatives to the *kihamba* regime and a new world of wealth and succession was all well and good, but what about the effects on the *kihamba*-based family life at the heart of Chagga social life?

Reproductive change for Chagga occurred on at least three related levels during the twentieth century: there were shifts in total fertility, the timing of childbirth, and the social conditions under which women were having children. The last issue is most significant for this discussion because it is linked to the dislocation and relocation of both men and women off and away from the mountain. While the relative contributions to growth rates of in-migration, high or rising fertility, and decreased or decreasing mortality cannot be assessed, it seems evident that Chagga were indeed having a great many babies and that these babies were surviving. By the 1950s, the Northern Province (which included Kilimanjaro) appears to have been the fastest growing area in the entire Tanganyika Territory, and Chagga were by far the youngest population in the Territory at the time (Tanganyika Territory 1957).[27] Even though age at marriage and the age at which women were having their first births were rising, fertility remained high in Kilimanjaro compared with elsewhere in Tanzania.[28]

As young men who needed to establish households were squeezed out of the *kihamba* zone onto land at the base of the mountain, social hierarchies weakened. Mobility and urbanization were the watchwords of the changing life situations of those who, fifty years before, would have been the leaders of the *kihamba* regime. Men moved to distant cities and traveled for business. By 1957 there were anywhere from one to several thousand Chagga in residence in every other region of Tanganyika but one, making them one of the most widely distributed ethnic groups in the Territory. All this for members of a cultural group that was known to stigmatize any land off and away from Mount Kilimanjaro as uniformly unfit for habitation by decent human beings. The cumulative effect was that, by 1988, Kilimanjaro had the greatest number of net lifetime out-migrants of any mainland region; out-migrants, mostly men, outnumbered in-migrants by more than 2.3:1.[29]

Many who remained on the mountain prospered from the peregrinations of their kin. Yet when they were interviewed about the past thirty years of local population history, older people intoned, as if they were dirges, stories of the exodus of men. After the World War II, out-migration picked up considerably and reached its peak in the 1960s and 1970s. Most of the migration was to Moshi, Arusha, or Dar es Salaam, with some moving to Mombassa or Nairobi. At this time, Kilimanjaro had the highest migration rates among young men in Tanzania (Barnum and Sabot 1976:108). While rural incomes stagnated (largely owing to the vagaries of world coffee prices), urban wages increased, and migration to Moshi rose sharply. Even those who maintained a toehold on the mountain were increasingly forced to take up some kind of income-generating activity that kept them off the mountain for long periods of time, and many found themselves among the growing number of daily commuters to Moshi town. Table 3.1 clearly establishes migration as characteristic of younger men in the 1960s.

Table 3.1 Percentage of Men Migrating out of Kilimanjaro Region, 1967

| Age Group | |
| --- | --- |
| 20–24 | 26.7 |
| 25–34 | 11.4 |
| 35+ | 2.6 |

Source: Barnum and Sabot (1976:108).

One-fourth of all men aged twenty to twenty-four migrated from Kilimanjaro, and the educated seemed to pour out of the region. Nearly 80 percent of those between twenty and thirty-four with one or more years of secondary education departed rural areas. Overall, rates of out-migration declined with age, tapering off to less than 3 percent for men aged thirty-five and older.

Moshi town was the primary destination for many young people. The draw of better wages made moving to town a more attractive option than staying relatively idle on the *kihamba* or working on a plantation.[30] By midcentury, Moshi had become a significant force in local population change and the regional colonial economy.[31] Migrants living in poor conditions in the growing town, however, had it rough. By 1929, the rail yard section of town (a focus of African settlement) was considered by city government to be a "hotbed of undesirables" (executive officer of Moshi Township Authority, quoted in Green 1986: 39). Migrants to this area constantly faced the threat of having their houses demolished owing to oppressive zoning laws. They contended with numerous pressures (such as being forbidden to garden in town) to join the wage labor force. Whatever the opportunities there, urban conditions were not pleasant for migrants, and by the 1930s Moshi began to take on some of the characteristic social and environmental ills of a modern city, with complaints from both Africans and Europeans about crowding, pollution, public drunkenness, and prostitution.[32]

Although these dominant demographic themes centered on male experience, they should not elide the fact that single women also underwent dislocation and urbanization, some of which, no doubt, was voluntary and some of which was not. The disruption of agricultural life courses for women is something more often associated with the economic upheavals of the 1980s, yet unmarried women were seeking opportunities in Moshi from at least the 1950s onward. Local leaders did not favor their increasing mobility and debated the daily flocking of women and children to town in local newspapers. They even proposed legislation designed to curtail their movements. In December 1954, letters were published in one paper which clearly linked urban space, female mobility, and uncontrolled sexuality. The letters complained about "girls leaving rural areas and moving to towns, and getting all sorts of diseases" (quoted in Meghji 1977:43). Nevertheless, from the late 1940s onward, women were employed in town and appear to have been able to make independent living arrangements. Meghji interviewed a number of women who went to work at a coffee factory in Moshi during the 1950s. One of them stated simply that "she likes town life as one could meet a lot of people and go to different interesting places. She likes going dancing or to films on weekends. She has different boyfriends who take her out. . . . She likes staying with her auntie because she does not interfere with her life" (1977:113–14).

People often described *tamaa* among young women, as well as young men, as a product of this type of modern life and the volatile mixture of lost culture, poverty, and the temptations of city life. Said one accountant in Moshi: "Many women these days have great *tamaa* for things. First, it's poverty [that drives them to link sex and desire], then others feel a great pleasure in sex. Their paternal aunts and mothers should be guarding them better, but they don't. Religion has lessened in value for women . . . they are exposed in school, work, they mix with many people who believe in different customs. Therefore they all sleep together randomly. Even marriage doesn't have the standing that it did in the past."[33]

From the 1950s to the 1990s, Moshi town grew apace with other urban areas and became crowded with young people from northern Tanzania and beyond. Between 1948 and 1967 its population more than doubled, and by 1972 it became the most predominantly male city in Tanzania, with an overall sex ratio of 128 males for every 100 females (Claeson and Egero 1972:15). Moshi also had the highest proportion of unmarried adults of any urban area in Tanzania. With three-quarters of the male population in their early twenties and single, Moshi easily acquired a reputation as a young man's town (Table 3.2). Surely there was no shortage of boyfriends to entertain Meghji's informant from the coffee-curing factory and her female co-workers. Between 1957 and 1988, the resident population of Moshi increased more than ten times to 96,631; two-thirds of this increase was accounted for by those born in Moshi itself and (mostly young male) migrants from elsewhere in the region.

A comparison of the age, sex, and occupational structures of both rural and urban communities reveals the disproportionate pressures on young people. The majority of Chagga still lived on the mountain.

Table 3.2 Percentage of Single Adults in Moshi by Selected Age Groups, 1967

| Age Group | Single Men | Single Women |
|-----------|-----------|--------------|
| 20–24 | 75 | 22 |
| 30–34 | 16 | 7 |
| 40–44 | 10 | 3 |

Source: Claeson and Egers (1972:10).

From their perspective Moshi was often viewed as a dubious and gendered location that subverted culturally honored ideas about the way men and women should live. For men, the point is not so much that they were becoming separated by great physical distances but that they increasingly seemed to be located in spaces that were socially and culturally remote from those inhabited by their parents and the mothers of their children. Thus, while Moshi seemed to offer the desirable option for Chagga of residing in town while maintaining close proximity to family, it quickly acquired a dubious role in local consciousness of population dynamics.

Most of the rural oral demographies collected came from the ward of Mbokomu, a few kilometers from Moshi town. In the early 1990s, the roads and paths that climbed the mountain were lined by what were effectively female-headed households. The adult population in residence was predominantly female and married; a quarter or more of these women had been left on the land with their spouses' children, almost as placeholders in the *kihamba* regime's still functioning system of succession.[34] In the 1970s, of 106 men with children, from a neighboring ward, 23 percent were residing in an urban area (Swantz, Henricson, and Zalla 1975:21). The majority of them were in Moshi, with Dar es Salaam and Arusha as the next most frequent places of residence. Another 10 percent worked in locations other than the rural wards, leaving only slightly more than half whose employment did not depend on mobility. Despite the rapid out-migration, by the 1960s population densities in Mbokomu and surrounding areas had reached over 240 per square kilometer, among the highest in rural Kilimanjaro (Thomas 1967). In the decade between 1978 and 1988, the population of reproductive age in Mbokomu grew by 15 percent, but the age and sex structure in the ward remained virtually unchanged, with a constant disparity of roughly 15 percent more women than men among people aged ten to fifty.

Figure 3.1 compares the sex ratios of men to women by age group in Mbokomu and Njoro (an urban ward where many people from Mbokomu went to stay). It is essential to bear in mind that persons who may be enumerated as urban residents in a national census not only are frequently highly mobile, but they also consider themselves true residents of rural areas where they actively maintain relationships. They merely "stay in town" (-*kaa mjini;* see Setel et al. 1996). This is not to suggest that urban and rural differences do not exist, but to emphasize that the dynamics attributed to "urban life" may be partly contingent upon the social exigencies of where people are when enu-

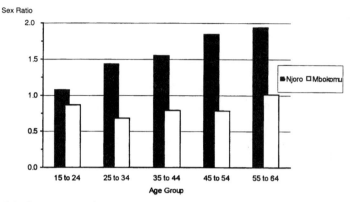

Figure 3.1. Comparison of sex ratios (M/F) for adult population (15–64), Njoro and Mbokomu Wards, 1988. (Source: Bureau of Statistics 1990:289, 310)

merated in surveys. Furthermore, supposed differences in urban versus rural behavior may be exaggerated or diminished by different tendencies in reporting an urban or rural location as one's "home" or area of "residence." Differences are not intrinsic to people by virtue of where they might be enumerated.

Mobility and migration, hallmarks of African population dynamics in the twentieth century, demand that urban versus rural distinctions be thoroughly contextualized. Figure 3.1 shows the relative surfeit of men in town and their comparative deficit on the mountain. Looked at in terms of the relative age and sex composition of the adult population, the town appears to have become almost the opposite of the *kihamba* zone.[35]

Even though Moshi was positioned as the emerging source of modern evils, easy access to town from the mountain meant that those who remained in core lineage lands did not reside in a rural idyll. Exposure to the kinds of institutions that influenced the lives of people in urban areas did not always necessitate a distant move and permanent migration. Population densities in several locations of Kilimanjaro climbed above a thousand per square mile by the 1960s. For those who did sustain a mountainside existence, many social networks remained intact and access to the colonial institutions in which people desired to participate—the church, the school, and the clinic—continued to expand. In 1958, for example, one "rural" parish in Marangu with a population of nearly four thousand was served by a health center, six schools, two women's clubs, and a large mission with its own schools and was the location of a teacher-training center. Such conditions prompted Moore to invent the term "rururb" to describe Kilimanjaro in the following manner: "Kilimanjaro today is a curious rururb, not only a rural area with an urban population density, but an area with pastoral, agricultural, and kinship values it cannot fully support. The pressure towards emigration from core lineage territories is continuous and intense, and greatly affects not only the emigrants, but those who literally succeed in holding their ground and maintaining core lineage life" (Moore 1986:223).

As we have seen, throughout this century there were many men for whom this increasing pressure proved irresistible. They were the ones for whom, in the first decade of the epidemic, AIDS was such a deadly paradox. The men were pushed off the mountain by land scarcity and economic stagnation and pulled to the town and the market by desires both modest and magnificent; their journey of dislocation from the *kihamba* became emblematic of the moral demography of Kilimanjaro. Over the years, the cultural logic that had long linked sexuality to ordered social reproduction in fixed locations on the mountain had to be stretched to accommodate the shifts in domesticity of those who could not be physically provided for on the mountain. The strains from this process began to show most clearly when men began to return home to die from AIDS, their devastated bodies the portentous signs of dislocated and disordered desire.

Suddenly, a visit home from a long-absent spouse raised the specter of infection with HIV, and the moral demography of Kilimanjaro quickly became a moral epidemiology of infective manhood against a background of vulnerable, pliant womanhood.

## Acquired Spousal Deficiency Syndrome

Men who belonged to older cohorts of migrants were often portrayed as villains in the demographic narratives of those who remained more closely connected to the land. These moral demographies were most frequently articulated by cultural elites (such as community or religious leaders) and by rural women.[36] They may be paraphrased as follows: After the 1960s or 1970s, even a primary education was a ticket out of Kilimanjaro for young men who desired a new kind of life. If and when they returned, they might receive a small section of *kihamba* land, build a house, and perhaps marry. Often they stayed long enough to watch the completion of the house and have one or two children, whereupon they would depart once again to pursue business or employment in locations away from the mountain. Over the years the visits of many men back to Kilimanjaro became more and more sporadic. Eventually, having established families in Dar es Salaam, Mwanza, or elsewhere, many men focused their attention on their new lives—and often on new wives. Not infrequently, men would bring offspring of nonmarital unions home to be raised on the *kihamba*. In the age of AIDS, the sexual activities of these men while away from the mountain brought the epidemic to the doorstep of the *kihamba* home.

By the time AIDS began to emerge in Kilimanjaro, 25 percent of men between twenty and twenty-four years of age who had migrated out in the late 1960s (Table 3.1) were in their mid-forties and fifties. Men in this cohort stated that marriage, sexuality, and reproduction were ever more disconnected from an idea of *kihamba*-based production and increasingly tied to long-term migration. Lines of inheritance, however, have remained important. Thus wives generally did not accompany their spouses when they moved but were required by them to stay on the *kihamba* to protect interests in land and to care for children and parents-in-law. Periods of spousal separation became increasingly long, and over time the remittances of many migrant men tapered off. The economic hardships of the 1980s placed added strains on geographically and economically stretched households. Women in Mbokomu claimed for twenty-five years that men had grown accustomed to avoiding marriage and diminishing their parental involvement (Freyhold, Sawaki, and Zalla 1973:273). Although many men have been geographically no further away than the residential sections of Moshi, their removal from daily life on the mountain was seen by some as total. "Even when they're here, it's like they're not here," said a woman named Martina, whose situation is discussed below.[37]

The absence of men corresponded to a disintegrating sense of fulfillment among women in maintaining the integrity of rural households, or even of marrying in the first place. In the dialogue below and the three cases that follow, the absence of "trust," *uaminifu*, which many people believed was essential to good human relations, expresses how desperate conditions had become.

> Philip: What has changed to make conditions between men and women so bad?
> Esta: Our culture hasn't changed as such, but it has completely faded away. The youth no longer stay around, and thus they don't know or practice the customs. There is no more initiation training and they don't know the proper cultural ethics for living.
> Philip: So how are things now?
> Gloria: There used to be much more trust between women and

men. That disease [i.e., AIDS] is bad; it shows the condition of trust between women and men. We have to get the fathers involved [in AIDS prevention], not just the girls and the women. It takes two people working together to protect against AIDS. It depends on love and trust. In the current atmosphere there is very little trust.

Philip: How did these circumstances come about?

Gloria: These days, the condition of the economy is such that men are only concerned with their immediate families; before we were concerned with everyone. They travel so much, and we don't stay together. It decreases our togetherness. They only come back once in a while.

Philip: So what about the women who are left here?

Rosy: The women have surprised themselves—and the men too— by developing a really keen business sense. When the women get money, it sometimes builds a wall between the sexes. The men sometimes just don't know how to adjust.[38]

In this brief exchange several important themes emerged. First, the removal of young men from the mountain was clearly associated with a sense that local culture has "completely faded away." Gloria connected AIDS directly with this process of dislocation by stating that "that disease" was a barometer of gender relations. Prevention, she felt, could only be accomplished in the context of a profound reconciliation. Last, Rosy pointed out that women's self-reliance and their ability to assist in supporting families had, paradoxically, often become a barrier to good gender relations. That such self-reliance should be threatening to men is not surprising. It made the implicit statement that men, whose adult capacity was once absolutely central to cultural practices of social and biological reproduction, were in danger of becoming superfluous to the daily lives of their lineage and nuclear family members.

All of these trends point to a complex and shifting set of interests in social reproduction and domesticity, and ultimately in fertility and sexuality. Unfortunately, quantitative data for examining this issue retrospectively are unavailable, and there are scant ethnographic data that document what must have been an increasingly emotionally charged range of considerations about having children. Nevertheless, there are some indications about the fertility-related responses of men and women during this time.

By the late 1970s Kilimanjaro was poised on the brink of a decade of economic misfortune (discussed in the next chapter), along with the rest of Tanzania and several other African countries undergoing recession and structural adjustment. In essence people in Kilimanjaro concurred that the recession of the 1980s brought a hard life (*maisha magumu),* exacerbating the vulnerability of youth to dislocation, increasing their desire, and profoundly affecting sexuality and reproduction for older adults. In the face of these economic conditions and the lengthening absences of men, childbearing for women began to acquire a bitter set of contradictory meanings, and sharp, unprecedented gender differences in fertility desires emerged.

It is extremely difficult to estimate the demographic impact of ten years of economic decline in African countries that shared in this period of hardship. It appears, however, that delays in the timing of some births could be linked to economic conditions; having another child had become too expensive (Working Group on Demographic Effects of Economic and Social Reversals 1993). There were exceptions. In some areas, such as parts of Nigeria, high fertility persisted under conditions of economic uncertainty (Fapohunda and Todaro 1988:572). Certainly there was great consensus among informants in urban Kilimanjaro, however, that people were having fewer children. In rural areas, though, the gender politics surrounding sexual and reproductive decision making were not so straightforward.

The "hard life" that emerged in the 1980s had different ramifications for and prompted different fertility-related responses from men and women of different ages. Economic uncertainties were far more than child related, and the notion of child-related "cost" had many noneconomic connotations. Women, for example, faced a shrinking marriage market for the first time; marriage, which once could be all but taken for granted, was becoming delayed, less of a certainty, or something to be avoided altogether by choice. Once people were married, long absences affected men's and women's thoughts about fertility in different ways. Some men, particularly those who were compelled to migrate and who were economically successful off the mountain, saw large family size as part of a symbolic restatement of their prosperity which otherwise may have remained largely invisible to those at home. Women, meanwhile, felt increasing burdens of caring single-handedly for parents-in-law and children. Conflicting reproductive objectives emerged within families; by the early 1970s there were reports of women hiding the use of contraceptives from their husbands and being beaten if discovered (Freyhold, Sawaki, and Zalla 1973:79). The vulnerability felt by these women in the age of AIDS is addressed below.

When, as the protocols of conducting research dictated, I asked a local official for assistance in contacting women in Mbokomu whose husbands had left them for long periods of time, he shrugged his shoulders and made a sweeping gesture that seemed to encompass the whole ward. "Where would you like to start?" he said. It is not surprising that women in these trying circumstances became extremely anxious about their own health once knowledge of the growing AIDS epidemic began to reach them, or that this concern would be channeled through local ideas about dislocation. Elsewhere in Africa, research has borne out their fears. High rates of HIV seroprevalence in much of Africa have been linked with dislocation and disruption due to labor migration (Hunt 1989; Obbo 1993). In Uganda divorce and long-term or indefinite separation among couples were found to be associated with a twofold increase in the odds of being HIV-positive compared with those who reported being currently married and (presumably) co-resident with their spouses (Nabaitu, Bachengana, and Seeley 1994: 244). While similar data do not exist for Kilimanjaro, many women who had been left indefinitely on their husband's *vihamba* in Mbokomu were seen—and saw themselves—as especially vulnerable in at least two regards. First, they were subject to the sexual demands of husbands whenever they might return to the mountain. Such vulnerability was voiced as a source of acute anxiety by those who attended a series of AIDS education workshops run from 1991 to 1993 by the Health Education Department of the Northern Diocese of the Evangelical Lutheran Church of Tanzania.

Second, "left" women engaged in affairs of their own. Frequently they represented their own infidelity (usually called *uasherati, zinaa,* or *kutembea nje,* in Swahili) as resulting from emotional vulnerability born of loneliness and the need for companionship. Concerns were frequently voiced about the increasing hardships of rural life driving women to engage quite openly in remunerative sexual relationships, called *umalaya* (a term which described both promiscuous sex and commercial sex). Although data about extramarital sex among women in rural Kilimanjaro are scant, it certainly takes place; medical staff from a rural hospital, for example, stated that it was not uncommon for married women to seek abortions during their husbands' absences of many years.

Women explicitly linked the fear of contracting AIDS to the erosion of gender relations within marriage and their own understandings of demography and development. During one of several small-group discussions held with the women of a community development committee, women discussed the demographic roots of AIDS in the village. Women who were left at home said they were promised the moon and left with nothing. The self-reliance women had developed, they

reasoned, was threatening to men and further poisoned gender relations in such a way as to impede communication and sour the happiness of the few visits home. Women assumed that their spouses were
sexually active while away; this went nearly without saying. Having
been educated about the growing epidemic, they felt threatened with
infection and powerless to communicate with their partners and so to
protect themselves. The lives of their men away from the mountain
were black boxes they dared not seek to look into with too many questions for fear of a beating.

### Three Cases

The situations of the three women whose cases are presented below
all represent different permutations of the "acquired spousal deficiency
syndrome" that preceded AIDS. One woman, named Happiness, was
getting virtually no support of any kind from her husband and rarely
saw him. She was expected by her husband's lineage, however, to be-
have as though the marriage were meeting her needs. The steps she
took to become more self-reliant brought about charges of adultery,
verging on *umalaya* prostitution, charges which a lineage meeting absolved her of but which she was vague in denying to me. Another
woman, Martina, was duped by her husband. He promised her a monogamous union and a church wedding. She got neither. In fact he
was already married before he brought her from western Tanzania to
Kilimanjaro. He left her on the *kihamba* to ponder her pregnancy, her
plight, and her hostile and equally surprised co-wife. He visited once
every year or two, and there was constant strife in the marriage.
Martina secured her position with members of her husband's lineage
through her fertility, her diligence as a farmer, her status occupation
as a teacher, and her clever manipulation of cultural mechanisms to
leverage support from her affluent spouse. He, however, continued to
add to his fertility and his number of reproductive partners as his
wealth increased, clearly increasing risk to his other wives and himself.
The third woman whose case is presented, Mariamu, had a husband
who was also successful and also made no secret of his infidelities,
many of which had resulted in the birth of children. Her position in
the household and lineage, however, was somewhat more precarious
because of her infertility. In order to maintain her security, Mariamu
cared for her husband's "outside" children and her father-in-law and
tolerated the sexual demands of her husband during his visits home.
This was an extremely unpleasant sacrifice of dignity for her, as there

was clearly no hope of having a child of her own and all her affection for her husband was long gone.

Happiness, Martina, and Mariamu spoke of their unmet expectations of adult life and marriage based on notions of trust, mutual understanding, mutual assistance, and respect. Women pointed to their husbands' children by other women or co-wives as evidence that it is in the "constitution" or nature *(maumbili)* of men to have sexual relations with several women (see chapter 4). Conversely, married women were acutely aware of the pressures on them to maintain the appearance of fidelity. Women who spoke with female research assistants or with me about sex outside marriage were sometimes incredulous, sometimes ambiguous. One woman simply said, "After what I just told you, do you think I have any energy left over for that? I'm exhausted all the time, and not the slightest bit interested; I have no desire at all." Another spoke in the abstract, explaining that "women here are so lonely. They go along to drink *mbege* and when they've had a bit they are easily seduced."

### Happiness

I met Happiness at a water tap near her home where she was filling a bucket containing bananas that she grew and used to brew *mbege.* The homestead of her husband, Kessawe, was set on five acres of *kihamba* land at the top of a ridge and looked down into the valley upon acre upon acre of banana plants and coffee trees. There were two houses and a cattle stall, or *banda,* on the *kihamba.* Happy and her three children were living in one house, and her husband's grandfather stayed in the other. The house was in poor condition; the walls were cracked and loosely patched with mud. Happy was thirty-seven years old at the time. She was tall and thin and wore a faded and tattered *kitenge* cloth wrapped over her dress. Kessawe had been living in Shinyanga for many years with his second wife, who was not a Chagga, and had a family there as well. He visited Kilimanjaro very sporadically; it had been four years since his previous visit. His last extended stay on the *kihamba* was in 1985, when he left Happy pregnant with her youngest child. Fifteen people, most of them children, depended on the produce of the five-acre *kihamba,* the four goats, and three cows, and the income from Happy's *mbege* business. Happiness felt that her position was strengthened by caring for Kessawe's grandfather and by having the sympathy of her father in-law. On the other hand, she had the enmity of her husband and mother-in-law. After Kessawe's grandfather died, she felt that her ability to continue on the land would become much less certain.

> [Has he sent money home?] When I gave birth he sent me six hundred shillings. That's the only money for the children he has ever given me. This house used to be in good condition. Now look at it. It's falling apart. And you know why? Things were so difficult around here that I started to brew and sell *mbege* to get what I need to live on. His mother went off to Shinyanga and told him I'd become a prostitute—that I'd been fooling around—because I'd started this business. She told him to divorce me. He came back and tried to drive me away. He broke the windows and the doors. I protested to his father, who realized that I was only trying to survive. Then he had to sacrifice a goat, and put the blood on the door, and the windows where he had broken them. Then he went to pour *mbege* in the *kihamba,* on the graves.[39]

Happiness insisted that her mother-in-law had falsely accused her because of the suggestion of adulterous behavior surrounding women's production and consumption of *mbege* in rural areas, not because of anything she had actually done. "Do you think that women around here are especially vulnerable to having affairs because of being left by their men?" I asked. "When women go to the market, or when they simply go to the beer shop after working all day, they may go without any money. The man then buys you the beer. Finally, you owe him. He claims his due; you should pay for that beer. If you've already drunk, you can't refuse. The result of that is AIDS."

### Martina

Martina lived down the path from Happiness. Unlike Happy's residence, Martina's house was in poor condition because her husband had never finished the construction. Her husband, John, whom she met in her hometown in western Tanzania, persuaded her to accompany him home to his *kihamba,* where he promised her a proper church wedding. By the time she found out that John already had a wife, whom he had married in a church wedding, Martina was pregnant with their first child. After the birth of the child, John returned to Lake Tanganyika to run his lucrative bar and guesthouse. Although Martina had full-time employment as a schoolteacher, she could not support her family on that salary alone. In addition to farming the *kihamba* for coffee and bananas, she rented a two-acre field, or *shamba,* to grow maize for home consumption. During the rainy season she had to leave home before daybreak in order to reach the *shamba*, have enough time to sow, weed, or harvest, and return before dark. Martina had also tried a variety of *miradi* (projects) such as keeping a dairy cow, selling cloth, and running a kiosk to boost her income: "[And now?] When I first came, there was so much love between us. There was enough. I got the things I needed. Now it's gone. Chagga men don't really care about their children. Last year he came home and stayed for five weeks. He'd come by the house once or twice after school to see the children, but he didn't even sleep here. He stayed with his first wife. When he came he gave me ten thousand shillings. When that finished, there was no more. Big deal! I need twelve thousand as it is just to buy food for a week."[40]

Martina was not so concerned about her position on the land because she knew that she had rights through her children. Their right to inherit protected her access to the house and the *kihamba*. Although secure in one sense, Martina felt a growing fear as she learned more and more about HIV/AIDS. In 1993, John had sixteen children for whom he acknowledged paternity. Ten of them were by three women recognized to be his wives, and six were by women "on the side." On one hand, Martina clearly lamented the state of her marriage and the lack of closeness with John. Yet in the face of AIDS, she almost came to regard this estrangement as a blessing in disguise, since it acted to dampen the sexual side of their relationship.

### Mariamu

Mariamu lived near Martina and was the second wife of a man whose father had had a great deal of power under the last *mangi*. The family had many acres of *kihamba* land and several fields under maize cultivation. Unlike most of the rural Kilimanjaro population, her family was Muslim. Mariamu lived with a senior co-wife and several children of their husband, Suleiman, in a homestead that consisted of a mud-brick structure that housed three cows, Mariamu's mother-in-law's room, and the cooking fire. The rest of the family slept in a separate cinderblock house. Mariamu was infertile, the result of an ectopic pregnancy that nearly killed her. Like Happiness, she had found a modicum of security in caring for her husband's kin. Her father-in-law tried to strengthen Mariamu's position with the family by "giving" her one of several children Suleiman had fathered outside marriage and had brought home to raise. The mother of Daudi, the boy given to Mariamu to foster, was rumored to have died of AIDS. Mariamu felt that what she failed to provide her husband with her own fertility, he took out of her in labor. Despite her infertility, she did not fear greatly for her rights on the *kihamba* and felt she had secured her position through her hard work and status as foster mother. Mariamu was well respected and had good standing with most of her husband's clan elders. Though Suleiman had refused to give her her own *kihamba* because she was infertile, he was not in a position to drive her away. I asked her about her marriage and her experience of trying to develop a source of income for herself through caring for the cows.

> [So what is marriage like for you here?] The Chaggas oppress their women more than other groups. If you get married in Chagga-land, you'd better count on relying on yourself. It's been like this since the last century. Just ask the grandmas around here; they don't tell you the good things about their husbands, only the bad. [Is there trust between men and women?] Chagga men totally mislead you. The first year is wonderful—and then the leopard shows his claws. They become tyrants. After the first child you will be amazed. Oh boy, you'll be tired. [And what about planning things for the future?] Give me a break—he doesn't even stay here! No, there's no discussion of the future. When I married, I counted on understanding one another in the home in order to help *both* families—his and mine. When you see how things are really going to be, you really get depressed.[41]

Beyond the obvious indictment of men and their conduct in marriage, these narratives convey disillusionment, disappointment, and burden without reward. They speak of anger and vulnerability to the ravages of "that disease." Since the advent of AIDS, children like Suleiman's Daudi, born elsewhere and brought to Kilimanjaro to be cared for, were not just the embodiment of the moral demographic of dislocation; they were explicitly seen by women as the living evidence of their own exposure to the risk of death. This made the Christmas pilgrimages back to Kilimanjaro a difficult time for married women. Referring to the rumors about Daudi's mother, Mariamu told me often that she thought it distinctly possible that her husband had infected her with HIV. After one interview, during which she seemed especially concerned about this possibility, I asked her if she wanted me to help arrange a counseling session for her at the regional hospital so that she could have an HIV test. She declined, explaining that it did not matter. Knowing or not knowing her serostatus would not change her life, she said. She knew, in her words, that she was not "a threat" to anyone else, and besides, she pointed out, she would have to repeat the procedure after each visit from her husband. Other women who expressed fear of being infected were even more afraid of confronting their husbands. Better they remain silent, risk death, and preserve the marriage, they openly said, than risk the stigma and upheaval of trying to refuse sex or demand the use of condoms. Over the course of a year and a half of residence in Kilimanjaro, I attended the funerals of several women who had believed themselves (and had been believed by others) to be infected under these kinds of conditions. I also attended rites for men who resembled the husbands of these women and who had come home to die, men who many felt represented the "first wave" of the local AIDS epidemic.

## Risk, Marriage, and Mobility in Tanzania

Although Chagga women have not been alone in their concern about marital stability, mobility, and risk, investigations by epidemiologists into these issues have not been thorough. Again, the problem stems from the oversimplification of the variables used in survey research. As the next chapter will discuss, sexual culture in Tanzania is much richer than static categories of spouses, co-wives, casual or cohabitant partners, prostitutes, clients, and barmaids suggest. Major studies of HIV epidemiology in Tanzania have not deeply investigated polygyny, informal polyandry, or other forms of partnership. Nor have they explored the links between nuptiality, mobility, partner separation, and risk (Barongo et al. 1992; Kapiga et al. 1994; Killewo, Dahlgren, and Sandström 1994; Mnyika et al. 1994; Mnyika 1996). Most of these studies do contain some information on travel and urban residence but appear not to have data on duration of spousal separation or on forms of relationships more culturally specific than "married," "cohabiting," and (occasionally) "polygynous."

Studies of sexual behavior that include number of partners, which are common, do not provide any information about more complex forms of relations and social context, and they almost always ignore fertility. Sexual research that leaves fertility and infertility out of the picture misses a critical opportunity to link these variables to sexual risk and HIV. This includes such massive efforts as the international Knowledge Attitudes and Practices survey conducted by the WHO's Global Program on AIDS (Cleland and Ferry 1995). The failure to address these interrelated issues has often been quite intentional; while aware of cultural variation, epidemiologists have been satisfied to lump nonmarital relations into the category of "casual" or "multipartner" relations and let it go at that (e.g., Hunter 1993:66). Yet "the com-

plexities of conjugal partnerships . . . are crucial to our present concerns
for understanding STD/HIV transmission" (Caraël 1996:59); these intricacies, as Caraël has shown, relate to cultural dimensions of both
nuptiality and nonmarital sexual unions and the social conditions under which these relations are maintained.

Even if these considerable shortcomings are put aside, it is still difficult to assess the risk of women married to migrant husbands, let alone
to migrant husbands themselves. Between 1984 and 1987, 100 cases of
AIDS were diagnosed in Kilimanjaro (Howlett, Nkya, and Mmuni
1987). The picture they began to paint of "the AIDS patient" was of a
young, well-traveled man, resident in urban areas outside the region
and of middle to upper socioeconomic status. Of these 100 persons
with AIDS, most were men (73 percent), about half of whom were
married (53 percent). Nearly all of the 27 women with AIDS (80 percent) were single, divorced, or widowed (1987:4–5). These figures are
roughly similar to those for the first 212 reported cases of AIDS in Tanzania as a whole (Mhalu et al. 1988:54).[42] In Kilimanjaro, most of the
people with AIDS named places outside the Kilimanjaro region as their
place of residence (59 percent), all of them urban locations. By far the
most common occupational category among the AIDS ill was business (23 percent), followed by farming (10 percent). As Howlett et al.
(1988:5) wrote, "Almost all of patients were middle or upper class and
they mostly worked . . . in urban Tanzania. Many had travelled exten-
sively." Studies that rely upon cases from hospital-based data, however, are heavily biased by patterns of facility usage and access that
are often strongly related to the prevalence of social characteristics
such as sex, economic status, and urban residence (most major hospitals in Tanzania, including the Kilimanjaro Christian Medical Center
[KCMC], are located in urban areas). In the context of the AIDS epidemic, the problems of bias or underreporting due to differential usage
of health facilities among the ill are compounded by the clinical challenges of correctly identifying the disease to begin with (Evans 1991:
1261).

Community, or population-based, studies of HIV in Tanzania conducted in the early 1990s yielded contradictory results on the question
of marital status, travel, and HIV risk. These data are difficult to interpret, however, for one's relationship status may well change radically
between the time of infection and the time of participation in a survey.
Thus, in Arusha region there was a fivefold increase in risk of being
HIV-positive associated with being separated or divorced for both men
and women (Mnyika et al. 1994:1479), while men in Mwanza who were

either separated or widowed had more than three times the risk (Barongo et al. 1992:1526).[43] Similar findings come from a longitudinal cohort study in Uganda, where those who were divorced or separated had a twofold increase in risk of infection. This prompted investigators to insist that the instability of relationships in communities where HIV is spreading must be taken into account in the design of intervention strategies (Nabaitu, Bachengana, and Seeley 1994:244). Although one assumption might be that separation or divorce could increase exposure to HIV infection, we cannot know the relative timing of these events (infection and separation) from cross-sectional epidemiologic surveys and must consider conditions under which either state might contribute to entering into the other.

Other studies reached different conclusions about the link between relationship status and HIV risk. In Dar es Salaam women in "cohabiting" relationships were at significantly greater risk of being HIV infected; being single, divorced, or widowed did not add to risk of being seropositive (Kapiga et al. 1994:303).[44] Kapiga et al. reported significantly elevated risks for married women in Dar es Salaam who claimed only one partner and who reported that their husbands had had extramarital sex during the previous five years. Men's reports of female infidelity were not included in the analysis. Data from rural Uganda reveal an extraordinary difference in risk between married and unmarried men and women. Relative to single men, men who were currently or had ever been in any form of relationship or marriage were roughly twenty times more likely to be HIV-positive, while women in relationships were from two to seven times more likely to be infected than women who were single and had never been married (Serwadda et al. 1992:985).[45]

Overall, "travel" does seem to be related to increased risk, but very few data are available on reasons for travel, frequency of journeys, or time spent away from home areas. Again, however, cross-sectional studies cannot inform us about the relative timing of migration and infection. For example, simply because someone is in town when he or she is determined to be HIV-positive in a serosurvey does not mean that this person was infected in an urban area. In the Tanzanian studies, the only travel that appeared to be consistently associated with increased risk of HIV infection was intraregional travel to capital cities, while in the Uganda study only travel to the national capital or outside the country was associated with elevated risk. In rural and semirural areas of Mwanza, women were 1.7 times as likely to be seropositive if they had visited Mwanza town in the two years prior to the study;

there was no statistically significant association of risk for men who traveled (Barongo et al. 1992:1526). Similarly, in Kagera region, travel to Bukoba town was significantly associated with being seropositive, while traveling outside the region could not be shown to carry added risk (Killewo et al. 1990:1084). For reasons stated above, duration of urban residence is ambiguous in its association with risk of HIV infection; some STD studies have indicated that long stays relate to increased risk (Caraël 1996:60), although Kapiga et al. (1994) stated that newcomers to Dar es Salaam had higher rates of seropositivity than long-term residents.

In sum, it is almost impossible to extrapolate from this mosaic of cross-sectional epidemiologic studies. The vulnerability of the *kihamba*-based wife and the urban migrant husband may well reflect a set of circumstances that has rendered women more vulnerable to HIV infection than others. However, this cannot be proven from the available data.

## The Women Respond

Even if epidemiologists did not understand the complexities of their situation relative to other women, there was no doubt that Happiness, Martina, and Mariamu and others like them had reason to suppose themselves at risk. These women did not remain passive in the face of their concerns; they were much more resourceful than men in channeling their energies into an organized response to AIDS. Martina and Mariamu were among a small group of women who formed the initial membership of KIWAKKUKI, the Kilimanjaro Women's Group against AIDS (see Setel and Mtweve 1995). This community-based response to AIDS has been centered in Moshi town but has established chapters in several rural areas.

KIWAKKUKI has been unique in Tanzania as a democratic forum where women of diverse economic, educational, and social backgrounds have joined together to set an agenda for local AIDS activism. Most important, in the women's view, it is accountable only to the group's members themselves. Members pay dues, elect the leadership, and set the organization's objectives. Men may be honorary members, but may not vote or hold office. According to KIWAKKUKI (which represents a much more diverse set of women than Happiness, Martina, and Mariamu), AIDS was first and foremost an issue of gender relations and women's status and demanded active intervention in order to ensure the humane treatment of those with the disease.

Since 1991 it has run a support group for people with HIV, operated home visiting programs, educated its membership, and begun income-generating activities. Out of four AIDS service programs begun in Kilimanjaro between 1990 and 1993, KIWAKKUKI alone remained a significant presence into 1999. Yet these women have had difficulty in squarely confronting the issue of those who see themselves at risk in marriage. During the first years of its existence, there was little sustained discussion in KIWAKKUKI of how to contend with the threat that absent husbands were perceived to pose to the health women. Nor did the group address the general topic of women's status.

The difficulty in addressing the questions of risk that these women perceived may indicate a tacit acknowledgment of the complexities of their situations. In just over two generations, an enormous gulf had emerged between cultural expectations embedded in *kihamba*-based models of personhood and the conduct of interpersonal relations, and the actual ways in which men and women were engaging with contemporary life. Conventional *kihamba*-based lineage structures had undergone huge stresses, of which women often bore the brunt. The perceptions of heightened vulnerability among rural women represented a paradoxical knitting together of an unraveling cultural experience. The gaps between cultural narratives about population dynamics and demographic realities, between (m)oral representations and embodied experience were libraries of experience out of which emerged stories of an attenuated cultural crisis in social reproduction and, eventually, about the risks of AIDS.

Reflecting on the condition of the women in rural Kilimanjaro who shared these concerns often gave me occasion to despair of my male friends, to doubt their earnest protestations that AIDS had changed their way of life, and to hold them accountable for what Aud Talle has called "sexual irresponsibility" in the age of AIDS (Talle 1995:28). But what have been men's own experiences of being uprooted and almost literally cast off the mountain over a generation ago? How had their struggle to make a virtue of necessity become manifest in spousal neglect and fears about AIDS, a transformation of virtue into deadly vice? As we have seen, the dynamics of dislocation and desire have been largely, though not exclusively, stamped with the discursive mark of the declining quality of Chagga manhood.

The experiences of young men (and women) in and around Moshi constitute an alternative, more subversive, and more contested representation of desire and moral demography in Kilimanjaro, one which casts AIDS as a paradox of gender and development (Setel 1996). In

Uganda, Obbo has called the predicament of youth in the face of the epidemic "the ignored voice of the young" (1995:89). In the decades before the epidemic, the individual bodies of men and women circulating in and out of Kilimanjaro were like the bearers of a marker dye in the arteries of a growing social body. They traced the pathways of new possibilities in the redefinition of desire. Desire often appeared bonded to colonial institutions, new commodity forms, and the decaying political-economic structures of an independent Tanzania under structural adjustment and, eventually, epidemic disease. In this unfolding experiential demographic, discourse about individual desire and the repositioning of persons was mapped onto an inchoate, nondiscursive dislocation and relocation of the bodies of young people. While narratives of the twentieth-century population process are retrospective and highly synthesized, the movement of people in time and space has been an ever-incomplete process with a shifting center of gravity. The particular population dynamics upon which local demographic narratives were based told no stories in and of themselves. Rather they represented complex lived processes onto which stories have been grafted, stories of men and mobility, women and abandonment, and the increasingly desirous taste for new things.

## CHAPTER 4

# Personhood and the Pragmatics of Desire

## A Person-centered Approach to Representing Relationships

The concept of desire bridged concerns about AIDS and risk in Kilimanjaro. Desire was woven into local stories of demographic change and structural vulnerability among dislocated men and their *kihamba*-resident spouses in middle age, and about young people, whose dislocation is more recent. Worries about AIDS and covetous desire, about the pathology of *tamaa*, were shared more or less universally across the social spectrum and were central to the evaluation of the sexual deportment of adult men and women young and old. This is because desire was basic to shared concepts of moral character *(tabia)*, personhood *(utu)*, and sexuality. In fact some degree of desire was necessary to life itself: suicidal depressions were said to result from the "cutting of desire" *(-kata tamaa)*. Concepts such as *tabia, utu,* and *tamaa* were inherently subject to evaluation by one's family and social group. Thus there was a large degree of consensus over what they were, but debate over what they *meant* as individuals made assessments of one another and explained them to an anthropologist.

The concept of personhood, and the cultural shaping of the person throughout the life course, have been important themes in Africanist research since the 1930s (Riesman 1986:71). Yet the theory employed in studies of personhood, beginning with Mauss's own (Mauss 1979: 75–86), and in more recent studies of embodiment have made a fundamental, and ethnocentric, category error. They have almost all located the concept of person within the concept of mind, and hence within a phenomenological model of meaning and cultural experience closely associated with the Western concept of self (Mauss 1979; see also Csordas 1988; Riesman 1986; Rosaldo 1980).

Again, moral character and desire were central to representations of sexuality and personhood in Kilimanjaro. They were not, however, just part of a mentalist concept of culturally shaped persons and selves, but were eminently bodily—embedded in the patterns of action by which members of Kilimanjaro society recognized and reacted to one another as social persons. This is an important point: *Persons were signified through the uses of their bodies.* Their actions—their bodily practices—were not pre-inscribed with a fixed set of meanings. Rather, meanings were hammered out in an ongoing negotiation of relational contexts. As Fortes perceived when working among Tallensi in the 1940s, even "normative" notions of personhood "are accessible to discovery primarily by reason of their realization in the customary or institutionalized activities of people. . . . It was only by observing and conversing with the common man, so to speak, that one could see how the ideas and beliefs relating to such abstract notions as that of the person were channeled through his daily activities. *They were more commonly exhibited in action and utterance than formulated in explicit terms"* (1987:247–48; emphasis added).

While things as seemingly abstract as cultural concepts of personhood might appear far afield of the practicalities of the fight against AIDS, they are not (see, e.g., Taylor 1990; Setel 1995c). Nearly all parties in Kilimanjaro discussed risk, male-female relationships, and the meaning of reproductive and sexual action in reference to specific examples of personal behavior. In other words, the qualities and capacities of individual men and women confronting and confronted with particular situations were central to local discussions about AIDS. The AIDS educator's cookie-cutter abstractions of sex, sexual contact, and risk were virtually meaningless without being related to the context of some sort of story about people. In these stories, the actors were recognizable as possessing certain kinds of *tabia* and different kinds of *tamaa,* and as being in varying positions of risk.

This emphasis on situations was apparent in the countless conversations about male-female relations in Kilimanjaro that began with the phrase *"kwa mfano"* (for example), followed by the narration of an actual or hypothetical situation. Cultural consensus on this score was all but absolute. At virtually every AIDS education speech I attended, and in almost every conversation I held about AIDS prevention in Kilimanjaro, Tanzanians explained that AIDS had been brought by the excesses of *tamaa* and that it could only be prevented if young people were to obey the edict to "correct themselves" (*-jirekebisha*) and "change their moral character" (*-badilisha tabia*). The relevance of understanding personhood and moral character in reference to AIDS prevention in Kilimanjaro could hardly be made clearer. From a local perspective, the cause (covetous desire) and cure (changed moral character) of AIDS were that simple, and that complex.

As I discussed in the previous chapter, Chagga had a clear understanding of the ways in which impersonal, large-scale forces acted upon their lives. They discussed the effects of these forces in specific terms of transformations in local models of personhood and desire and tied them to changes in patterns of sexual action and the collapse of domesticity. During the *kihamba* regime a sense of "proper" personhood was rooted in a cultural semantics of action based on ritual and imitation. Similarly, in contemporary contexts of male-female relations, *tabia* and *tamaa* were *only* revealed through action. Thus these concepts allow us explore how actors conceived of their sexual relationships. They also provide insight into how mundane, taken-for-granted elements of personhood were embodied in the idiom of sex, and how bodily praxis within male-female relationships constituted habits of meaning central to local notions of personhood.

There are a number of interpretive challenges in carrying out the important task of distinguishing "sex as it is practiced and sex as it is discussed" (Caldwell, Orubuloye, and Caldwell 1992:1179). Despite the emphasis placed on conduct as the key to unlocking sexual meanings, in the action-attuned conversations of sexual relationships, the most overt deeds often seemed more ambiguous than the faintest of whispered intentions. This was true no less for informants who provided relationship histories than for the anthropologist who elicited them. On one hand, the relative roles of *tamaa* and *tabia* and the overall significance of the relationship to the lives of informants seemed contingent and indeterminate. On the other, there was enough patterning of experience and of differences in salience of moral character and desire in partnerships to allow informants to participate in the construction of a lexicon of relationship terms and types.

The precision of meaning that I sought in assessing sexual meanings in the context of relationships was not a preoccupation that many informants shared. For them, contemporary sexuality stood somewhat outside what they felt to be the cultural domain. Kilimanjaro did not possess the degree of formalized sexual culture and language found in the Caribbean (Yelvington 1996:315ff.). For Swahili speakers in northern Kilimanjaro, the concept of culture, *utamaduni,* is often close to that of a rule book; it is ordinarily used to refer to constellations of ideal forms of customs, traditions, and rites that guide the formal dimensions of living. Within this sense of culture, Chagga (unlike many groups in

East and Central Africa; see, e.g., Ahlberg 1994:230; Caldwell, Caldwell, and Quiggin 1989:197) appear never to have had a positive cultural emphasis on sexual pleasure; the topic was either referred to in an oblique and ambiguous manner or was cast in a negative light. None of the accounts of male initiation, or *mregho,* speak of teaching that husbands were entitled to sexual pleasure or that wives experienced desire, nor are there songs recorded from Kilimanjaro, as there were among other strongly patrilineal agrarian groups in East Africa, that spoke of women literally taking matters into their own hands if sexually neglected (Håkansson 1990:192). For women, circumcision was aimed, in part, at *quelling* desire. The Chagga *shiga* training, unlike the *unyago* initiations of many neighboring groups like the Pare or the Bemba *chisungu* initiations of the 1940s and 1950s (Richards 1956), did not include instruction on techniques for giving sexual pleasure to men such as the erotic hip movements called *kucheza* or *kukata kiuno.*

The most technical discussions of sex in both male and female initiation focused on the quality of the result (i.e., a pregnancy) rather than the pleasure of the process. Even the older alternatives to bridewealth marriages, such as "opening a hut" or bride capture, were spoken of as different paths leading to domestic objectives and were not referred to as ways of channeling desires. Where the lessons allude to sexual desire, it was usually in a nonmarital context and was referred to in a negative way. Desire was portrayed as something to be avoided through modest dress, as something irresponsible, immature, and dangerous to one's health and reputation (e.g., Raum 1939:560). Nevertheless, as discussed in chapter 2, there were opportunities for young men and women to flirt and to assert their preferences in the selection of partners. As long as it was possible to "not know" about desire-driven sexuality, it was clearly tolerated under certain circumstances.

The continued semantic placing of the sexual outside the cultural did not mean that people were unable to express their desires for or experiences of pleasure; on the contrary, sexual pleasure and the satisfaction of desires were common topics of conversation among friends. The sexual and reproductive worlds of young adults were alive with options, risk, love, and emotional and material interdependence. This rich texture may not have been explicit in local moral demographies, but it informed private thought and action. Nevertheless, what informants considered "culture" was either silent or hostile on these matters.

Again, then, we must be explicit about whose concept of culture is being used in the analysis. How, indeed, can one provide a cultural analysis of sex that both maintains and explains the distinction made about this very concept by informants themselves? How can we show the way in which culture allowed Chagga to place sex outside culture? Following Rosaldo, I do not assume "that all individuals within a culture are the same, all 'socialized' to be the ideal 'persons' of their society [but] rather . . . insist that the reproduction of a given form of social life demands such continuities in discourse as would permit a shared and sensible frame for the interpretation of daily practice" (1980:223). This requires a contingent model of culture that goes beyond acknowledging contradictions between ideology and practice. It must approach an extreme constructionist model of culture in which the very concept itself can be seen as a product of the anthropological endeavor. We may accept that people do act in the world according to some core of pattern and predictability within onion-like layers or, as Daniel puts it, "signs of habit" that are often reduced to ideas of "cultural norms." Nevertheless, we may also assert that culture is "spun in the communicative act engaged in by the anthropologist and his or her informants, in which the anthropologist strives to defer to the creativity of his informants and self-consciously reflects upon the [deferred meanings] inherent in this creative product" (Daniel 1984:13).

## Moral Character and Desire in the Life Course

For people in northern Kilimanjaro, *tabia* was intimately connected with how people judged all adult action, including sex. It was thus central to local ideas about the spread and control of AIDS. Tanzanian AIDS educators, for example, fairly browbeat their audiences, beseeching them to "effect changes in their moral character." While an explicit discourse that employed notions of moral character might have been expected in religious settings, it was common throughout daily life and in the context of secular health education. It could not have been otherwise: *tabia* was held to be the aspect of personality that motivated all significant action. *Tabia* was identified as a set of inborn tendencies that were related to gender and changed during the life course. It was specifically connected with how one performed work and behaved toward others.

*Tabia* related to several other culturally shaped components of the person. Together, these formed interconnected layers of being that developed in the individual as she or he grew and matured, and ultimately yielded an adult, *mtu mzima* (literally a whole or complete person). A "whole person" in Kilimanjaro consisted of embodied qualities revealed through action in the context of human relations over the life course. In a highly simplified form, a person was thought to be made up of aspects such as *ufahamu*, consciousness or understanding, and *akili*, applied intelligence. These became apparent early in life through the ability of a baby to demonstrate awareness of its environment, and a child to direct its energies intentionally. All people also possessed *roho* (soul, heart, or spirit), which became known, usually in early adulthood, through deeds that displayed sincerity, duplicity, cruelty, or kindness.[1] A person's body, *mwili*, consisted not only of flesh, bone, and blood, *nyama*, *mifupa*, and *damu*, but also of *mishipa*, "vessels." This term referred not only to veins and arteries but also to the "channels of consciousness or understanding," *mishipa ya ufahamu*, in the head, *kichwa*, and brain, *ubongo*.

All people were possessed of characteristics explicitly relating to the set of concepts Westerners consider to make up sex and gender. Maleness and femaleness were rooted partly in the immutable characteristics of *maumbili* and partly in the concept of *jinsia*. *Maumbili* was a concept that referred to a combination of one's physical shape, male or female sex, and the innate tendencies of having a physical body with those sexual characteristics. English speakers in Kilimanjaro translated *jinsia* as "gender relations," while non-English speakers used a cognate term, stating that *jinsia* referred to *mambo ya kigenda*, "matters of gender." Sexual *tamaa* was thought not only to be a product of environment but also to be an environmental exacerbation of natural urges from one's *maumbili*. *Maumbili* was also that aspect of a person's composition that was generally thought to provide men with more sexual drive than women. Although one's *maumbili* was fixed, *jinsia* was an explicitly relational concept that connoted the way in which men and women were socialized or habituated to interact with one another. As participants in an AIDS workshop indicated, *jinsia*, rather than *maumbili*, was an appropriate entry point for interventions designed to improve gender relations.

## Tabia *from Birth to Adolescence*

The career of one's *tabia* begins before birth and is rooted in biological notions of heredity and the cosmological agency of ancestors. Striking  personal qualities, either positive or negative, can reemerge in infants as their clan legacy of the *tabia* from the ancestors. One's *tabia* could come through either parent's line. Some educated Chagga women stated that there was a strong biological component of *tabia* that began at conception, when "male and female hormones mix together in the mother's womb." In practice, *tabia* was a concept that showed many subtle gradations, although people often operated with a simple dichotomy of good and bad *tabia*.[2] An infant or young child between birth and about two or three years of age possessed both *ufahamu* and *tabia*, but only after a child could engage in some form of reciprocal action did its *tabia* begin to be apparent to others.

Rituals performed in infancy and early childhood officially located the child in the clan, and protected and fostered its development. In addition to guarding the physical well-being of the new person, a major goal of these rituals was to provide the proper cosmological bedrock for the *tabia* of the new person. Rituals of this nature that were widely practiced in the early 1990s included: the burying of the umbilicus, shaving and disposing of the first hair, and the "beseeching of the name" from the ancestors.[3] The consequences of neglecting any of these rituals for the child might be serious febrile illness and convulsions (*degedege*; often a manifestation of cerebral malaria), mental illness, or death.

The gendered properties of *tabia* emerged in childhood. The *tabia* of girls was said to be far easier to influence for the good than that of boys, because girls naturally felt *haibu* (shame). Feeling shame reduced the desire to do ill, and so could be useful in "training out" bad *tabia*. The love shown to children or the atmosphere around the household might also influence the *tabia* of a child. "It's time to teach children love," urged a psychiatrist at an AIDS education seminar run by the Catholic diocese: "A child with love will have sensitivity [*huruma*], and a child with love and sensitivity will have a good *tabia*."[4] Similarly, the young father of a three-month-old boy explained that "if parents share with each other, love each other, and stay together faithfully, it's hard for the child to become ruined [*-haribika*]."[5] Children who showed especially bad moral character might be punished in a number of ways, including being reprimanded or beaten. Particularly in cases of bad *tabia*, however, the innate forces of biology and ancestry were often thought to win out in the end. Young parents watched for signs of bad *tabia* in their children so that they could undertake to correct them before the children became accustomed to antisocial behavior. An especially ominous sign of the beginnings of bad *tabia* was to sneak money from one's parents; this was also a sure sign of excessive *tamaa* at an early age.

Other environmental factors resulted in the development of one kind of *tabia* or another. For example, education (in the sense of both formal

and religious schooling) played a large role in guiding *tabia*. A car mechanic with a young son explained that "a child hasn't ripened [*hajako-
maa*] and is too small to know that stealing or sneaking money from
his parents is bad. But once he has some intelligence [*akili*] and he goes
to confirmation class or to Koranic lessons, they stress moral values
and he can know that these things are bad and cut it out right there."[6]
While environmental influences were thought to be important, there
was no general agreement about whether the village or the town was
preferable for raising children and guiding their moral development.
The detractors of city life decried the mixing of people of diverse ethnic
backgrounds, the crowding of people of all ages in a single dwelling,
and children's exposure to bad influences like videos. Those who believed town to be preferable insisted that people in rural areas were
much more prone to suffer the ravages of alcohol abuse. Too many
people in the village were "ignorant" and "backward," they said, and
children in town were more likely to stay in school and be studious
than those on the mountain.

The importance of imitation in the development of personal moral
character has been an enduring theme in Kilimanjaro. It has also been
part of American folk models of personal development since the end
of the nineteenth century, when concern over children's "role models"
first became widespread, and included discussions in the 1990s about
violence on television and sexual explicitness in popular music lyrics
(World Health Organization 1992:41–42) and the influence of peer
groups on character development (Harris 1998). Throughout childhood
in Tanzania, the models that a young person had to imitate were
thought to have a determining effect on her or his *tabia*. Young working
adults stated that the propensity to imitate could be seen very clearly
by watching children's responses to videos. The perceived effects of
videos on children in Moshi are a clear example of how the mimetic
faculty, the act of imitation, served to "empersonate" the bodies of the
young. During one visit to a group of friends working at a soda-bot-
tling plant, the conversation came around to the topic of videos. I asked
one young man if he thought videos might play a role in forming *tabia*
and *tamaa*. In his reply, he stated that somewhere in the sensibilities
of children "subtle changes that you are not aware of" become internal-
ized through an imitative response to videos: "The children see *everything* on those videos. The parents put them on and leave the children
alone. The children imitate the moral character of what they see [*-iga
tabia*] on the video. You see this a lot in Dar, where people are imitating
the songs and dress style of people in places that they have never been

to. It's in the head. In the intelligence [*akili*] there are changes that take place—subtle changes that you are not aware of. People have gotten used to this *tabia*. It builds a certain nature of desiring things [-*tamaani*]. First you fear it, then you get used to it, and then you start to want it. There are films that show embraces, kisses, and even sex right out there in the open. These videos give you the desire to have sex."[7]

### Adolescence and the Stirring of Desire: "They Are the Complete Opposite of Us"

Adolescence and young adulthood *(ujana)* are crucibles for the development of qualities of *tabia* that remain with a person for the remainder of his or her life. For older adults it was thought that *tabia* was extremely difficult to change, because one has "become used to it" for so long *(-zoea)*. Men and women who were considered to be elderly *(wazee)* were said to have a fixed and immutable *tabia*.[8] During adolescence, *tabia* could be very difficult to alter, a belief that fit with stereotypes of young men, *vijana*, as both stubbornly fearless and shameless.[9] Puberty and the process of physical maturation *(-balehe)* were said to accompany the urge to become sexually active. As with *tabia* itself, external forces influenced this stirring of desire. If not properly channeled, desire could lead to precocious sexuality; if properly directed, one would become hardworking and trustworthy.

One young married man explained that "to mature brings the desire to be with a girl at all hours of the day and night. You also give up a childish *tabia*, and start to like work, and so become more trustworthy in the eyes of your parents."[10] Similarly, for young women, an adolescent *tabia* could lead either to proper comportment or to impropriety expressed through an interest in beer and men. Mariamu in Mbokomu explained that "once a girl starts to get her period, she doesn't listen any more. She does what she wants. At this time she is very changed. It is a tricky time for girls. Once they pass through it they can either end up being gentle [*mpole*] and respectful, or she can go talking to boys in the clubs and drinking beer."[11]

The expectations that young people begin to assert their independence made adolescence and early adulthood a precarious time. Many adults felt that adolescents did not yet have the maturity to negotiate their feelings of desire and would succumb to the temptation to follow the examples of those with bad *tabia*. Young women often spoke about the sensations of desire in these terms:

[Would you say that, overall, *tamaa* is a good thing or a bad thing?] *Tamaa* is good, but it can cause you to risk a great deal. For instance, if desire has already taken hold of you, you can't stop it until you get a man. If you don't it will go on for days. [When did you first start to feel it?] *Tamaa* started in me since I started to have sex. I have more now than when I was small. It's okay to feel this if you're already officially engaged, but when it happens to me, I try to think about something else or go to sleep. If I do this, I generally don't run into problems.[12]

I asked two older women in Mbokomu about where *tamaa* came from and when it emerged into one's consciousness. They explained that "*tamaa* comes from deep inside the body. Young women today, they really want to try this thing [i.e., sex]. Especially our children; they don't have good upbringing. They are the complete opposite of us. Girls today look for wealth [*utajiri*]; they don't look for goodness or beauty. They do this in order to buy nice clothes and to feed their children well. 'If there's money,' they say, 'why look at anything else?'"[13]

Wasted sex and easy money were the two most commonly evoked signs of the excesses of *tamaa*. I asked a twenty-nine-year-old building contractor from Moshi whether he could share any experiences from his own life to illustrate how *tabia* was reflected in actions related to *tamaa*, even at a very young age. In response, he gave the following account of his brother, whose bad *tabia* and vulnerability to *tamaa* began early in childhood when he filched money from his parents: "My brother was chasing girls very early on. He started to sneak money from my father when he was about eight years old. Then he started chasing girls. He was often in jail. When he was out, he would chase money. If he got money, he'd take two or three women per day. He'd get them at the bar; they were barmaids. Then they would go to the guesthouse. He's been like that since he was about eighteen or twenty, and now he's just over thirty."[14]

*Tamaa* was like a barometer of one's *tabia* in its encounter with the external world. Alcohol, money, and the opportunity for sex brought turbulence to the heart, while "good work" calmed the waters. "Beer is beer. Once you use it, it's no longer your own intelligence," was a commonly heard sentiment among women. This meant that inebriated women were easily seduced; that the moral character of women, normally safeguarded by the intelligence (*akili*), became susceptible to unrestrained expressions of *tamaa*. Money and alcohol were certainly *tamaa*-inducing for men. One young man from Mbokomu said that after he collected his payment for smuggling goods from Kenya, he took his money directly to his wife, who sold cloth in the market; he did not want it in his pocket because it brought too much *tamaa.* There were differences of opinion about whether money brought *tamaa* to women, but in general it seemed that the closer one got to city life, the more *tamaa*-inducing effects there were of money for everyone. When it came to desire, said market women in Kiboriloni, "*kichokozi ni pesa*" (the little provocation is money). Ill-gotten gains were like an irritant that inflamed desire and provided the means for the unrestrained consumption of alcohol and indulgence in sex.

In discussions of gender, *tabia, tamaa,* and development, women were often portrayed as being prone to the influences of money and desires encountered through living an itinerant life. An AIDS educator from the zonal referral hospital implied this when giving his own version of the history of the epidemic's emergence in Kilimanjaro: "During the 1960s and '70s they didn't have much promiscuity [*uasherati*] here among the Chagga. It wasn't their *tabia.* But recently—by the end of the 1970s—women were more and more engaged in businesses that meant they were traveling. They got power and influence, and became promiscuous through their business success."[15] Thus *tamaa,* in nearly all aspects, was thought of as a natural capacity responsive to a number of influences from the social environment, any number of which could lead to risky behavior.

*Tamaa,* however, must be distinguished from two other concepts related to desire in a narrower, interpersonal sense: *nyege,* sexual excitement and uncontrolled lust, and *wivu,* the jealousy one might feel toward persons, but not toward objects. The term *nyege* captured the sense of intense eroticism of sexual contact itself, the ardor of sexual arousal. As one thirty-four-year-old man stated, "I mean your private parts are already stimulated . . . *tamaa,* well, you can even have '*tamaa*' for a watch, but you can't have 'nyege' for a watch! [So *nyege* is *only* of the body, and *tamaa* is not?] Not *tamaa.*"[16] While *tamaa* required some sort of reasoning process, *nyege* was an unreflective need for sex; rape and male-male sex among prisoners were often thought to be the products of *nyege,* but not of *tamaa.* While adult men and women of all ages (except the very old) experienced *tamaa, nyege* was related to the bodily strength of youth. *Nyege,* or variants of it, may be a widely shared part of the cultural "process of passion" in East Africa and Central Africa (see World Health Organization 1992:25). Groups of adolescents from six countries in the region who were asked to construct narratives of sexual encounters frequently indicated that the young couples in their stories were overwhelmed by a sudden surge of lust (1992:26). This feature of interpersonal relations, the WHO points out, may have implications for the ability of those experiencing the rush of *nyege* to exert control over situations in which they may be at risk.

*Wivu*, which I shall gloss as "jealousy," was more difficult to distinguish from *tamaa* than was *nyege*. *Wivu*, as most people used the term, was a generally more insidious sentiment than *tamaa*. As we have seen, *tamaa*, if properly directed and controlled, could be very productive, a valuable trait. *Wivu*, however, was rarely so. As the individual who spoke of *nyege* above stated, "I think *tamaa* is good if it doesn't exceed the desired limits, because it will help you to generate an income, to build a nice healthy, educated family. . . . It will also attract you to building a good house or to buying a car. But *wivu* will just lead you to stay in doors and in the end brings quarrels to the house because there is no desire for development. There will be no peace in the house. Every day you will have problems, and problems bring quarrels. . . . Another way of saying this is that someone who has *wivu* doesn't want someone else to get development."[17]

Desire was thus a layered and complex concept deriving from a number of forces aside from one's *tabia*, including one's physical and psychological constitution, one's upbringing, the wider environment of the village, city, or market, and one's vulnerability in particular situations. It was also distinguished from pure lust and jealousy. The various forms of personal desire, such as that for a good life, the desire of the body, the desire for money—to name a few kinds—were closely interrelated. Again, *tamaa* was seen as a form of desire that implied a will to possess something that one did not have. This was why many felt that two people who had given themselves in marriage did not experience *tamaa* toward each other; it would have been nonsensical to desire in that way (*-tamaani*) something they already had. Even those who said *tamaa* was necessary for marriage often described it as coming into play after a enforced period of separation.

## Desire and the Array of Male-Female Relationships

AIDS transformed the bodies of both suspected and confirmed sufferers into icons of disordered desire, unlocking the doors of culturally supported silence surrounding the plurality of coexisting sexual forms in Kilimanjaro.[18] AIDS rendered these relations subject to public scrutiny and concern to a degree far beyond that preceding the epidemic. To this point in the text, I have emphasized the role of *tamaa* in the local exegesis about contemporary male-female relations. It shall soon become apparent, however, that there was a great deal more at stake than the satisfaction of desire. *Tamaa* was an important axis along which young people gauged sexual culture in Kilimanjaro, but it was not the only one. *Tamaa*—with all its conceptual nuance, and with the power of epidemic etiology bestowed upon it by AIDS educators, teenagers, grandparents, and bar workers—must be seen in the context of the spectrum of concerns within the day-to-day world of male-female sexual relationships in Kilimanjaro.

In the 1990s, the array of nonmarital and unsanctioned sexual relationships that had emerged into the blank zone in explicit cultural discourse gave sexual life the appearance of randomness. Indeed, the word "random" *(ovyo)* was often applied to the sexual behavior of young people whose presumed promiscuity was characterized euphemistically as "walking about randomly" *(-tembea ovyo)* or simply "wandering" *(-zururazurura)*. As Ahlberg (1994:226) found among Kikuyu, however, "The openness with which sexuality is expressed does not necessarily mean that sexual activity is indiscriminate." Similarly, the lack of formal cultural guidelines for contemporary nonmarital relationships in Kilimanjaro did not prevent them from bearing a degree of systematicity. To be sure, these relationships were not formulaic; most aspects of sexual relationships were subject to the personal interpretation of the actors directly involved. In this way they were layered with a sense of structured indeterminacy; they worked precisely because there were many gray areas that allowed individual and situational interests to be negotiated. Each example of the various types of relationship examined below illustrates how, within a sexual culture of silence, conventional types of action could be reproduced imperfectly and yet remain recognizable to actors involved. Through the manipulation of cultural concepts of moral character and desire, sex was brought into relationships in an implicit and ongoing process of self-definition for young men and women. The tactical use of ambiguity in "rules" for contemporary male-female relations was central to the ability of young people to develop their sexual identities in this manner.

There are many ambiguities in the accounts of relationships presented here. They stem partly from the artifice of the ethnographic encounter and partly from the context I have just outlined. However much consensus there was about disordered desire and dubious moral character in the sexual lives of *others,* the *personal* meaning of these categories was highly contingent. The appearance of cultural systematicity within the semantics of action in sexual relationships should not be overstated. Elsewhere, with regard to fertility, I have discussed how men in Papua New Guinea used superficially similar information to reach opposite conclusions about whether small or large families were preferable, or reached similar conclusions about fertility goals using widely divergent rationales (Setel 1999b). In a similar way, men and women in Kilimanjaro presented very different motivations and rationalizations for engaging in what seemed otherwise to be similar kinds of relationships. And yet the quality and character of relationships were often defined only in retrospect, and just as often, upon their retelling, a different rationale or agenda emerged.

I make these points in order to stress that my analysis of the cultural aspects of sexual relations does something that my informants did not: it asks that desire and sexual pleasure be examined as something eminently culturally organized and recognized. Writing of ethnomedicine in Hausaland, Last (1992:393) faced a similar conundrum in asking and answering the question, "How much do people know, and care to know, about their own medical culture?" In the plural medical culture of northern Nigeria, where many healing traditions were present, Last was ultimately left describing medical culture there as a "nonsystem." There were no common sets of expectations about the kinds of knowledge and skills that "traditional" healers would use or employ; there was not even consensus about the meanings of medical terms and words for illnesses. Yet this nonsystem thrived, not as a clear-cut set of treatment alternatives but, from the cultural insider's point of view, as a large set of potentially "appropriate ones—appropriate, this is, to where one happen[ed] to be" (398). Similarly, in the sexual culture of Kilimanjaro, there was an acknowledged range of patterned action in male-female relations that could be meaningfully discussed as an "array" of relationships, but there was seldom much consensus about formal or informal guidelines for conducting them. This meant that although people had a conception of subtleties within more embracing categories of involvement (like "boyfriend" or "living together"), women and men did not go about saying things like "I'll have a crypto-polyandrous relationship with these two, but an informal polygynous union with him" or "I was a 'sugar daddy' with her, but a steady boyfriend with the other."

This points to the role of secrecy in this sexual culture. Under the *kihamba* regime, certain types of concealment and secrecy (about bodily states of being open and closed) were key to sexual and reproductive culture. So, too, in the twentieth century was secrecy important to the maintenance of the system. While young men might brag to one another about their conquests as young men, secrecy was important to women in most situations and to men on many occasions. Furthermore, many women who became aware of a partner's infidelity (some of whom had ended a relationship because of it) insisted they were not distressed so much by the infidelity itself, which was a tolerable expression of male character, as by the disrespect and ignominy they suffered as a result of the infidelity's becoming discovered and discussed. As long as a relationship remained private and secret, it naturally remained outside the purview of cultural discourse on proper moral character. Those involved indirectly could, within certain bounds, even define their relations in ways that were "appropriate to where they happened to be." Given this pervasive secrecy, it is not difficult to see how the emerging AIDS epidemic was like turning on the lights in a room long kept intentionally dark.

An array of relationships in Kilimanjaro of the 1990s can be discerned and described. A simple taxonomy of relationship categories, however, would be wholly unsuited to understanding their significance to those who participated in them and to a depiction of the forming of normative, yet ultimately ephemeral, patterns of sexual action. This is not to say that some distinctions between different types of relationships cannot be usefully made for the purposes of social, epidemiologic, and demographic understandings. From the standpoint of a cultural analysis, however, a rigid taxonomy would lead to artificial rigidity, excessive idealization of types and oversystematization—a loss of nuance for which survey researchers of AIDS have been criticized and of which they are aware (Ankrah 1989; Dare and Cleland 1994). A taxonomic approach would remove the important essence of "deferred meaning" that was so much a part of the retrospective self-presentations of informants and of their experiences in the moment.

The short case studies below demonstrate the personal emotions, aspirations, and struggles of young people in the process of negotiating adult life. Although most of the cases are used to illustrate discrete and acknowledged categories of relationships, they also demonstrate that relationships evolved from one category to another. Some who were involved in relationships that implied no initial commitment may have been testing each other out as possible spouses. In such instances, the early phases of a relationship were not necessarily seen as part of courting unless a marriage resulted; they were affiliations with their own sets of expectations. This was owing, in part, to the fact that crises often arose that either spelled the end of the relationship or forced its transformation. Such crises included a young couple's being discovered by their parents, a pregnancy, infertility, deepening financial dependency between partners, or a proven infidelity.

Table 4.1 presents a thematic matrix of relationship categories elicited from informants (for comparisons with Haiti, see Allman 1980).

Table 4.1 Male-Female Relationship Matrix

| Type of Relationship | One Must Desire (-tamaani) One's Partner | Partner Must Have "Good Character" (tabia) | Partner Assumed to be Faithful (uaminifu) | Importance of Receiving Food, Gifts, and/or Money | Importance of Fertility | Importance of Being Provided with Shelter | Do Partners Cohabit? | Must Relationship Be Kept Secret? |
|---|---|---|---|---|---|---|---|---|
| *Malaya* (domestic prostitution) | | | | | | | | |
| Female perspective | Unimportant | Unimportant | No | Very important | Undesirable | No | No | Very important |
| Male perspective | Very important | Unimportant | No | NA | Undesirable | NA | No | Very important |
| *Kuuza baa, kufanya kwa gesti* (bar girl, guest-house worker) | | | | | | | | |
| Female perspective | Unimportant to somewhat important | Unimportant to somewhat important | No | Very important | Undesirable | No | No | Very important |
| Male perspective | Very important | Unimportant | No | NA | Undesirable | NA | No | Very important |
| *Uhuni, uasherati, kuzurura* (promiscuity, "streetwalker" prostitution, an adulterous liaison) | | | | | | | | |
| Female perspective | Very important | Unimportant to somewhat important | No | Unimportant to very important | Undesirable | No | No | Very important |
| Male perspective | Very important | Unimportant to somewhat important | No | NA | Undesirable to somewhat desirable | NA | No | Unimportant to very important |

*Starehe* (entertainment, "one-night stand," short-term affair)

| | | | | | | | | |
|---|---|---|---|---|---|---|---|---|
| Female perspective | Very important | Unimportant to somewhat important | No | Unimportant to somewhat important | Undesirable | No | No | Very important |
| Male perspective | Very important | Unimportant to somewhat important | No | NA | Generally undesirable | NA | No | Unimportant to very important |

*Awara* or "sugar daddy"

| | | | | | | | | |
|---|---|---|---|---|---|---|---|---|
| Female perspective | Unimportant to somewhat important | Unimportant to somewhat important | No | Very important | Very undesirable | Generally no | Occasionally, if provided with shelter | Very important |
| Male perspective | Very important | Very important | Yes | NA | Generally undesirable | NA | Occasionally, if he provides shelter | Very important |

"Sugar mommy"

| | | | | | | | | |
|---|---|---|---|---|---|---|---|---|
| Female perspective | Very important | Unimportant to somewhat important | Yes | NA | Undesirable | NA | Occasionally, if she provides shelter | Somewhat important |
| Male perspective | Unimportant to somewhat important | Generally unimportant | No | Very important | Undesirable | Occasionally | If provided with shelter | Somewhat important |

*continued*

Table 4.1 (*continued*)

| Type of Relationship | Desire | Character | Faithfulness | Gifts or Money | Fertility | Provided with Shelter | Cohabit | Secrecy |
|---|---|---|---|---|---|---|---|---|
| *"Nipe-nikupe"* ("you give me, so I give you") | | | | | | | | |
| Female perspective | Very important | Somewhat important to very important | Ideally yes, but often no | Very important | Generally undesirable, but may become so | No | No | Somewhat important |
| Male perspective | Very important | Very important | Yes | NA | Generally undesirable | NA | No | Unimportant to somewhat important |
| *Ndoa ya kienyeji* ("traditional marriage"—bride capture, coercive elopement/rape) | | | | | | | | |
| Female perspective | Unimportant if coerced, very important if consensual | Unimportant if coerced, very important if consensual | Unknown | In order to placate woman if coerced | Undesirable if she is coerced, desirable if consensual | Yes | Yes | Not if she is coerced, plans kept secret if consensual |
| Male perspective | Very important | Very important | Unknown | NA | Very desirable | NA | Yes | Plans kept secret |

*Kimada, nyumba ndogo, "little house"*

| | | | | | | | | |
|---|---|---|---|---|---|---|---|---|
| Female perspective | Somewhat important to very important | Somewhat important to very important | No | Very important | Undesirable to very desirable | Yes | Occasionally | Not very important if Muslim; important to very important if Christian |
| Male perspective | Very important | Very important | Yes | NA | Undesirable to very desirable | NA | Occasionally | Not very important if Muslim; important to very important if Christian |

*Kurithi (levirate)*

| | | | | | | | | |
|---|---|---|---|---|---|---|---|---|
| Female perspective | Unimportant | Unimportant | No | Occasionally | Undesirable to somewhat desirable | Yes | Seldom | Unimportant |
| Male perspective | Unknown | Unknown | Yes | NA | Unknown | NA | Seldom | Unimportant |

*Urafiki, mpenzi, mchumba* (boyfriend or girlfriend, lover, engaged to marry)

| | | | | | | | | |
|---|---|---|---|---|---|---|---|---|
| Female perspective | Very important | Very important | Ideally yes, but often not | Somewhat important to very important | Undesirable | No | No | Somewhat important to unimportant |
| Male perspective | Very important | Very important | Yes | Somewhat important | Generally undesirable | No | No | Somewhat important to unimportant |

*continued*

Table 4.1 (*concluded*)

| Type of Relationship | | Desire | Character | Faithfulness | Gifts or Money | Fertility | Provided with Shelter | Cohabit | Secrecy |
|---|---|---|---|---|---|---|---|---|---|
| *Kuishi pamoja bila kufunga ndoa* (long-term cohabitation) | | | | | | | | | |
| | Female perspective | Initially very important | Initially very important | Ideally yes, but often not | Important | Usually very desirable | Yes | Yes | Not secretive |
| | Male perspective | Very important | Very important | Yes | Somewhat important | Usually very desirable | NA | Yes | Not secretive |
| *Ndoa ya serikali* (civil wedding) | | | | | | | | | |
| | Female perspective | Initially very important | Initially very important | Ideally yes, but often not | Initially very important | Very desirable | Yes | Ideally, but not necessarily | Not secretive |
| | Male perspective | Initially very important | Initially very important | Yes | Unimportant to somewhat important | Very desirable | NA | Ideally, but not necessarily | Not secretive |
| *Ndoa ya kanisa, kiislamu* (church or Islamic marriage) | | | | | | | | | |
| | Female perspective | Initially very important | Initially very important | Ideally yes, but often not | Unimportant | Very desirable | Yes | Ideally, but not necessarily | Not secretive |
| | Male perspective | Initially very important | Initially very important | Yes | Unimportant | Very desirable | NA | Ideally, but not necessarily | Not secretive |

The rows are arranged according to what are generally the relationships of youth (with the exception of *malaya,* which cuts across ages for men) versus those of later adult life. Several of the relationships mentioned had historical antecedents or were contemporary permutations of unions that had existed since at least the turn of the century.[19] There are numerous gradients at work within this schema. These are represented by the split rows, which generalize to female and male perspectives, and the columns, which give a summary statement about the salience of *tamaa, tabia,* faithfulness, the exchange of money or gifts, reproduction, shelter / cohabitation, and secrecy for each category of relationship.

### First Relationships: **Starehe** *and Sugar Daddies*

The first explicitly sexual experiences of young people often involved members of the same sex and were spoken of in terms that suggested the innocent inquisitiveness of pubertal and prepubertal children about changes and new sensations in their bodies. Many young men masturbated during puberty, often while playing or swimming in the company of other boys their age. Before menarche, girls eight or nine years old might explore each other's bodies while sleeping with friends or cousins of the same age or stimulate themselves using a variety of objects. Informants did not consider activities of this nature to be problematic; they were portrayed simply as part of growing up. When it came to beginning one's intimate life with members of the opposite sex, however, matters quickly became complicated.

First experiences with members of the opposite sex were often arranged through third parties and frequently involved either a schoolmate or a friend of a sibling. The interested boy usually, but not always, initiated contact. A classmate, sister, or brother was enlisted to deliver a love note or a small gift. Often there was an exchange of notes leading up to an encounter. At other times young people were more spontaneous and silently agreed to slip away from a disco or party in order to be alone. These early assignations, whether in the market, at school, or at dances, were shrouded in secrecy and represented some of the more familiar ways younger people flirt or become more intimately involved (see Gutmann 1926:68,129; Marealle 1952:61; Shann 1956:26). The following text, written in the mid-1980s to an informant while the girl was in primary school, indicates some of the conventions that applied to the seduction of partners through intermediaries and notes. A friend of the recipient's older brother wrote the note.

Salaam:

I hope you are fine since we last saw each other. I want in this letter, first to thank you for responding to the little talk we had yesterday. To answer your concerns—you are worried that your mother will know. That's not likely. Maybe, unless you cause it to happen yourself. We can do it without people knowing. I also don't want people to know; it will be our secret. So, now, if you agree, I ask that we do it tomorrow (Thursday). In the evening, as we saw each other yesterday. So, if it's okay, I want you to answer me before you go to school. And I want the answer to be good! If we meet often, we might easily be discovered. Please send a quick answer.

Thank you.[20]

These kinds of relationships, usually referred to as *starehe*, "recreation" or "partying," or by the English cognate *kampani*, "company," were the first sexual experiences involving intercourse for many young people.[21] For girls, losing one's virginity was called *-vunja bikira*, "to break the hymen," but most young women referred to the episode by saying that they "were taught sex," *nilifundishwa sexi*. Men referred to their entry into sexual life simply by saying that they "started to sex" (*-anza kusexi* or *-anza kufanya mapenzi*) at a certain age.[22] Many *starehe* relations were single episodes or a series of encounters over a short period of time. Some, however, lasted many years. In such cases, the partners had little contact other than when they met to make love. In rural areas, *starehe* relations often occurred between acquaintances. In Moshi, they might occur between strangers, but there was usually some sort of social connection that allowed the parties to recognize each other as a "friend-of-a-friend," for example; sex between complete strangers fell into another category of relationship, *uhuni* or *uasherati*.

When discussing their earliest relationships, men generally distinguished their *starehe* partners from their first girlfriends. Boys who had the opportunity to have *starehe* partners in primary school were considered fortunate by their peers. While girls tended to keep the advent of their sexual lives as quiet as possible, male peers gained status with one another through having their conquests become known. What tended to emerge was a form of status competition among a network of male friends in which they lowered each other's status by seducing one another's former *starehe* partners or girlfriends. While male informants cited this status competition, along with the satisfaction of *tamaa*, as the most important motivation for having a *starehe* relationship, female informants cited the satisfaction of desire as the main reason they chose to participate.

While it was assumed that a main appeal of *starehe* was to satisfy the naive sexual desires of people just starting to become sexually active, a *starehe* partner's *tabia* was said not to be important unless the couple continued to see each other. In fact, the practicalities of *starehe* often prevented the partners from even having long conversations; their ability to meet depended on secrecy, and they were rarely at an age at which they lived independently. Thus they were forced to meet in locations where they had to be quiet in order to avoid being discovered. The decision to continue with a partner was based on two main criteria: the amount of sexual satisfaction that each partner experienced, and whether or not there was compatibility. Brief *starehe* relationships were easy to keep secret if the parties so desired and were the most convenient way for young people to be sexually active. Partly because they were often so spontaneous, they implied no commitment whatsoever by either party. There was no expectation of faithfulness *(uaminifu)* or exclusivity.

Small gifts to the female partner, which were expected tokens of affection and concern in other relationships, were sometimes seen as essential but were sometimes completely dispensed with. One informant, a twenty-year-old man, recalled how he had to learn the ropes in his first sexual encounter, when he was in his early teens. "'If you *starehe* with me, how much will you give me?' she asked. I was surprised. I asked her if that money was needed at home. 'No,' she said, 'but I will have given you something, and you will not have given me anything at all.'"[23] For girls, *starehe* relations could begin at a very young age and might or might not lead to long-term relations. Vero was twenty in 1993 and had had nine sex partners, some of whom she referred to as *starehe* some as *rafiki,* or boyfriend (discussed below).[24] She was working as a domestic servant, had no children of her own, and was the last-born child of a large family living on a *kihamba* in rural Kilimanjaro some distance from Moshi. At the age of nine she had learned to masturbate and had received the attentions of a persistent older boy who had sent her many love notes. After accepting what she said was the tenth note, she agreed to meet him for sex. When asked why she agreed, Vero stated that she was flattered by his attentions, that he dressed well, and used "sweet words." At first the relationship was just *starehe,* but after eleven years, Vero said she was still having sex with Robert when he came home from Dar es Salaam, where he had moved. Although Robert gave her gifts, she insisted that she did not remain involved "because he took me shopping. I just liked him." Vero's second encounter was another example of *starehe* sex that did not lead to any longer-term connections. She narrated it in the following way.

> One night I was coming home from buying milk. Terence came up to me along the way and said, "How's it going?"
> "Fine," I said.
> "Where have you gotten lost to?"
> "I'm around . . ."
> "Now, what about it, my friend . . . I've been trying to . . . um . . . find you, but someone said you'd gone to stay at . . . I don't know . . . your grandmother's, your uncle's . . . I'm begging you to show me "the garden of love" [*shamba la mapenzi*] just a little bit, my friend . . ."
> "Aaah. I don't have time now. Wait here till I take the milk home. I'll take the milk home and you wait right here."
> "Come on. Just put the milk down here, what's the problem? We'll only take a short time."
> "OK."

While, as the name implies, *starehe* relations may have been good fun for young people exploring sex and romance, the sexuality and fertility of young people were perceived to be an issue of great concern across Tanzania by the 1990s (Tumbo-Masabo and Liljeström 1994). Available demographic data suggest that the majority of young women and girls, such as Vero, over whom such concern was expressed were probably born within marriage (Bureau of Statistics 1973). By 1996 in urban Moshi, in contrast, a majority of men and women had their first children prior to formalizing a union (Setel et al. 1996). Even for young parents of the 1970s, however, social values about the appropriate age and life conditions for commencing fertility had changed a great deal. Reported births to those who were aged twenty to twenty-four in the 1970s had dropped 40 percent since their mother's generation (calculations based on Bureau of Statistics 1973:203, 225), and in the same year in which Vero began showing boys the garden of love, abortion-related admissions to hospitals in Dar es Salaam increased dramatically (Mpangile, Leshabari, and Kihwele 1993:21).[25] By the time Vero and her young adult friends reached the ages at which most of their own parents had begun to reproduce, the age at which most women were beginning to have children had risen still higher, and with it the age at marriage.[26]

As parents in Kilimanjaro were well aware, delays in marrying and childbearing did not imply a corresponding postponement of entry into sexual life.[27] Rather, by attenuating entry into adulthood (through marriage, ideally after the completion of secondary education), the delays served to emphasize the consequences of the transgressive sexual activity of young people. In 1992, the national median age at first intercourse for twenty to twenty-four-year-olds was reported to be 17.1 for women and 16.9 for men—roughly a year and a half lower than the median age at first marriage (Weinstein et al. 1995:54). In Kilimanjaro, adolescents appear to have become sexually active at a somewhat younger age. Among primary school students with a median age of fourteen, roughly two-thirds of the boys and a quarter of the girls reported having engaged in sexual intercourse (Klepp, Ndeki, and Mliga 1994). Yet the age at first birth among women in Kilimanjaro was comparatively high in the national context; rural Kilimanjaro had the lowest rates of childbirth among women aged fifteen to nineteen in Tanzania (13.8 percent; Bureau of Statistics 1993).

The effect of a rising age at marriage and a corresponding increase in the age of first birth was to lengthen the period between one's sexual debut and time at which men and their partners could be considered to have formed a recognized union. At the same time, the penetration of Christianity and Islam has had profound effects on morality expressed about premarital pregnancy across Africa (Lesthaeghe, Kaufmann, and Meekers 1989:329; Ahlberg 1994:228–33). In Kilimanjaro, where Christianity in particular found enthusiastic acceptance, premarital pregnancy was seen as among the gravest of problems facing youth. Given the difficulties many men had in establishing themselves in the kinds of domestic arrangements or businesses in which they felt ready to marry, it is not surprising that many people, including young women themselves, feared the consequences of an early pregnancy. The widespread changes in domestic life and nuptiality served to throw into stark relief sexuality which once might have been managed in such a way as to censure the precocity of the fertility while reintegrating young people into a sanctioned union. Instead, young adult fertility was increasingly portrayed as precocious in a way that indicated bad *tabia* and a proclivity to engage in promiscuous sex. The AIDS epidemic heightened these anxieties further.

When a pregnancy occurred, the consequences fell more heavily on young women. Men might deploy the concepts of *tabia* and *tamaa* in such a way as to give themselves an escape route. "If she had the kind of *tabia* to *starehe* with me, she must have other partners—so how do I know the child is mine?" went the reasoning. Children born to unmarried women not only pointed to a rupture in the "proper" ordering of adult life but also raised new and disturbing questions about inheritance, filiation, and responsibility in an era of attenuated individual/

kin group relations.[28] Fertility outside a stable union could also reduce a woman's prospects of getting married or stabilizing an independent domestic life. As Haram (1995:42) found among Meru in neighboring Arusha region, such women faced a double bind: those with children were stigmatized as having been "spoiled" (*ameharibika*) or, if offered marriage, might decline since these offers might entail a prospective husband's refusal to care for the child of another man (see Freyhold, Sawaki, and Zalla 1973:177). The best that some of these women could hope for was an informal polygynous union which offered freedom but little security (see below).

In practice, then, the commonly voiced fears about increasing teen-age pregnancy arising from a pandemic of *starehe*-type sexual relations did not necessarily reflect an increasing prevalence of the phenomenon of younger women having children per se, but of children born before the establishment of a stable union or before paternal support for a child had been secured. Although by the 1990s ages at first birth had been rising for a long time in Tanzania, the fertility for the majority of a random sample of men and women in Moshi town did precede the establishment of a stable union (Setel et al. 1996).[29] Nevertheless, the denial of paternity among those giving birth before marriage may have been a rarer occurrence than feared. In 1996, roughly 2 percent of sampled women in Moshi town whose first birth preceded a stable union reported ever having difficulty in getting the genitor of any of their children to acknowledge paternity (Setel et al. 1996), and among women presenting at hospitals in Dar es Salaam with complications of induced abortion, the denial of paternity was not frequently mentioned as a reason to seek pregnancy termination (Mpangile, Leshabari, and Kihwele 1993:25).

As the case of Ishindi illustrates, however, it is reasonable to expect that younger women with younger partners (i.e., partners with access to fewer resources) may be more likely to experience problems in obtaining support in the case of pregnancy.[30] Ishindi was a twenty-year-old woman from Kibosho, on the mountain slopes above Moshi town. She had eight siblings and was the oldest of the children remaining at home; the others had all moved to Dar es Salaam. Ishindi became sexually active at the age of twelve, and had a child when she was nineteen. The infant was born premature and died after three days. The child, she says, was the result of *starehe*. Ishindi pursued the man she thought was the father, but he refused to acknowledge the child was his. Actually, she was not certain herself who the father was; she had had three different partners at the time. Ishindi pursued all of them, thinking one would either marry her or help her get an abortion. None of them offered to marry her or to provide her with the funds for an abortion. "When I had sex it was just *starehe*. I didn't think a baby would come—that that would be the result," she said. Nevertheless, Ishindi managed to gather TSh 12,000 for an illegal abortion, and made the necessary arrangements.[31] Upon examining her, however, the doctor told her that she was too close to term and refused to terminate the pregnancy.

In Kilimanjaro, concerns over the sexuality of young women were highest for schoolgirls. Since a discovered pregnancy meant automatic expulsion, schoolgirls were under pressure to guard their parents' investment in their education (Stambach 1996a). Because of the investment made in them, if they became pregnant, they were seen as more likely to compound their transgressions by attempting to procure an abortion. Not surprisingly, in Tanzania, the younger and the poorer a woman, the more likely she was to resort to unsafe means of pregnancy termination. Although teenagers accounted for 14 percent of abortion-related hospital admissions in Dar es Salaam, they represented nearly a third of those whose admission resulted from an unsafe abortion practice; a quarter of these girls were primary or secondary school students (Mpangile, Leshabari, and Kihwele 1993:28). Unsafe practices included invasive procedures by healers with no formal training, abortions performed by poorly trained staff of public hospitals or private clinics, or abortions self-administered by using sharp objects or ingesting substances like chloroquin phosphate. This last method was also a favored way of committing suicide, as the following text indicates. This letter was written by Upendo, a woman in her early twenties, to her friend in Moshi in 1993.

> Dear Laura:
>
> I think you are well, sister. Everyone here at home is well. The purpose of writing this is to explain to you something that I will do. I should grind up a bottle of chloroquin and drink it down because I am anxious about my life. See, the way I feel now isn't good; I feel like someone who is pregnant. So if you possibly can, come to Arusha to assure me whether or not it is so. You see, I watch for my period every month—even right now I should be having it—but things are not good. I beg you, if you can even borrow the bus fare and I won't fail to find some way of getting you what you need to get home. I beg you, do it fast. It's that, my sister, I'm in form two, and as if that weren't enough, I cannot bear to bring this shame upon my home.
>
> Don't tell anyone why you'll be coming to Arusha. I will explain to you how it all happened. I beg you, don't delay because there

is no one else I can speak to about this. Also, if I see that my condition is just getting worse and worse, I will swallow chloroquin; there's plenty of it in the stores. It's not that I'm trying to scare you. I'm telling you the truth. And if you should find that I've already swallowed it, then good-bye beloved sister. You know, we really got along with each other, you and me. We listened to each other and respected each other. Just pray for me to God that he forgive me. And if you should find that I have already died, don't tell anything to anyone. I should just die with my child. We'll see each other, my beloved sister, in heaven, God willing.
It's me, the one with the problem,
—Upendo M.

P.S. Don't cry for me, sister, because all of this I have been brought by my own intelligence [akili] that doesn't work. Move fast so that you at least see me before I am dead. You should take at least one pair of my shoes to remember me by in your life.

I never had sex since I was born. But this one day, the first time I've ever done it, the enormity has gotten me. Good-bye, sister.[32]

While girls such as Upendo and Ishindi may end up in dire straits, boys in secondary schools gained enough independence when living away from their families to begin asserting themselves sexually, and generally enjoyed themselves. Many found it easy to sneak out of the school compound on weekends or bribe the watchmen with cigarettes or money for *mbege*. Saba, who was born in Old Moshi, was twenty-nine years old and worked at a fiberboard plant in Moshi.[33] He was married and had two children; the whole family stayed together in a small room in Moshi town. Saba was the fourth child of ten, only one other of whom had remained in Kilimanjaro region. His father was a farmer who supplemented his income by working as a driver and auto mechanic. Saba finished form four at a secondary boarding school in Old Moshi in 1984 and then studied manufacturing at a vocational center for two years.

At secondary school, Saba stayed with two roommates who were older and more sexually experienced than he was. They taught him about sex. Saba and his friends categorized girls into three groups: town, school, and village. According to this scheme, the most desirable were said to be town girls, the most available were village girls. Once or twice a month he and his friends had enough pocket money to take a bus from Kiboriloni market to town in order to *starehe*. They would arrive at the bus stand in the center of town late in the afternoon. After passing by the movie house to see whether a new film was playing, they headed to the Sidecar Club in Njoro ward near the rail station in order to look for young women.

[So which girls were most desirable?] The girls from Moshi were desirable because they were experienced. The Chaggas don't have *unyago,* so the girls really don't know how to have sex. The good partners were the Hehe, Haya, Sukuma, and the Pare. [And where in town would you find them?] We would go to the club and start talking to the girls. [So how would it go?] We would try to get them drunk and invite them to the movies. The girls from this part of town were always available because they were always looking for money to buy things for themselves or to drink or go to the cinema. After that we knew where the guest houses were that we could go to. Early in the morning we'd escort the girls back to their neighborhood and we'd go to my roommate's brother's house to sleep for a few hours. [And girls from the village—how would you find them?] The ones [from the village] who would take you were about fifteen years old. You could find them along the paths while they were cutting fodder, and so on. We knew our way around up there, so we'd try and talk them into it. If they agreed we'd just slip into the bushes, the bananas, the coffee, whatever. These girls knew their days so they didn't get pregnant. Sometimes they would tell us "I'll be at Kiboriloni at a certain hour." We'd meet there and go straight to a guest house. [And the girls at school?] The school girls were day students, and they were a pain. They are the ones who looked at you to see if you had money. If she accepts, you buy her some peanuts or a soda, and you suggest something—a place to meet. She can agree, refuse, or make her own suggestion. [And with these friends, were you looking for serious relationships, or was it just for fun, or . . . ?] All these goings on were *starehe.* They knew we were in secondary school, and they didn't expect anything from us. They knew we didn't have anything in our pockets.

Adolescent females, especially those with a need for assistance with school fees, were seen as vulnerable to the material persuasions (*vishawishi*) and sweet talk (*maneno matamu*) of "sugar daddies" and younger men with means. The stereotype of the sugar-daddy relationship was one in which a wealthy older man provided gifts or paid school fees for a much younger woman. The large gifts aided in the seduction of the young woman by tempting her to accept a suitor much older than herself, and presumably one who was not sexually desirable. For his part, the man presumably got access to a virginal school-girl whose supposed pristine condition was a guarantee that he would not acquire HIV from her. Naturally, the concern was that the vulnerable schoolgirls would either become pregnant and/or infected with HIV by their partners.

The extent to which such stereotyped young woman–older man relations formed as large a part of the sexual culture in Tanzania as many parties feared has been questioned (Leshabari and Kaaya 1995; Nnko and Pool 1997), although it does seem clear that such relations do exist. Mpangile et al. found that among a sample of girls aged fourteen to seventeen seeking abortions, 20 percent stated they were made pregnant by a boy also in his teens, 30 percent said their partner was over forty-five years of age, and among the students, 20 percent reported ever having had a partner over the age of forty-five (Mpangile, Leshabari, and Kihwele 1993:28). Those who have looked deeper into relations that superficially fit the sugar-daddy type have found that they may represent an investment by a man in the education of a woman he desires to establish a formal or informal polygynous union with (see case study in Haram 1995:35–37) or that the men involved are often younger and less well off than commonly thought (Nnko and Pool 1995).

In Kilimanjaro relations between very young girls and older men were sometimes referred to as *awara,* or *hawara,* a term that could also applied to other situations (see below). It should be noted that a large age gap between sexual partners was not an innovation in Kilimanjaro; indeed a significant age gap among marriage partners in a growing population is one of the only ways to sustain both universal marriage and polygyny. Gutmann described a number of situations in which an older man might acquire a much younger woman as a wife (although such arrangements seemed to contradict other supposed norms of the *kihamba* regime and may not have implied that this marriage included a sexual component). By the 1970s, however, such relations were commented upon as a social problem in rural Kilimanjaro (Freyhold, Sawaki, and Zalla 1973:177). Girls were said to be attracted to the money or gifts made possible by married men, some of whom might promise marriage in the event of pregnancy. It appears, however, that the social and legal sanctions against such men were so mild that few families pursued the matter if the ostensible father refused to honor his commitment.

The case of Abdul and Niri is one in which several of these themes emerged.[34] At the age of twenty-six Abdul started a sexual relationship with Niri, who as eleven at the time. He was hardly the stereotypical sugar daddy and could not be said to have dazzled Niri with riches. Abdul was a builder but had not had steady work since 1990. After briefly being well off enough to support himself, he had been reduced to living with his mother and surviving on *kibarua,* or casual labor. Abdul strove to keep his relationship with Niri secret, but when it was discovered, a crisis emerged. From Niri's family's perspective, the main concerns were Niri's youth and the partial payments of bridewealth they had received from another man, not the fact that there was a large difference in ages between Niri and Abdul. This case also demonstrates the kind of crises that often emerged in less formal relationships, forcing them either to end or to move from one category to another. Niri received a beating from her brothers when her relationship was discovered; she then fled back to Abdul's home, where he agreed to let her stay the night. This was a significant act; when a woman spent the night at a man's home under such conditions, she was often acknowledged to have had a "traditional" wedding, *ndoa ya kienyeji*. While this escalation of formalization in Abdul and Niri's relationship did not last, traditional weddings often lead to the establishment of long-term unions.

Abdul first began pursuing Niri after seeing her selling fish outside her parents' house in another part of his neighborhood in Moshi town. He initiated contact with her by dropping a fifty shilling note into her basket as he passed by and telling her to go buy a soda with the money. "For a long time," he says, "I didn't tell her anything more. I kept doing this until she got used to me. I just kept it up until one day I told her that I really liked her and so forth. The way she laughed, I could tell she'd agreed but was ashamed to say 'yes' straight out." Soon after that Abdul took her to his house, where they had sex. "Her parents heard she was at my house," he explained. "They came and found us there. 'We don't want a lot of words,' they said, 'we just want this girl to return home.' She did, and her brothers beat her terribly. She fled to my house, and I told her that she could stay until morning. That was that. I sent my father to her house the next day to tell them not to look for her because she was with me. Her mother said, 'Look. First of all, she is still too young. But second, she is betrothed to someone who has already paid half of the bride-price. It just can't be.'"[35]

Nevertheless, Niri continued to visit Abdul, and when she was twelve years old, she became pregnant by him. At this point, although he was twenty-seven, Abdul had no independent means. He was no longer employed and had not yet succeeded in obtaining a plot and beginning to build his own house. Therefore, he needed the support of his father in order to marry Niri, as he wished to. Abdul's father refused to provide assistance, accusing Niri's parents of having acted improperly when Abdul had first proposed marriage. Abdul was thus unable to marry and no longer saw Niri. Although he acknowledged his paternity for the baby, and knew that she was living with her maternal grandmother, he wanted nothing to do with her. "The child was a baby girl," Abdul said, "and I don't want her. What would I do with her?"

Abdul's case suggests, as Mpangile and colleagues found (1993), that the "sugar daddy" probably misrepresents the character of a great number of relations between older men and much younger women or girls. Furthermore, the fact that Abdul and Niri's relationship transcended *starehe* sex and that Niri's parents' main objection had to do with her betrothal to another man suggests the need to consider the risks to very young women and girls and how to protect them—particularly in conditions of poverty. Niri was put at risk not only by the attentions of Abdul but also by her parents' acceptance of bride-price payments for her.

### Stigma and Exploitation: Barmaids and Guest-House Workers

Since early on in the sub-Saharan AIDS epidemic, epidemiologists have paid a great deal of attention to urban African women engaged in commercial sex as a "core risk" and "core transmitter" group in the spread of HIV infection (see Kreiss et al. 1986; Mann et al. 1987; Piot et al. 1987). Others have focused on women in economically marginal occupational categories for whom sex trade was an ancillary activity (Mhalu et al. 1991). Social scientists were quick to point out that the value-laden Western concept of "prostitute" as employed in these epidemiologic studies added little to our understanding of the sexual and economic lives of women in African cities. This tendency muddied clear thinking about risk with ethnocentric notions of stigma and promiscuity and exaggerated the pervasiveness of "prostitution" in the Western sense in African sexual cultures (de Zalduondo 1990). Indeed, the cash nexus in contemporary African sexuality has generated a host of historical and contemporary case studies of commercial sex work and, at the margins of commercial sex work, debates over the general transactability of sex (e.g., Larson 1989; White 1990; Pickering and Wilkins 1993; Weiss 1993; Haram 1995).

In Kilimanjaro, people generally referred to prostitution as *umalaya*, although this term could also be used to refer to the sex life of someone thought to be promiscuous. Although women in commercial sex work in East African cities engaged in several forms of prostitution (White 1990:13–21), in Kilimanjaro they were usually grouped together under the term *malaya*. Many informants classed *malaya* prostitutes together with barmaids, though there seemed to be several differences between the two groups. These differences extended to their apparent risks for HIV infection. Self-identified *malaya* prostitutes in Moshi, who numbered fewer than 100 in the late 1980s and 1990s, had substantially higher HIV seroprevalence than bar workers (Nkya et al. 1987:63; Nkya et al. 1991). Women engaged in *malaya* work reported having between ten and twenty sexual contacts per day, earning from TSh 80 to TSh 100 per contact during the late 1980s (Nkya et al. 1991:2). This contrasted starkly with the type of commercial sex work that took place among barmaids and guest-house workers.

Women working in guest houses in Moshi town and at the markets of Kiboriloni and Himo often came from outside Kilimanjaro region and were far away from their families. Those who came from Kilimanjaro attempted to keep the nature of their work secret from their families. "This work is not something to enjoy; just staying alive is more trouble than its worth. This work has absolutely no respectability," said Alice, a twenty-two-year-old Chagga woman who was trying to keep her presence at the guest house a secret from her parents in Uru, near Old Moshi.[36] Alice was the third of eight children. Her father had a *kihamba* in Uru and a *shamba* below Moshi town. When she was small, the family depended on her father's coffee and maize; in 1991 her parents and three younger siblings were depending on Alice's income from working as a barmaid. Her two older brothers had moved away and were contributing little to the household.

Before working at the bar, Alice worked as a domestic servant for a family in Moshi. She had just finished primary school, and there was no work in her home village. As a domestic servant, she was paid TSh 1,500 per month, plus room and board, and found the pay and workload intolerable.[37] At the bar, she earned TSh 4,000 per month, plus her room. In addition, she earned another TSh 1,000 to TSh 3,000 from the one or two "boyfriends" she took every month. In the border town of Namanga in Arusha region, long-term relations between a bar worker and one or more boyfriends sometimes existed. These were classed as another variant of *awara* relationships (Talle 1995:24–25). This type of *awara* relationship entailed the provision of shelter, and money for food and clothing, in exchange for exclusive sexual access and other domestic services. Bar workers in these relationships, Talle found, might "steal" from their *awara* boyfriends by having casual relationships when their boyfriends traveled. They also might abandon an *awara* relationship if it did not suit their needs and opt for more profitable occasional one-night partnerships. These relationships resembled those between Alice and her boyfriends. The woman would be provided with beer and food for the evening and be given between one and two thousand shillings after spending the night with her partner.

Given the rate of partner change for these bar workers, the risks of such an existence were clearly substantial (although Talle found it difficult to obtain estimates of numbers of partners [1995:25]). Women in Alice's position were very vulnerable to exploitation, partly owing to laws meant to protect casual labor from exploitation.[38] Certain statutes dictated that casual labor could only be hired on a three-month basis, after which time employees were entitled to benefits. Furthermore, if dismissed before the end of the third month, casual workers could not be rehired at the same establishment for several months thereafter. Women who had no other options often reached an understanding with the guest-house management that allowed them to earn a small income off the books, occupy a room at the guest house, and supplement their income any way they were able.

From the perspective of most men, sex with bar girls was seen in very straightforward terms as an outlet for *nyege* and *tamaa*. Bars were places infrequently visited by couples and even more rarely by a married man and woman together. The atmosphere of a bar, which might or might not be attached to a guest house, somehow heightened the sensations of desire for men. Perhaps this was because these locations were focal points of forces people associated with excesses of *tamaa*, such as alcohol and conspicuous consumption of luxurious food items. The aspect of *tamaa* relating to the commodification of a traditional world was also part of the bar scene. These encounters parodied bridewealth transactions; in both cases beef and beer were exchanged for sex. The "proper" transactions were between clans for long-term access to reproductive sexuality; in bars they were exchanges between individuals for the gratification of immediate need and desire.[39] Sex with women in these locations, I was often told, was of the no-holds-barred variety. Bar girls had not only sold their sex, but they had sold their dignity and right to respect. Sexual positions, such as "folding" (*-mkunja*) a woman, that were spoken of as titillating "styles" for both partners in *starehe* sex were used to render paid partners prone and to degrade or "fix them" (*-mkomesha*). Even the most transgressive of sex acts, anal intercourse, *ulawiti*, was not considered out of bounds with a woman for whom one had paid.

### *Lovers:* Urafiki *and* Nipe-nikupe

Ahlberg (1994:233) notes that contemporary African youth are confronted with four distinct "moral regimes" in public discourse about their sexuality: the religious (which she limits to the Christian), the traditional African, the administrative/legal, and the more secular romantic love. Yet ultimately youth are left stranded in a no-man's land of social values and sexual action that leaves them cognizant of cultural dogma but beyond the reach of a systematic or coherent set of sexual values. AIDS educators, family-planning proponents, parents, and community and religious leaders readily support three of these moral regimes: the traditional, the Christian, and the administrative/legal. All of these bar premarital sexual activity, discourage sex education, and forbid abortion and contraceptive use by unmarried young people. Yet these adult-supported values operate in a vacuum and lack sufficient regulation and control mechanisms: "The adolescents therefore live in a highly paradoxical situation of prohibition, silence, and confusion on the part of the adult world" (1994:234). Young people, Ahlberg observes, choose the fourth option, that of romantic love. This domain of sexual values "dictates that sexual activity is all right so long as people are in love, regardless of their marital status. The 'romantic love' moral regime . . . leads to a form of sexual activity characterized by serial monogamy, where loving relationships occur in quick succession between female and male adolescents of the same age group. . . . While the relationship lasts, adolescents may not practice safe sex, simply because they consider themselves at no risk: their relationship at that particular time is firm and involves just one faithful partner" (1994:234).

Among young people in Kilimanjaro, as among primary school students in Mwanza (Nnko and Pool 1997), this notion of romantic love was prevalent but was tempered with suspicions about the hidden acquisitive motives of girls and the deceitful, lust-driven motives of boys. The two kinds of relationship that were most commonly experienced by young people were friendship (urafiki) or lover (mpenzi) relationships, and what I have termed nipe-nikupe ("you give me, so I give you").[40] In day-to-day conversation the major distinction made between these categories had to do with whether or not the partners felt "true love" toward each other. Young people used the English phrase or—by removing the ambiguity in the Swahili verb kupenda, to "like or love"—kupenda sana, to "love very much." In this case, the significance of material and sexual transactions between partners was downplayed, and emotional reciprocities and compatibility were emphasized. Nipe-nikupe, which appears to have been part of the urban sexual landscape since the 1970s, was simply an heuristic used to indicate an ongoing sexual relationship in which financial and material support of the female partner (usually in the form of clothing or cosmetics) was an important display of commitment, affection, and entitlement.

Young men often spoke with a sense of sympathy for and responsibility toward their partners. When the economic dimension of *nipe-nikupe* predominated, however, a woman could be said to be doing it "as a business," *kama uchumi*.

Women in *nipe-nikupe* relationships, however, were rarely considered on a par with bar workers or *malaya*, because the former group "feel ashamed," *-ona haibu*, about their situation. Young women who became involved in *nipe-nikupe* were often trying to establish independent lives; they relied on inadequate salaries in order to support not only themselves but also their younger siblings, their own children as single mothers, and/or their parents. While *starehe* relationships offered fun and recreation, in *nipe-nikupe* and *urafiki* relationships young people engaged in more serious forms of reciprocity and intimacy. Compatibility became an important psychological component of these kinds of relationships, and they were not quite so secretive—perhaps because they were often considered to be a form of courtship. *Urafiki* or *mpenzi* (lover) relationships developed over time and often included a long initial period of socializing and mutual scrutinizing. During this time, the prospective partners would "study" each other *(-soma)*.

> [Now, what are the first stages of a relationship?] It's better if you study him first. If you do that, you learn something about his *tabia* and whether he is a liar or whatever. If a guy comes around in the afternoon, a woman might tell him to come around later for more "study." [And how do you know when you've "studied" enough?] It's hard to get the opportunity to study someone enough. Usually, you have to take your chances and see if it works out.[41]

*Urafiki* also involved the kinds of gifts given in *nipe-nikupe*, such as clothing, shoes, cosmetics, food, entertainment, and money. Older secondary school students in *nipe-nikupe* and romantic friendships often received help with their school fees, books, and other materials. They did not have to seek out or accept the attentions of much-older men. The support did not extend to the provision of shelter, however, and the partners did not cohabit. Men who were especially interested in a long-term relationship with girlfriends occasionally discouraged them from using contraception both as a demonstration of trust and fidelity and in hopes that the woman might become pregnant. In *nipe-nikupe* and friendship, fidelity was expected of both partners, but it was also understood that many men had *starehe* relationships "on the side." It was common, for example, for a young man who lived in Moshi to have a girlfriend on the mountain whom he saw once or twice a month;

while in Moshi he might well take *starehe* partners to "decrease his *tamaa*" (*-punguza tamaa*).

Boyfriends and girlfriends who said that they believed in true love spoke about love, commitment, and faithfulness in ways that their peers in superficially similar relationships did not. From the woman's perspective, a partner who showed true love was often spoken of as being gentle (*mpole*), respectful (*ananiheshimu*), compatible (*tunaele-wana*), and trustworthy (*mwaminifu*), in addition to being physically attractive. From the male point of view, a desirable partner was pretty, well brought up (*mwenye adabu*), gentle, soft spoken, and obedient. *Nipe-nikupe* relations were characterized by a greater emphasis on the man having paid for the right (*haki*) to exercise his pleasures with regard to his partner's social movements, her dress, and the use of contraceptives, including condoms, in their sexual relations. While *mpenzi* relationships often implied that neither party was married, they did occur extramaritally. A pregnancy resulting from an *mpenzi* or *rafiki* relationship usually transformed the terms by which the partners referred to each other. Ostensibly, it also changed the expectations they were entitled to have of each other. As one woman put it, "When we started out, he was just my '*rafiki*'—he's *rafiki* before you give birth. Once you've had a child with him he's '*bwana*' and you are '*bibi*.' When we marry we'll be husband (*mume*) and wife (*mke*)."[42] Partners who intended to marry but had no children referred to each other as *mchumba*, which implied a state of betrothal.

Sharifa was twenty-two years old and worked as a tailor. She was from Tanga and moved to Moshi after finishing primary school to live with her older sister in a house in Somalitown, near the central market.[43] She had one close female friend, Yasmina, who lived next door, and on many evenings the two would sit in front of Sharifa's house talking and laughing about life, work, and men.

> [Do you have a boyfriend now?] These days having a boyfriend is more bother than fun. I haven't been with anyone since last year, when I was working at Sifa's Fashions. I liked that guy a lot, but he went to Botswana. He has a wife and a child. [Did she know about you?] Yes. [How did you meet him?] Before we started going out, I asked people who knew him what he was like. He was a Chagga from Marangu, and is now a doctor in Dar es Salaam. He was here for a while on leave. He came to Sifa's Fashions one day; that's where I met him. [How long before you slept together?] We knew each other two months before we started sleeping together. He'd stop by the shop on his way home to Marangu in the afternoons. [So what did you do together?] We'd go on outings to

Moshi Hotel, to Arusha, to the National Park. Before we started being friends, we'd just go for the day and come back. [How often did you see each other and stay together?] We saw each other every day and spent the night together about once a week. [Did you talk about AIDS?] Before we started sleeping together, he said we have to know and trust each other, and so he said we should go get checked. He took my blood one day at a guest house. He has friends in a lab somewhere. [What about him?] He didn't take his own blood as far as I know. [And did he tell you the result of your test?] He didn't mention it again, so I asked him and he said there was no problem. I was still nervous, so he brought some paper from the lab. Even after that I was nervous for a week or so, but then I forgot about it.

Gloria was born in Tabora and moved with her parents and six siblings to a growing residential section of Moshi called "Soweto" in 1974.[44] She finished secondary school in 1988 and since then had been working at a bank. Gloria was the middle child, and two younger siblings remained at home. Her father had retired, and her mother did occasional work as a tailor. Gloria's social life consisted of casual friends at work, a "*besti*" (best friend of the same sex), and her boyfriend, Jon.

[Will you tell me about your boyfriend? Is he a "permanent"? Does he help you out with things?] I do have a "permanent" boyfriend, and yes, Philip, he helps out. [How did you meet?] He came here from South Africa to study at the Health College, and was a friend of a family friend. That's how we met. [How long have you been together?] Nearly two years. [Do you think you might marry?] We don't have any plans to marry. [How will you know if you want to?] Many times boys from Moshi approach you and say "I love you," and so on, but they're not being honest. [Is it important to have a boyfriend?] I can stay a long time without a boyfriend. Jon, for example. We just hung out together for six months before anything happened at all. Jon is honest, open, and faithful. That's what I like about him. [Do you use anything to prevent getting pregnant or to stop AIDS?] Most of the time when we are together we use condoms. Those who don't use condoms say it's because they can't feel anything, but it's all in their mind. They're stupid. You can avoid so many things, not just AIDS. Boys here, they think they have rights with a girl over *everything,* so even if a girl wants him to use a condom, he can refuse. I don't like that.

### Informal Polygyny: Kimada *or* Nyumba Ndogo

In Kilimanjaro there was a precedent for a form of polygyny, called "opening a hut" (Gutmann 1926:176), that did not involve the payment of bridewealth. In the early 1990s, however, many stated that this type of relationship had been brought in more recently from the coast. Elsewhere in East Africa, this type of informal polygyny appeared to be increasing (Larson 1989:20). By definition, *kimada*, or *nyumba ndogo* (literally "small house"), relationships took place between a married man and a single woman. In some cases, fertility was a desired part of a *kimada* relationship and in others was considered by both partners to be a liability. Women who were in *kimada* relationships were often said to be divorced and were caring for the children of their former husbands. Men who had a *kimada* and who wanted to have children by their partner usually accepted responsibility for the children privately, although they did not always publicly acknowledge their paternity. They provided *kimada* partners and their children with food, money, clothing, and shelter. Though she was not always expected to work to contribute to this ancillary household of the man, a *kimada* was often a business partner. She might live in her partner's rental house and act as a superintendent and rent collector, or run a kiosk or used clothing business for which he had provided the capital. Tina, a single mother in Kiboriloni whose close friend was a *kimada*, explained why *kimadas* were becoming more popular with women and men alike.[45]

> [Is it difficult to marry if you are a *kimada?*] These women don't marry because they don't want to. If you taste the sweetness of being a *nyumba ndogo*, you don't want to marry. [Why not?] It's freedom, a place to stay, and the protection of having a permanent partner all rolled into one. [Is this common?] Here in Kiboriloni, *kimadas* are an open secret. My boss had one next door here. Women who are Muslims, it's easier for them to be installed as a *kimada*. It's not so much a secret for them; they can show they have become a *kimada*. The Christian women hide it because they fear being accused of adultery in church if the wife finds out. [How do they hide it?] The men don't hide it very well. They say, "I'm going to Dar for two days," when really they're coming to Kiboriloni to stay with their *kimada*. [Why do men take a *kimada?*] This is their form of *starehe*, and it satisfies their desire. Also the ones who are wealthy, their financial position makes it possible and somehow necessary for them to have these arrangements. Thus they only pick women who really know sex. [What is the benefit to the woman?] She gets freedom, money, shelter, material support, and clothing. She is not in it because of her own desire, love, or the *tabia* of her partner; it's the money. The money confuses her until she forgets to ask about marriage.

As Tina implied, *kimadas* were not recognized as wives, although as part of the conventions of a *nyumba ndogo*, they might refer to their partners as "husband"—particularly when the two had had children together. *Kimada* relations were also one way in which single mothers could expand sources of support for their families without fear of having to relinquish their children or arrange for them to be fostered. The principal risk that a *kimada* ran was that she had no real security; all her property belonged to the *mume* (man) who had provided it and who could evict her for any reason at any time (see Haram 1995:43–44). Her bargaining chip, especially with Christian men, was to threaten to reveal her existence to her partner's wife. While such a revelation would reflect badly on her, the social consequences could be worse for her partner, depending on his status.

### Forms of Marriage: Kienyeji, "Sealed" and "Unsealed"

In the early 1990s, two "traditional" *(kienyeji)* forms of marriage that were part of the *kihamba* regime continued to be recognized in Chagga communities on the mountain—though many Chagga consider them "backward." These included leviratical unions and elopement/abduction, or bride capture. The cultural rules for bride capture, however, had changed since the early 1900s, when Gutmann stated this kind of union had become exceedingly common. Whereas the "lifting up of the girl" had once required some sort of sanctioning authority (usually that of the *mangi*), women of the past few generations had become the victims of abduction that had no social sanction. Although this practice was not looked upon favorably by the government or the church, many Chagga insisted that the practice was not uncommon, and many informants were personally acquainted with women who had been "taken" in this manner. One young woman explained how in 1992 she had been abducted by a complete stranger while on her way to work; he kept her in his house overnight and declared that she had become his wife. She had no intention of remaining with the man, but her parents recognized the union over her objections and demanded customary payments of beer and livestock as a fine.[46] Among others who spoke about their marriages under these conditions, it was apparent that while traditional marriages gave legitimacy to the abduction of women, it could also serve as a form of elopement in which both parties agreed on what was to take place. Leviratical marriages were rarely spoken about. They were seen as a source of shame to women; an anachronistic and "pagan" *(pagani)* custom that many "civilized" clans would not enforce. In some cases, women who were subject to the exercise of leviratical rights by their affines were concerned about sexual and reproductive

demands placed on them. One widow, for example, tried unsuccess-
fully to obtain birth control from a clinic and later had a child by one
of her husband's brothers.[47]

Two other types of marriage were much more common. These were
referred to as marriages that were "sealed" (-funga) and those that were
not. An unsealed marriage existed between partners who had cohab-
ited and reproduced, and afterward referred to themselves as married
and called each other "husband" and "wife," without an official ceremony to legitimize their union. The case of Devota illustrates the kind
of conditions under which unsealed marriages could emerge.[48] Devota
was twenty-eight years old and was born in the Rombo district in East
Kilimanjaro. Her parents divorced when she was very young, and her
father had raised her. When she was sixteen years old, Devota was
raped by a soldier who was home on leave. She did not report the
assault, and later discovered that she had become pregnant.

> When I discovered that I was pregnant, I realized that I would
> have to stay home. My father was furious, but there was nothing
> I could do. I didn't even understand what sex was, and I certainly
> didn't see that soldier again. He went back to the army, and until
> today we haven't crossed paths. My father drove me from the
> house, and sent me here to Moshi to look for my mother. I went
> to people whom we knew, and asked them to help me beg her
> forgiveness and that she should receive me. She resisted and
> fought, but finally she agreed to take me in. I stayed with her until
> I gave birth to a baby girl in February 1981. I continued to stay
> with my mother and help her with the housework and to raise my
> child. Today my daughter is in standard seven, and she still stays
> with my mother.
>
> In 1984 I met a young man called Thomas. I liked him and he
> liked me. We made love from time to time and eventually, later
> that year, we decided to live together. I informed my mother that
> I'd be living with my lover because I didn't want to "bear at home"
> [kuzalia hapa nyumbani] again. She tried to refuse, but I thought that
> I had better decide myself that I was going to move from her place.
>
> I got pregnant the first time with him and gave birth to a girl in
> 1985. We continued to live happily together, and in 1988 I got a
> second child, a boy. In 1990 I got the third, also a boy. In matters
> about the "marriage," we share things together well. Until today
> we are staying together just fine.
>
> But every time I remind him about a proper wedding, he gets
> angry and says, "What do you lack?" In this I don't understand
> him. If I complain further, he leaves and goes his own way. I asked
> a priest to come and call on him once, but the priest refused and
> said that it was usually better if the man comes to a decision on
> his own.

I do business here in town. I sell out of a little kiosk, and look after things here at home. As for my *tabia*, I've decided to stay with one man. As for him, well, I can't be positive, but I haven't gotten any information that he's got anyone else. Anyway, finally, just the other day Thomas himself asked me to pray for him that even he will someday agree to live inside of his religion [i.e., seal the marriage].

There are three ways of sealing a marriage; to have a government marriage or civil wedding *(ndoa ya serikali)*, a Christian church wedding, or a Muslim wedding. Of these, government marriages had the least status, and it was often implied that they were an easy way out for couples who wanted to give their unions legitimacy. Because neither the Lutheran nor the Catholic church (the two largest denominations in Kilimanjaro) granted divorces, civil weddings were also an option for men and women who had separated permanently from previous spouses married in a Christian ceremony. Christian men who had married in church might also agree to a government marriage with their *kimada* partners, especially if they had had children with them. In line with old formulations, readiness for marriage on the part of men depended in part on markers of a prosperous productive life, including having been given a section of *kihamba* (or, in Moshi, readiness to purchase a plot) and beginning to build a house. Men in their twenties and early thirties seldom were in a hurry to marry. Once they did decide to do so, however, the process could often be completed in a matter of months.

A marriage sealed by a church or in an Islamic ceremony was set apart from all other male-female relationships. Yet entering into marriage had become more problematic for men and women at precisely the time that HIV was beginning to emerge. In Moshi, some women expressed reluctance to marry or were increasingly inclined to dissolve marriages, a phenomenon seen in several places in Africa and linked to women's assertion of more control over their life courses (Bledsoe 1980; Stambach, forthcoming). One twenty-three-year-old unmarried woman likened marriage to sexual slavery.

> [Is getting married important?] It is not so important because men, once they have installed you in their houses, they think "that's that." They've got you. All the time they "sex" you, and marriage is like slavery. Men just make women into slaves around the house. You wake up in the morning, all you hear is: "Hey, you! What's-your-name! Bring my wash water! Bring my food!" Ach. I'd rather stay unmarried than hear "Hey you! Do this and that!" all the time.[49]

For men, entering into marriage had become a difficult prospect, but for those concerned about AIDS, it was one they considered seriously. In the 1990s, people stated that fear of AIDS was beginning to cause men and women to "respect their marriages more," and by 1996 even women who had previously regarded their husbands as hopeless philanderers were quick to acknowledge that the epidemic had brought about changes in their husbands' *tabia*. Men cited a number of obstacles to entering into marriage. The ones most commonly mentioned were an inability to purchase a plot in town, lack of access to land in the village, and the lack of proper housing or of the money to build. Lack of resources for bridewealth, which retained great symbolic if not economic significance, was seldom mentioned as a deterrent.

The meaning of sex within marriage was entirely different from that in any other kind of relationships. In marriage, the erotics of "stylistic" sex (i.e., in various positions) were left behind. Most people stated that *tamaa* was simply not part of marital sexuality. "When you have sex with your wife, ideally, it is for love and for children. It is respectful. With a girlfriend there is a sort of love, but it's more about mutual understanding [-*elewana*], a lot of *tamaa* and a lot of *starehe,* and release. With a wife, *tamaa* doesn't enter into the picture."[50] Positions that unmarried couples used to heighten sexual pleasure and excitement were unthinkable acts to engage in with husband or wife. Several men who went from having *starehe* partners and girlfriends to being married men during the period of fieldwork described a dramatic change in the character of sexual activity after marriage.

Many people felt men and women were delaying marriage more in Kilimanjaro than elsewhere in Tanzania. Certainly this was the case in Moshi. Table 4.2 shows the marital status of 360 men aged fifteen or older, from a 1996 census in Moshi, compared with those from the national sample in the 1994 Tanzania Knowledge, Attitudes, and Prac-

Table 4.2 Marital Status of Men Aged 15+ in Moshi (1996) and Tanzania (1994)

| Marital Status | Moshi[a] | Tanzania[b] |
|---|---|---|
| Never married | 50.0% | 35.0% |
| Currently married | 34.7 | 55.7 |
| Cohabiting | 8.3 | 4.2 |
| Separated/divorced | 2.8 | 2.9 |
| Mean age | 31.4 | 35.3[c] |

[a] Source: author's census, Korongoni Ward, Moshi 1996.
[b] Source: Weinstein et al. (1995:51).
[c] Calculated from 1988 census (Bureau of Statistics 1990).

tices Survey (Weinstein et al. 1995). Many of the differences between the Moshi and national samples can probably be explained by the younger age structure of the urban area. Nevertheless, in demographic terms, the perception that there were fewer married men overall than elsewhere in Tanzania was correct. In Moshi, half of all men aged fifteen or more had ever been married or been in an unsealed cohabiting relationship. At the time of the census, 34.7 percent were currently in some form of sealed union, compared with 55.7 percent of men nationally. Once the decision to marry was acted upon, men did not usually enter into a sealed marriage without transferring some or all of the agreed-upon bridewealth to the families of their spouses. Among married men in Moshi, nearly 90 percent had a sealed marriage in which full or partial payment of bridewealth had already taken place. Only a few (10.7 percent) had yet to begin bridewealth payments. Among all men, the proportions in cohabiting relationships in Moshi were twice those of Tanzania as a whole (8.3 versus 4.2 percent), while the proportion divorced or separated was virtually the same (2.8 in the Moshi sample and 2.9 nationally). Among all men in Moshi, 8.3 percent were in polygynous unions, almost the same proportion as men in Tanzania as a whole (9 percent; Bureau of Statistics 1993:131).

## Two Extended Case Studies

The cases of Helen and Rahman, together with the shorter cases presented above, illustrate the way in which male-female relationships have met the needs and desires of young people in different ways and at different times of life. With varying degrees of importance, sex, desire, the evaluation of moral character, and transactions at once symbolic and material were necessary to these relationships but did not define them. Women and men alike sought sexual pleasure, but the quality of relationships in which sex took place was linked to other considerations such as compatibility, trustworthiness, or the desire to marry. Furthermore, as these extended case studies are meant to show, the meaning of sexuality to young people in Kilimanjaro was not a matter of selecting from a menu of relationships and adopting a set of expectations and behaviors consonant with one's selection. The meaning and salience of both nonreproductive and reproductive sexuality was experienced by actors as part of unfolding life courses, with desire and moral character as part of the broad charter for action and choice.

Over a period of nine years Helen had experienced sex as part of a loving relationship with a man she felt committed to and lucky to get.

Sex was also part of a nonmarital relationship in which she felt both pampered and mentored in almost a fatherly way and a means of satisfying physical desires and *nyege* through casual encounters outside this relationship. Finally, sex in her *kimada* relationship was a means for obtaining stability in her personal life, access to business contacts, protection (so she thought) from HIV infection, assistance with housing and living costs, and a child. Rahman had experienced a similar range of personal meanings with regard to sex, relationships, and desire in the eleven years since he had become sexually active. These cases offer an opportunity to see over time the connections that young people made between their personal projects of becoming adults, their sexuality, and the mutable formal parameters of "types" of male-female relations. In addition, they represent two different trajectories: Helen, who married young, divorced, and had maintained a great deal of independence in her sexual life, and Rahman, whose sexual life was filled with casual liaisons and who moved quickly from a committed relationship to a sealed marriage.

*Helen.* Helen was thirty years old and the firstborn of her father's eleven children.[51] Seven of the children were born to Helen's mother, and the other four to women to whom her father was not married. Two of Helen's siblings now lived in Dar es Salaam; two others lived in Moshi. Her younger sister, Adela, was staying with Helen in a rental house in the Majengo area of Moshi. When Helen finished secondary school she planned on taking up a place at university to study pharmacology. She had fallen in love, however, with the successful brother of a friend, Beko, who convinced her to marry him and travel with him to Finland on a government posting. He promised Helen she could find a place to study while they were abroad. She explained that "at the time I was twenty-one, and he wasn't staying in Tanzania much. He traveled a lot, and we wrote each other. I had other boyfriends, but not the kind you sleep with. If you sleep with them, you call them *mpenzi*, but they were not *mpenzi*. I was a virgin until I was twenty-three years old. Beko wrote me love letters. He was much older and had a lot of money, and I was just overwhelmed by him. He was a professor at the co-operative college and traveled a lot, and that lifestyle really appealed to me. At that time in Tanzania we had a lot of problems with the necessities of life, and when he traveled, Beko brought back loads of stuff like clothes, shoes, money, cloth—things that were really important."

Helen did not succeed in getting into university in Finland, and she and Beko had not yet sealed their marriage. Helen was twenty-five when she and Beko returned from Finland, and when Helen became pregnant, she insisted on sealing the marriage: "We moved back to Moshi and just about that time I got pregnant. I insisted that we get married, so we had a government wedding. We did this so everything would look proper. After all, I wanted to work, we were living together, and I wanted to seal the marriage so that it would be officially known that I am his wife. I didn't want a church wedding because I wasn't sure I wanted to be with him forever—you see he had started to get very nasty. This was because I discovered his secret. He already had a wife and had children with her, but they split up. He tried to hide this all from me."

After Helen discovered his deception, and after she had a miscarriage, her marriage lasted only three months. Beko had begun drinking heavily and became abusive. Helen looked back on her decision to forgo university with regret, seeing it as a lost opportunity to build her capacity for self-reliance: "I should have stayed in school. I had plans for myself, and if I'd finished my degree here at least I would have had some way of depending on myself whether or not he was around. In my family, education is stressed more than marriage, and my family had tried to refuse the marriage because he was taking me away from my studies. They were right. In the end I left him because of his bad *tabia*, and because of my parents. I went to stay with a girlfriend I was working with. I bought a bed and found a room—the one where we're sitting right now. I started all over. I started to depend on myself. For myself, I might want to marry again, but I doubt I'll be able to. The problem is the *tabia* of men. They are all liars in marriage."

Helen started two small businesses in addition to her work in a government office. Soon the sideline businesses were making her rich. She opened a kiosk in the front of her rental house and was one of the first women to go into the used clothing, *mitumba*, trade. Helen was able to buy bales of clothing at a special price through her government connections. As she stated, "I bought them for fifteen thousand shillings and sold them for thirty thousand. I bought five bales at a time, and they were gone in three days. I made three hundred and sixty thousand shillings a month from *mitumba* and eight thousand, two hundred seventy-five on salary!" Once she was able to prosper through her own means, the meaning of both family and male-female relationships in Helen's life changed dramatically. She paid school fees for siblings and cousins, built a house for her parents on *kihamba* land her father allocated her, and felt particular pride in being able to state that "I bought everything myself." Men were there for company, and Helen said that "I had any kind of *starehe* that I wanted": weekends in Nairobi and the company of men when she wanted it.

At this time Helen also began a more formal *mpenzi* relationship with an American man who was in Kilimanjaro with a development project. At first, she stated she was not especially interested. But he showed both good character and his desire to be with her, "because he brought money and gifts and one holiday he brought nice people, nice guests over to visit." Their relationship lasted three years. "That guy helped me a lot. He helped my parents, he paid school fees, and he had a lot of really good ideas and suggestions that helped me develop myself with respect to business and work. He was even going to teach me computer, but time ran out. I loved him like a father, and I was satisfied because I didn't lack anything."

After her American lover, Helen stayed by herself for a long time. She described her life in terms of hard work, exhaustion, and diminished desires. This connection between work and desire will be examined in depth in the next chapter. As Helen put it, "I was by myself for a long time. If I'm by myself, I work a lot and get exhausted. I get tired. I just forget about sex and . . . well, if there isn't anyone nearby I just put it out of my head. It's part of my consciousness [*akili*]. If you are tired, your body relaxes and so your mind relaxes. Plus all the time and bother that's involved [with having a sexual relationship]. I can't have a real boyfriend now because I don't have the time to chase around. Sex is *starehe*. It's like drinking beer. So you have to find a suitable place to do it. Somewhere that fits. I can't do it at home now because my little sister is living here."

Ultimately, Helen entered into a *nyumba ndogo*, or *kimada*, relationship with a banker, Freddy. She also had occasional *starehe* partners on the side and, because she feared AIDS, she always insisted they use condoms. Helen began a *nyumba ndogo* relationship for several reasons. First, she took time to "study" her partner's *tabia* and found him agreeable and a pleasure to be with. She did not agree to sex for the first six months of the relationship. Second, the profits from her *mitumba* business had radically declined after many women in the region began to flock into the trade, flood the market, and compete for business. Helen saw in her *kimada* partner a way of obtaining access to resources and contacts that might start her off in a new business. Third, Helen was very concerned about AIDS. She did not hide the fact that she enjoyed sex and felt that in addition to these other benefits, a stable partner was good protection and did not necessitate the bothersome use of condoms. Last, Helen desired a child but had no interest in re-marrying. As a *kimada*, or *nyumba ndogo*, Helen was aware that her position was tenuous, and she thought for more than a year about her partner's wishes to have a child before consenting. All these reasons were important to Helen; she did not emphasize one over the other.

> What I have now suits me. He started coming here with another girlfriend, but she was sleeping around, so I told him about it. We were together about six months before we started sleeping together. He works at a bank and also advises me about money and business. He also helped me get a loan. He introduced me around, and now I can do a lot of business on my own. He's nice and gentle . . . but his wife! Yaie-yaie-yaie. If we see each other, she hurls abuse at me, "Helen you dog! You barbarian! You took my husband!" I just ignore her—that's how I'm fierce with her.
>
> I'm his *nyumba ndogo*. He trusts me and has certain rights here. We depend on each other. He consults me about things he does at home and at business. He pays everything here: rent, doctor, everything I need and use here in the house—even getting my hair plaited. He wants to marry me and have a child, and I'm seriously thinking about it. I can marry him and still stay here. I'm thinking about it very seriously, mostly because of AIDS. I'm frightened of it. I'd prefer to stay single; I don't want any one's laws over me, but I'm afraid of the temptations of boyfriends. So he wants to have a baby with me, and I think that would be quite OK. I was on the pill from 1987 until last year, but now I want a child because I'm capable of keeping it and caring for it well.

As it turned out, Helen was wise to base her agreement to have a child upon her own ability to care for it. Helen had a daughter, Laura, in 1994. When I returned to Kilimanjaro in 1996, I met Helen and asked how things had proceeded with her relationship. Helen explained that the birth of the child had precipitated a crisis in Freddy's marriage. His wife had come to Helen's house and destroyed furniture and dishes and had threatened both Helen and Laura. Freddy's response was to ignore Helen, and to start to take other extramarital partners more openly. Although he came by to see Helen and Laura from time to time, Helen insisted she was receiving no child support. Helen herself felt this position was not entirely unreasonable because, on the basis of the threats made by Freddy's wife, Helen refused to let Laura spend time with her father at his home.

*Rahman.* Rahman, a man in his late twenties, was driving for a tourist safari company.[52] He married in early 1993 and later that year was eagerly awaiting the birth of his first child. Rahman had been born in

Moshi, at Mawenzi hospital. At the time of his birth, his parents were living on the mountain, although they moved shortly thereafter, as his father was given about one-third of an acre of *kihamba* land to farm. His mother, who was not a Chagga, farmed peanuts and maize on a *shamba* plot near Moshi's huge sugar plantation. His father established a home on that plot and continued to reside on the *kihamba.*

Earlier, while he attended primary school, Rahman went to live with his paternal aunt in Tanga and later boarded at secondary school on the mountain. He began to be sexually active at the age of seventeen. His earliest sexual experiences were with masturbation, but shortly thereafter he slept with girls from his school. When he moved back to Kilimanjaro, he began going to Moshi town with friends on weekends, where they sought out Haya prostitutes on Mafuta Street. "They were in known houses, and they were just sitting outside. You just chose which one you wanted. You paid first, then you went inside, then sex, and then you leave. That's it. You'd just go up to them and say 'Hey, do you have the time?' They say 'yes,' and you just go. It was thirty to fifty shillings for service." Afterward, he and his friends would go to his aunt's house for a meal, spend the night, and then return to the village. These outings took place once or twice a month.

When he was eighteen, Rahman was offered a place in a teacher's training college in another part of Tanzania. Although his father wanted him to pursue his education, Rahman refused. He did not want to be a teacher; he wanted to be a driver. He learned how to drive from a relative, got his license, and found a job driving a tractor on a coffee plantation. During this period, Rahman had *starehe* partners and also had a steady girlfriend who lived near the coffee farm. Despite being with her for more than six months, he referred to her as *"kampani"*: "She was just company, though. We got together because one day when I was working, we were sitting together talking under a tree. She had a nice *tabia;* she was honest and smart. At first we kept it a secret, but then we were found out. We knew each other for a month before we started to sleep together. I was faithful to her, and I was jealous if I saw her talking to anyone else. I didn't get the impression that she wanted to marry me, and we didn't use anything to prevent her from getting pregnant."

Rahman left this job to join his uncle's car-hire firm. Although he was no longer residing in the village, if his routes for his new job passed near the farm, he would make a detour to find his girlfriend. As he began to earn a better living, Rahman met family obligations in a way that was seen as laudatory. Yet he also conducted his personal life in a way that echoed the concerns of those who perceived a threatening randomness in a local sexual culture driven purely by desire.

> I liked the work and it paid well. I drank with the money, and bought clothes and gave five or six thousand shillings a month to my father. I helped my younger sisters with school fees, and the rest of my money went into girls who were basically prostitutes. You'd just meet them and ask if they wanted to go out. You'd go drink, then to a guesthouse, and then you give her a thousand [shillings] in the morning. There were some of these girls I followed even though I knew they were taking other men. I'd do this two or three times a week, and I'd stay with one girl for a few days if I liked her, but as soon as she bothered me, that was it. I only ever bought them food and bottled beer. The desirable ones were either the pretty ones or the ones who knew how to "move their hips during sex." Some of them just lie there like a banana plant, but some—especially the ones who are circumcised—really know sex.[53]
>
> I was typical; there were a lot of guys like me going around. Those who went around like me were the smugglers and the drivers. We had a little gang. There were four of us. We did most things together; if we were in problems we'd lend each other money, or go with each other to the hospital.

Given the character of the sex life Rahman described, it is not surprising that the issue of pregnancy emerged on more than one occasion. Rahman's first child died. The second time one of his partners became pregnant, Rahman felt eager to accept the child, not so much as a father but more to demonstrate his adulthood and to see the living proof of his reproductive power. As he put it in the slang of the day, he wanted to see his "copyright." Rahman's partner, however, obtained an abortion. He felt this was motivated by jealousy on her part, and Rahman became violent toward her for having done it.

> There was another one with my child. Her name was Meredith, but she went and got an abortion when she saw me with another woman. I didn't want her to do it. I was giving her money. Anything she wanted I was ready to provide. I was happy when I found out she was pregnant; not because I liked her—she was an average girl—but because I wanted my copyright in the world. I beat her when I found out about the abortion. Why should she do such a thing? Actually, I think what made her so angry was that I slept with her friend. She was furious.
>
> Those days I wanted a child so that I would have a copy of myself in the world. I would have given that child everything. Everything. I wanted that child because it would have shown that I am a real man and not barren. It's not OK not to bear children. It's a

shame. People might think you can't get it up—that you're not
healthy [*mzima*]. Without a child, how could my family know that
I'm healthy?

As with Helen, there was a period during this stage of Rahman's life
during which he found casual relationships too much of a bother and
marriage out of the question: "I had not planned to marry at all in my
life. As I saw it, marriage was pure problems [*taabu tupu*]. Ladies are
very complicated, you know. I finally got fed up with the whole thing.
After that one got the abortion, I decided on my own that I would just
have one girlfriend. Not to marry, just to have sex—and not to live
together, either." Rahman, however, had not figured on Rehema. He
met Rehema during the course of his work, driving passengers between Shinyanga and Moshi. Rehema was Rahman's "true love." In
recalling their relationship, which lasted three years, Rahman never
expressed concern about using Rehema a means for producing his
copyright. Instead, he seemed focused on her *tabia* and soon determined he wanted to marry her. Rahman struck up a relationship with
Rehema immediately upon their arrival in Moshi.

> She was visiting her sister here in Moshi, and I took her right to
> the door. When I dropped her off, I told her I'd be back to visit
> later. I went back and we talked. We talked and we talked and we
> drank . . . finally she went home.
>
> Next day, same deal. We sat and talked and drank, and she went
> home to sleep. The day after that we slept together. She moved up
> here from Singida. I gave her the money to go back and collect her
> things. She was great. She was circumcised, and I liked everything
> about her. She was well brought up, she was a great cook, she had
> a good reputation and she was well liked. She knew how to get
> along in life, she was smart, she had a great body, and she was a
> Muslim. I would have married her totally, and I will love her until
> the day after tomorrow.

The marriage of true love, however, was not meant to be. Rehema
left Moshi unexpectedly with a man from Dar es Salaam. Although she
continued to write love letters to Rahman, he wanted nothing more to
do with her. Rahman attempted to understand Rehema's motives in
material terms. "She said she went with that Arab because of money.
I don't know. Maybe she had to do it to help her family. I don't know."
His relationship with Rehema, however, put Rahman in mind to marry
and heed his parents indirect warnings about AIDS and their more
direct criticisms of his "promiscuous" conduct. Rahman's parents assisted him with the money for the bridewealth and the wedding. Rah-

man agreed to have his mother participate in the selection of his bride. Together they chose a woman Rahman had known and been sexually involved with for many years, an old schoolmate and the neighbor of relations living in the coastal town of Tanga: "I decided on her because I had known her *tabia* since she was small. She's gentle, and she likes to listen to me when I tell her things. She's not stubborn, she's civilized, and she has good judgment—hey! That's it! I proposed in January. My mother went to Tanga to introduce the idea, and she came back with Safina as my fiancée. I paid a brideprice of small things. There was a *kanzo* for her father, about three thousand shillings, another cloth that was about fifteen hundred, two cows that cost ten thousand each, and later on two bed sheets."

In order to save on expenses, Rahman and Safina were married in a double ceremony with Rahman's cousin and his wife. Safina became pregnant during their first year of marriage. According to Rahman's beliefs, sex in mid-to-late-term pregnancy would have been dangerous for the fetus. Given his previous commitment to an active sex life, I wondered whether the enforced abstinence had prompted Rahman to seek out *starehe* partners. He denied it and emphasized that he was most interested in establishing a small tourism business and in securing the conventional foundations to a sealed marriage: acquiring a plot and building a house: "Although you can't have sex with your wife when she is pregnant, I have totally abandoned the wandering around. It has been easy. I just decided 'That's it. No more.' I was losing money like crazy. It was a total waste. I'm much happier now. It's very nice to be married. I don't look back at all. The money stays around. It's so different from before. Man, I used to get VD twice a year, and I lost lots of money. Now it's much better. I'm also happy now that I'm getting a child. Right now there are four who depend on me: my parents, one of my little sisters, and my wife. My main aim is to get some money together, find a plot, and start building. It's hard though. I really love Safina. What she says I listen to more than anyone else."

### Sexuality as the Cultivation of Embodiment and Personhood: Setting the Stage for Understanding AIDS

From an anthropological perspective, it is not possible to speak of sexual chaos in Tanzanian society in the age of AIDS, local lore notwithstanding. The epidemic cannot be blamed on the notion that people partner and separate purely according to whim and want, or that sex for young people has been amoral. Etiquette, convention, and choice surrounds even *stahere*, which is sex of the most casual and ephemeral kind. To be sure, there are many situations in which choice of partner and power to negotiate issues such as condom use are lacking for women: in cases of rape or among those whose commercial sex work arises primarily out of economic hardship, for example. Understanding such situations is critical for understanding the epidemic, but *starehe* and commercial sex work have never represented the predominant forms of sexuality in Kilimanjaro.

The "transactional nature" of sexual encounters and relationships in Africa is virtually an article of faith in the social demography and social research on AIDS across the continent, an "old saw" in which sexuality and marriage are seen as essentially commercial transactions (Schoepf 1992:355). Researchers point to several features of African life in order to demonstrate this. These include the institution of bridewealth as an enshrined mechanism through which female sexuality is transacted; contemporary relations among young people in which gifts are an expected and sometimes necessary component; and contemporary forms (like the sugar daddy and the *kimada*) that entail substantial financial support to a female partner. My account, however, questions the centrality of transactions conceived in those ways to the majority of male-female intimate and sexual relations. Simply because sex *can* often be transacted does not mean that it *must*. To emphasize so strongly this particular axis of male-female relations in Africa deflects attention from the fact that sex and marriage in the West are also "transacted" and distorts what sex signified to those whose personal lives are recounted here.

In its life as a "sign" in Kilimanjaro, as an experiential, conceptual, and symbolic entity embedded in the process of giving meaning to existence, sex was "never at rest" (Daniel 1984:42). As the cases of Helen and Rahman have shown, this restlessness in the signification of sex and sexuality was a product of the inherent tensions of meaning as persons negotiated desire (in both narrow and broad senses of the term) and character (of both themselves and others) through different categories of relationship. While the exact shape of each sexual relationship was highly contingent, a shared frame of reference remained in operation; sexual actions were defined against a grid of commonly held categories of social persons and the life course. Far from operating in a mode of sexual chaos, young adults made use of recognized forms of long- and short-term association to satisfy various emotional and material needs. Both in- and outside marriage, young people negotiated their own sets of standards and morality using a value system that amalgamated cultural concepts of personhood. The emergent forms of reciprocity involved in these relations can only be seen as "transactional" if this concept is expanded to include the symbolic as well as the material.

What, then, are the general lessons to be drawn from this analysis of contemporary sexual culture? With respect to the larger interaction of population dynamics and culture within which the AIDS epidemic is embedded, we may draw one set of conclusions. With respect to AIDS, and messages that might be used in the design of prevention programs or measuring risk, we may draw another.

To begin with, sex was not an activity that could be characterized as either recreational or "procreational," as either or *ovyo* or "proper." Sexual life in Kilimanjaro concerned much more than these polar objectives. Sex was part of the context in which young people expressed their moral character and desires and evaluated those of others. It was a situation in which to assert independence and in which dependencies and vulnerabilities could be, and often were, exploited. Many of these relationships (not just their sexual aspect) were hidden as much as possible from public view and were discussed only in vague terms. Regardless of type, many of them were also highly unstable by their very nature. It is this instability, perhaps, this sense of "muddling through" with available models, that accounted for confusion or disorder in the sexual worlds of young Tanzanians in Kilimanjaro.

Although we can make some general statements about the intimate emotional character of sexual culture, and about the larger demographic frame of reference in which sexuality was played out, there are few generalizations to be made about its more formal aspects. Historically, the development of one's character could be related to an ideal state of adulthood that culminated in becoming a "complete" person, which, by definition, included marriage and *kihamba* ownership (if not residence). By the 1980s, however, AIDS threw a spotlight on processes of change within sexual and reproductive life that had been in motion for generations. The recognition that accompanied AIDS belied the fact that much of the sexual domain, as practiced by young people themselves, no longer related in a meaningful way to a productive *kihamba* life. The next chapter will examine more closely the economic conditions under which modern sexuality developed, and how epidemiologies of AIDS became intertwined with them.

With respect to the question of AIDS and its prevention, it is clear that an awareness of AIDS existed among young people. As Sharifa and Gloria's cases indicate, this awareness (for some) had begun to affect both their perceptions of partners and their behavior. Furthermore, if we look back over the account so far, it should be emphasized that the international health community and policy-makers must be aware that the behaviors that spread the epidemic are the product of large-scale forces as much as they are of individual choice and character. This may not be comforting to those who harbor the naïve hope that social science will still succeed in identifying key "cultural risk factors" that can be easily addressed and are amenable to conventional health education, which targets individual behavior. When such ideas are seen in the light of how sexual life has been lived and experienced before and during the early years of the epidemic, it should be clear that Sweat and Denison's (1995) call for structural and environmental interventions must accompany any behavioral change campaign.

# CHAPTER 5

## The "Acquired Income Deficiency Syndrome"

> In 1988 the initials SIDA were used by women to stand for:
> Salaire Insuffisant Depuis des Anées ("Insufficient Salary for
> Years"), or Salaire Individuel Difficilement Acquis ("Individual
> Salary Acquired with Difficulty"). In anglophone countries,
> AIDS was the "Acquired Income Deficiency Syndrome."
>
> Schoepf (1992:37)

### Economic Collapse, AIDS, and Adult Personhood

There is no better way to represent the social and epidemiologic realities of AIDS in Kilimanjaro between 1984 and 1993 than to evoke
Treichler's apt phrase of "an epidemic of signification" (Treichler 1987).
In this chapter and the next, which conclude the analysis of the first
decade of AIDS in Kilimanjaro, I chart this process of signification on
the local stage. By the time AIDS arrived in Kilimanjaro social reproduction for Chagga had been undergoing a century-long crisis, a crisis
that simultaneously shaped the cultural and epidemiologic manifestations of the epidemic. Even before the epidemic began, cultural concepts of changing moral character, desire, and sexuality were filtered
through a misplaced nostalgia for the order of the *kihamba* regime.

Paradoxically, the *kihamba* regime itself contained many elements
that contributed to the emergence of demographic and economic conditions of risky sex and disordered domesticity. The sexual values of the
nineteenth century, which appear never to have been associated with
a stable social order, changed even more rapidly in the face of a development process about which Chagga felt increasingly ambivalent. Coffee wealth, education, and the embracing of colonial institutions and
Christianity brought many Chagga prosperity. Yet the demographic
consequences of migration, social mobility, and spousal separation
caused many to call into question the cultural and practical ramifications of development. The production of persons through the ordered,
domestic sexuality of the *kihamba* regime was a thing of the past for
many Chagga in the 1990s. What replaced it was a sense of loosened

control over sexuality, over the terms and conditions under which sex took place, how relationships formed and ended, and the timing of the birth of children.

These concerns could be seen in how people judged one another's moral character and in the way in which people went about the pursuit of their life's desires. From the late 1970s through the mid-1980s the tectonics of forces far beyond their influence brought economic growth to a standstill for many Chagga. Another series of shocks in the late 1980s and 1990s saw a precipitous fall in the standard of living conjoined to a new and devastating disease. During the first decade of the AIDS epidemic, people symbolically linked the disease both to the attenuated process of regional demographic change and to the fact that its arrival and spread entirely coincided with the intensifying effects of economic breakdown.

Thus AIDS should not be seen as a particular problem of African *sexuality*. For the values that inform contemporary sexual morality and practice are themselves partly a reflection of cultural responses to demographic and economic change. As Schoepf (1991b:95) has argued, "The explanation for African [AIDS] lies not in 'African sexuality' but rather in situations of risk produced by intersections of biology, political economy, and culture." To talk about sex was to talk about the performance of personhood. Yet personhood, which was so rooted in the agency of social reproduction, was being continually remade over the course of the twentieth century—largely in relation to the altered material conditions of productive life.

In many East and Central African contexts, the emergence of AIDS was associated in popular thinking with symbols of an imbalanced political economy and development. In Tanzania, the idea of an acquired deficiency of income translated into Kiswahili. The Swahili acronym for AIDS, UKIMWI, was twisted into "UKWIKWI," a disease characterized by excessive weight loss in one's pockets. Other slang names for AIDS such as *skanya*, the name of a weevil that eats bagged maize, or "*dudu*" (bug) played on the resonances between sex, food, money, and insidious misfortune. The *skanya* conjured an image of a hefty and valuable commodity, ready for sale or stored for security, being eaten away from the inside out by a small, seemingly innocuous, but silently persistent pest. Thus it could be quipped that the acronym AIDS stood for "Acquired Income Deficiency Syndrome."

During the years preceding the announcement of Tanzania's first cases of AIDS in 1983, people all over the country saw their standard of living plummet. Between 1979 and 1982, the average retail price index for goods and services used by urban populations had doubled (Cheru 1989:90); five years into the epidemic, workers were earning 65 percent less in real wages than they had made in the mid-1970s, and consumer prices had risen tenfold (Tripp 1989:606). Those at the bottom of the wage scale saw a 20 percent decline in real wages in just the first four years of the 1980s. By the mid-1980s Tanzania, along with other African countries, was suffering from pressures on productive life so severe that the costs of social reproduction, of starting and maintaining a family and contributing to the perpetuation of significant social institutions, simply became unsupportable for much of the population (e.g., Kerner 1988:50; Schoepf 1991b:97). Hardship was everywhere as the epidemic began. Between 1983 and 1986, more than four thousand cases of AIDS had been reported nationally (NACP 1991: Table 3)—a tiny fraction of those infected with HIV.

Although the combination of factors differed from country to country, several other African nations were in similarly dire economic straits. Many of the states that suffered during the "decade of decline" also had severe AIDS epidemics, a fact that prompted some to heap blame for much of Africa's HIV epidemic on the shoulders of the IMF and the World Bank (e.g., Lurie, Hintzen, and Lowe 1995). Worsening conditions of landlessness and urban poverty translated into conditions of deadly risk in the AIDS era and were exacerbated by north-south relations mediated through structural adjustment (Sanders and Sambo 1991:164).[1] In West Africa it was argued that AIDS arose out of a postcolonial legacy of poverty and debt and that Africans conceptually linked the disease to an industry of international development that had benefited only the very rich (Konoky-Ahulu 1989:179). From Sudan and Senegal to southern Africa a burgeoning, poverty-induced mobility of young people accelerated trends toward cultural change that many people associated with the spread of AIDS (Harries 1990; Ahmed and Kheir 1992; Enel and Pison 1992:250, 261). Regardless of informants' moral laments about contemporary sexuality, or the assumptions embedded in conventional demographic and AIDS research representations of young African sexuality, conditions in Moshi and elsewhere did not represent "the sudden break with traditional values that most observers assume" (Larson 1989:725). Rather, they represented a discernible outgrowth of social, demographic, cultural, and political-economic forces unfolding over time.

Some of those who attributed the severity of AIDS to structural adjustment (e.g., Lurie, Hintzen, and Lowe 1995) naively overlooked the role of African states themselves in bringing about conditions of hardship. Yet there is little doubt that north-south macroeconomic relations are connected to economic and social dislocation and drastic cuts in public-sector spending. In this way they have contributed to the conditions for the rapid spread of the epidemic. Schoepf's detailed studies of the effects of economic dislocation and AIDS risk among women in the Democratic Republic of Congo, however, suggest that a critique of political economy on its own is not sufficient for understanding AIDS in Africa. Political economy, she demonstrates, must be situated in closely worked analyses of cultural context and the local institutions that transform economic vulnerability into epidemiologic risk (Schoepf 1988, 1991a, 1991b, 1992; Schoepf et al. 1988).

The calamity of AIDS not only conjoined epidemic disease and economic decline, but it also corresponded to a particular response to this decline: the rise of the informal sector.[2] This response necessitated the dislocation and relocation of millions of women and young people, who made a transition from full-time agricultural production to part- or full-time participation in the exploding informal sector. All the while AIDS was creeping invisibly throughout a disarticulating Tanzanian social body. For young people, this alignment of structural forces proved to be a fatal and paradoxical bit of serendipity. At the moment environmental conditions for youth had reached their worst and many became enrolled in black market *(magendo)* and informal sector activities, HIV arrived. In local consciousness, excesses of desire, an accelerating reallocation of productive energies to the informal economy, and epidemic disease were sealed together in a powerful discourse that vilified youth and the inventive solutions young people were developing in order to survive. The following comments about youth, AIDS, and the devaluation of survival-oriented nonagricultural pursuits were made by the leader of a women's development committee in Mbokomu during a meeting about promoting microenterprises for young people through a revolving loan scheme: "We know how AIDS is caused—it shows the kind of bad moral character [*tabia mbaya*] that the youth have to start leaving aside. But it's hard for them since their work doesn't tire them enough. If they had proper work, like farming, they would be too tired to wander around. Business doesn't tire them enough. Farming, though, would wear them right out."[3]

In the early 1990s, this was commentary of the most usual kind. The image of young businessmen "wandering around" and "causing AIDS" as an example of a pervasive sense of loss of direction was symbolic of local understandings of the epidemic. According to local ideas about "business," those who were responsible for AIDS were shiftless and aimless, while those who succumbed to their charms were often said "to have forgotten themselves" (-jisahau). As women were dislocated from the kihamba zone, they too were tainted by the desires brought by business. An AIDS counselor from the zonal referral hospital emphasized the mobility and role of female agency in the origins of the epidemic in Kilimanjaro: "The people of Moshi are engaged in business . . . nearly the whole region . . . young people, adults . . . they do business and they don't stay in Moshi. They travel around to Kagera, to Dar. . . . This is the way that AIDS was brought to Kilimanjaro. They come home at Christmas. They come home from the border areas with Kenya. During the 1960s and 1970s, the Chaggas did not have much prostitution. It wasn't their tabia, but by the end of the 1970s, many Chagga women were engaged in business and started traveling. They gained influence and became promiscuous through their business contacts. Those women came from Moshi and traveled to Dar, Nairobi, and Mombassa to buy cloth, soap, cooking oil. There were many involved in this trade, this magendo, and even today many of them engage in sex at the Kenyan border in order not to be arrested."[4]

Among those who promulgated these stereotypes there was a cultural consciousness that no single social grouping any longer had authority over the proliferation of productive and reproductive practices, over the trajectory of social reproduction. It is hardly surprising, then, that AIDS should have acquired such strong associations not only as a disease of disordered sexuality and physical desire but also as a pathological manifestation of the course of social development in the region more generally. Throughout human history epidemics have often been blamed on others, on outsiders. To the French, syphilis was the "Neapolitan disease," and to the Italians it was the "French disease" (Becker and Collignon 1999:65); to nineteenth-century Malawians, syphilis was the "Arab disease," blamed on slave traders arriving from the Indian Ocean coast (Chirwa 1999). Epidemics have also been imputed to "others who are also the same" (Frankenberg 1992), that is, disenfranchised or marginal members of affected societies. In this respect, AIDS set no historical precedent (also see Brandt 1987; Chirimuuta and Chirimuuta 1989; Sontag 1989). This chapter describes the context in which the latter type of "inward-looking" censure emerged among Chagga. It also examines how this opprobrium was directed at some of the most vulnerable members of society, how and why this blame deflected attention away from the more complex realities of the epidemic, and how AIDS prevention itself was caught up in these meanings. Chapter 6 shows how epidemiologic narratives tied this "othering" of AIDS and common ways of living in the 1990s to conventional stereotypes of African sexuality and vulnerability and how, in turn, these stereotypes were also employed by Tanzanians in a harsh auto-critique.

The market, the town, and a stereotyped image of youth formed an unholy trinity in the representation of pathogenic social conditions at the onset of the AIDS epidemic. From the perspective of community and religious leaders in Kilimanjaro and from areas of Tanzania where the epidemic had first emerged, the economic mobility required for survival was demonized as the cause of epidemic. AIDS, mobility, commerce, urbanization, and the desires of youth gelled into an image of disordered development.

## The Informal Sector in Kilimanjaro

The economic crisis in Tanzania was precipitated in part by the failure of President Nyerere's *Ujamaa* socialism. The implementation of *Ujamaa* policies in the 1960s and 1970s concentrated enormous power in the hands of a poorly functioning and increasingly corrupt party/state bureaucracy. *Ujamaa* caused great social disruption through the forced resettlement of millions of Tanzanians into planned villages. The leadership also badly overestimated the ability of the peasantry to clear Tanzania's path to development with agricultural productivity through the intensification of the hoe-based farming system (e.g., Kerner 1988:605–6; Cheru 1989:3–7). The inherited colonial economy, which was dependent upon cash crops such as coffee and sisal, proved vulnerable to worsening terms of trade, falling commodity prices, and the oil price hikes of the 1970s embargo. The 1978 war to topple Idi Amin from the rulership of Uganda was another huge financial drain on government resources. Conditions for the Tanzanian citizenry were worsened further still by coercive aspects of emergency economic policies (Campbell and Stein 1992) and the country's participation in programs of structural adjustment that were negotiated with the International Monetary Fund (IMF) in the mid-1980s (Shivji 1992; Bagachwa and Naho 1995).

These conditions led to the swift expansion of Tanzania's so-called second economy (Luvanga 1996). Women and youth from all over Tanzania who had not previously engaged in trade began to move more frequently between rural homes, towns, and markets, hawking everything from roasted peanuts and cassava to smuggled soap. Those with capital started projects *(miradi)* such as home poultry keeping and urban dairy farming, while many wage-earning men in the government bureaucracy spent less than half their days at their offices, using the workdays to pursue other survival-oriented activities such as running their vehicles as illegal taxis. As the epidemic worsened, productive life moved still further away from local clan and lineage-based authority structures. Between 1980 and 1990, the informal economy became a major source of livelihood, income, and employment for the majority of Tanzanian households (International Labour Organisation [ILO] 1992; Luvanga 1996:1393). While 300,000 new job seekers entered the work force annually, the creation of wage employment in the mid-1980s was on the order of 30,000 positions a year; by 1989 only 9,500 positions were added (ILO 1992:16). By 1991, Tanzania's informal sector resembled that in several other African countries. Across the continent, it was estimated that the informal sector accounted for between 20 and 60 percent of urban work forces and approximately 20 percent of GDP (ILO 1992:1). Tanzania's national Labor Force Survey showed that informal sector activities accounted for 22 percent of the entire work force and nearly a third of GDP (Kerner 1988:2). The early explosion of the informal sector allowed some to make a great deal of money. Eventually, however, the markets became crowded with hawkers and, as happened in the former Zaire years before, economic involution set in (Schoepf 1992:360).

For Chagga, the upheaval of the 1970s and 1980s was the latest (and perhaps harshest) installment in a process of economic and domestic dislocation that had been under way for some time. The coincidence of the onset of AIDS and economic collapse branded the early years of the epidemic with the stinging reminders of male absenteeism from family and productive networks, and the growing need for female self-reliance in home lineage areas on the mountain. The consequences of gender imbalances in the population structures of rural communities exaggerated the effects of the sexual division of labor and heightened the paradoxes of AIDS and its association with disruption of the productive lives of reproductive adults (Table 5.1). This can be seen clearly when examining the sex structure of the working population of Moshi Rural District (where Mbokomu is located) by occupational category (Table 5.2). As the table shows, agricultural work was the predominant activity for both sexes, and unemployment was a serious problem for both men and women (about a quarter of the total population). Although roughly equal proportions of male and female rural residents were engaged in agricultural work (41.5 percent of men and 52.5 percent of women) or unemployed (23.5 percent and 30.9 percent),

Table 5.1 Comparison of Age and Sex Structures of an Urban (Njoro) and Rural (Mbokomu) Ward, 1988 (in percentages)

| Age Group | Njoro | | Mbokomu | | Difference | |
|---|---|---|---|---|---|---|
| | Men | Women | Men | Women | Njoro | Mbokomu |
| 15–24 | 52.0 | 48.0 | 46.4 | 53.6 | 4.1 | −7.1 |
| 25–34 | 59.0 | 41.0 | 40.6 | 59.4 | 18.0 | −18.7 |
| 35–44 | 60.9 | 39.1 | 44.3 | 55.7 | 21.8 | −11.5 |
| 45–54 | 65.0 | 35.0 | 44.0 | 56.0 | 29.9 | −12.0 |
| 55–64 | 66.0 | 34.0 | 50.3 | 49.7 | 32.1 | 0.6 |

Source: 1988 census (Bureau of Statistics 1990:289, 310).

Table 5.2 Main Occupational Categories of Moshi Rural and Urban Residents, 15–59, by Sex, 1988 (in percentages)

| Male[a] | | Female[b] | |
|---|---|---|---|
| Moshi Rural | | | |
| Agriculture | 41.5 | Agriculture | 52.5 |
| Business, commercial | 23.9 | Unemployed | 30.9 |
| Unemployed | 23.5 | Business, commercial | 8.2 |
| Skilled labor | 8.2 | Skilled labor | 4.8 |
| Other | 2.9 | Other | 3.9 |
| Moshi Urban | | | |
| Business, commercial | 43.0 | Unemployed | 34,4 |
| Unemployed | 26.7 | Business, commercial | 24.7 |
| Skilled labor | 16.6 | Agriculture | 23.9 |
| Agriculture | 8,8 | Skilled labor | 15.7 |
| Other | 5.1 | Other | 1.3 |

Source: Author's calculations based on 1988 census (Bureau of Statistics 1998:167–68, 178).
[a] Total male population aged 15–59 = 66,002 (rural), 34,791 (urban).
[b] Total female population aged 15–59 = 85,555 (rural), 28,033 (urban).

the predominance of women in the population meant that nearly two-thirds of the people in each category were female. On the other hand, among service providers, shop workers, and petty traders the situation was reversed. This sector was dominated by casual laborers and petty traders for both sexes and represented a great number of underemployed people of both sexes. It was also clearly the province of men. It was these petty traders for whom special scorn was reserved in Chagga moral demographics and local epidemiologies of AIDS.

AIDS began to bring out latent cultural associations between sexual pathology, mobility, towns, and trade. Through the 1980s, the sexual division of labor appears to have remained stable and did not vary by urban or rural residence. Nearly identical proportions of men and women were at work within each occupational category, regardless of where they lived.[5] The demographic basis of the stereotypes of entrenched young male dislocation and growing disruption of female life courses was rooted in the cross-cutting axes of age, gender, and location. In examining these figures, one must keep in mind that many people derived their livelihoods from more than one economic activity.[6]

In Moshi Rural District, the modal occupation of men was farming (41.5 percent). For every farmer there was a businessman or an unemployed youth (most of whom may be assumed to have been engaged in small business).[7] Yet less than a fourth of male farmers were under thirty years of age, while two-thirds of all petty traders and 86 percent of the unemployed were under thirty. This meant that young businessmen and their ilk outnumbered young farmers by nearly five to one, even though 40 percent of all men were engaged in agriculture. In Moshi Urban District, business and commerce workers (including tradesmen) and the unemployed accounted for more than two-thirds of male residents. In town, three-quarters of the small-scale traders and unemployed were under thirty, while only 15 percent of young men were engaged in the more "fixed" occupations (including skilled workers and shopkeepers).

For women, half of those residing in rural areas were engaged in agriculture, with another 30 percent unemployed. Fewer than 10 percent of women stated that they were engaged in commerce or business. In Moshi Urban, a third of women stated they were unemployed, while roughly half of all women were involved in either business or farming. Again, if we examine younger women relative to their elders, 80 percent of small traders and the unemployed were under thirty, while only 30 percent of farmers were of this age. The differences for young women were less marked. Although roughly 80 percent of the female petty traders and unemployed women were under thirty, younger women also predominated (61.7 percent) among those who were working as professionals, in offices, or in farming. These regional conditions varied somewhat from the national pattern. Although, as in Kilimanjaro, men predominated in the informal sector, two-thirds of them were over thirty years of age (von Troil 1992:13, 15). Thus in Kilimanjaro, younger men seemed especially susceptible to incorporation into the informal sector, thereby acquiring their "income deficiency."

## "Getting AIDS Is Like Breaking Your Shaft in the *Shamba*"
### (*Kupata Ukimwi Ni Kuvunja Mpini Shambani*)

From the foregoing discussion, it is not difficult to understand how urban and commercial space could become central to the cultural signification of AIDS in Kilimanjaro. The city and the market were closely associated with the harbingers of a new disease—small businessmen and women who epitomized "bad *tabia*" and "excessive *tamaa*." In these locations, young people operated in sociogeographic networks situated at the flashpoint of epidemic disease, demographic trajectories, and wider economic forces that determined their overall well-being. The movement of successive cohorts of young men and women off the mountain and into nonagricultural activities and urban spaces meant more than a relocation of young people; it fostered forms of young adulthood and sexuality that appeared to be entirely new, yet that played on familiar themes.

### *Town*

In the early 1980s urbanity was not only emerging as pathogenic of AIDS, it was officially scorned as economically subversive. The rising number of petty traders and business people in cities and towns was initially met with a coercive and derogatory response from the state. People in urban areas who did not have obvious formal sector employment were treated as virtual traitors to the cause of peasant-led agrarian development; many were forcibly removed to rural locations, where they were exhorted to take up their hoes. The change in status from rural peasant to urban trader symbolized not only a shift in economic mobility, but it was construed by the government as a betrayal of the Tanzanian socialist project (Kerner 1988:44). While making the move to urban life was not without its risks and costs (von Troil 1992), people flocked to towns such as Moshi, Arusha, and Dar es Salaam, moving the sense of control over sexual relations and young adulthood further and further away from the spheres of cross-generational and clan-based influence. For many young people with no secure or steady work in northern Kilimanjaro, city life meant using Moshi as a base from which they operated small business, trade and other activities in the informal sector. In some ways, theirs was more an urban-based existence than an urban existence per se.

In the early 1990s, the day-to-day atmosphere of Moshi's main streets bore witness to the jumbled experience of the thousands who sought subsistence in petty trade. Women and men three rows deep lined the dirt margins between the storefronts and the roadways, selling produce and imported commodities such as foam rubber thongs, soap, and toothpaste. The air was filled with the chatter of treadle-powered sewing machines and the clang of anvils as tailors and cobblers worked along the crumbling concrete sidewalks. In dusty side streets, *fundis* fashioned rubber bushings for auto and truck suspensions out of used tires, stringing them from trees like ornaments, while others scavenged copper wire from car motors or stolen lengths of electrical and telephone cable. Kiosks and *mbege* bars abounded. Many women operated unlicensed eating establishments out of their courtyards. Around the bus stand young men sat disconsolately on their empty pull carts waiting for the long-haul buses or lorries to arrive in town, and the chance to ferry a load for a few hundred shillings. Children walked along the bus platforms hawking biscuits, gum, cigarettes, candy, plastic toys and bangles, watches, peanuts, fruit, and boiled eggs.

In the evenings as the day's bustle faded away, women continued to serve food in their courtyards or in front of their houses, and as it grew dark, Zairean pop music blared from broken speakers. In Somalitown, where many Muslims resided, a few restaurants served meals, sodas, and tea late into the night. Along comparatively quiet streets, groups of friends would gather in front of houses, sitting on woven mats, drinking tea and soda, chewing *miraa*, and talking.[8] Young people moved around the streets in twos and threes, paying social calls on one another, trying to ferret out who was visiting whom, sharing new cassettes, or investigating which house had a good video on and a supply of soda and *miraa*. In the uptown bars, videos played on TV sets suspended from the ceilings in metal cages while women in threadbare dresses and beer-stained *khanga* cloths served *mbege* ladled into large plastic cups. Some settled in for a *kitochi* (literally "small flashlight') of *mbege* and a small plate of roast meat, while others made the rounds in search of friends, business, conversation, or company.

Such huge geographic-economic shifts from an agricultural life entailed changes in the organization of domestic life and so subverted the vestiges of ideal *kihamba*-regime forms. What Manderson (1996:96) called, in another context, "the pathogenic city" acquired new power as a landscape in which "geographic, spatial, and subjective" meanings connected to youth and AIDS were struggled over. During the first decade of the epidemic, the organization of domesticity in town symbolically subverted (if not perverted) valorized forms of productive and reproductive action. For example, the area of Moshi around the central market was characterized by a mix of businesses, single-family dwellings, and rental accommodation, *nyumba za kupanga*. The organization of these rental properties and the social conventions to which their inhabitants subscribed were emblematic of the relocation of young people away from kinship networks, permanent residential units, and social relations of the *kihamba* zone. Many young families had little choice but to rent a room in one of these houses if husbands or partners had not been given land or if their land was too far away from Moshi to make commuting practical. These dwellings also served as home base for young businessmen and -women who were often on the road several days each week, sleeping at guest houses or the homes of relatives or friends if they were unable to return to Moshi from their places of business. Young men often called their single rooms in *nyumba za kupanga* by the term *"geto"* (i.e., ghetto), a term that evoked their economic precariousness and social marginality.

In the 1990s, *geto*s were a feature of the village as well as the city and were seen as the locations in which unmarried young men living in close proximity to one another would talk incessantly about sex and encourage one another in sexual conquests. Young women avoided being seen going to a *geto*, for, as one friend said, "once she's entered, poor thing, she's already agreed." Yet young men have long resided together in Kilimanjaro. The building of *matengo* (singular: *tengo*, the older name for *geto* and one without ironic overtones) was an integral part of the life course, an intermediate station for young men on the way to occupying a house and *kihamba* of their own. *Matengo* were constructed by young men after initiation, and several age mates might reside there together, signifying their achieved adult status in the ordered *kihamba* world. Even after marriage, a man might decide to sleep in a *tengo*. The reassessment of the traditional form of the *tengo*, its acquisition of the pejorative nickname "ghetto," and its association with heightened sexual desire among young men show how the relocation of desire was associated with some common social conditions of youth.

For many *geto* dwellers such as Jackson, a seventeen year old who operated a shoeshine stand, living conditions could hardly be said to reflect the stereotype of the young man's *geto* as a den of iniquity. The child of Chagga parents, Jackson grew up in Arusha and left home after quarreling with his family. He had been unable to find work near his natal home and had moved to Mbokomu in order to participate in the large regional market of Kiboriloni. Jackson's *geto* was nearby the market and was nothing more than a hovel. "We sleep on gunny-sacks spread on the ground, and cover ourselves with more gunny-sacks. That's it. No mattress, no bed, no blanket," he explained. "We are like orphans looking for sustenance in the street. You know what we are called? *Wasoto*. That means our life is just to survive."[9]

Jonas and Lewis lived in rental accommodation in Dar es Salaam Street, in the center of Moshi. They were both engaged in small business work and eked out a living in the small pull-cart market. The social and demographic conditions in which these young men found themselves were precisely those that epitomized the characterization of risk and AIDS as an outgrowth of young adult lifestyles in popular representations of the disease such as "Hey, Listen!" In 1993, Jonas was eighteen years old and trying to make a living with his pull cart. After finishing schooling, Jonas began small business activities with his friends in a rural part of the Kilimanjaro. At first he sold roasted peanuts. Carrying a large, broad basket filled with nuts, he walked the streets of Moshi day after day selling bottle caps full of peanuts for TSh 10 each (about four cents). The income, however, was already enough to enable him to live on his own in a rental house. Then Jonas moved into the *magendo* border trade, which involved illegal activities such as smuggling beer into Tanzania from Kenya. At the time he was making about TSh 10,000 per week. After almost a year of these activities, Jonas was caught by customs officials. "You're closed down after something like that," he explained. Existence became much more difficult for Jonas after he was apprehended. He was still able to live with his friends in their rental house in Moshi, but barely managed to cover his rent out of the pull-cart work in which they were all employed. In our interview, Jonas reflected both about his present circumstances and what he hoped for and desired.

> I don't want to marry yet; girls here are only interested in satisfying *tamaa*. You take them to a guest house and waste your money. Still, I take girlfriends from time to time. [And condoms . . . ?] I don't like condoms and I don't use them. If you are nervous about a girl, you don't go with her. [So what do you do about *starehe?*] All these difficulties in life exhaust me, but when I let loose a bit, it refreshes me. Mostly, though I am always looking for something that can bring me a little more money.
>
> [What kind of woman would you like to marry?] I would marry a woman from any ethnic group, but she would have to be a virgin. Education is not important. Here in Tanzania now we follow *tabia*; it is foolish to chase after beauty. You have to watch out now, even if you are taking her just for company. You have to ask how her

*tabia* is. Now, these days, there are lots of diseases. If she's no good, you'll see it in her face, or what she wants. Expensive clothing shows bad character. These clothes cost a lot of money. The ones that want clothes that cost ten thousand shillings, well that's simply inhuman. [So you have no one at the moment?] Well, actually, there is someone. She is at home. When I go to visit my mother every four months or so, I also see her. I avoid the women in town here. They are loose; they like men too much. She has to have good *tabia* and to know that you have to stay with her a little while and study her.[10]

Lewis was eighteen years old and lived in a room in a rental house in the center of Moshi. As we spoke, he was stripping wire from engine coils, thick electric cables, and the steel belts from the insides of tires to sell as scrap. Lewis was the firstborn of four children of his father's second wife. The first wife had no children, so Lewis was given her to raise. Although Lewis's father had died more than ten years earlier, Lewis had not been permitted to inherit his part of the six-acre *kihamba* in Machame, where he was born and raised. His school fees were paid by his mother, although there was no way for him to continue beyond primary school. Lewis did not stay on the *kihamba* because his mother insisted that he learn a trade. After finishing primary school, he began a small business, selling food items out of a kiosk. Lewis would ride the bus to Moshi, purchase coconuts, tomatoes, and onions and then transport them back home for resale out of his shack. This business was profitable enough for him to begin building on the *kihamba,* even though he had not yet officially been given a section on which to farm. Lewis's mother had promised to designate his portion later that year because he was planning on marrying. Meanwhile, she had arranged an apprenticeship for him with an auto mechanic. Such apprenticeship arrangements were common and could be extremely exploitative. Apprentices were often paid half salary or less and might even be charged for learning from practicing mechanics or for "breakage" of materials used in their training. Apprenticeships frequently ended the way that Lewis's did—he was driven away after demanding two months pay that was owed him. Afterward he participated in the scrap metal trade, where I met him scavenging for copper.

[When did you come to Moshi?] When I was studying at Moshi Technical. I still lived at home, but I moved to town when my mother could no longer afford to send me to school. I came here to look for work. At first I stayed on Dar es Salaam Street with my uncle, but I didn't like it there because we didn't get along. I stayed

there four months, then moved out into a ghetto. That's where I
am now.

[You said you were planning to marry. Who is your fiancée?]
Her name is Mary, and she works at Coffee Curing.

[How long have you been together?] We are together now more
than a year. [What do you like about her?] I love her because she
has such good character. She is respectful and gentle. With Mary,
I depend on being able to exchange ideas with her about our future
life together. Because we've already decided to marry, we have to
think about the future. Right now our biggest plan is to build. We
are hoping that the proceeds from our farming will give us a start.
[Do you ever think of going out with anyone else?] I don't want
anyone else. After all, these days you have got to think, "Do I want
to live for a long time or a short time?" The surprising thing is that
so many people haven't changed. Doing this "wandering around"
is something that young people imitate from one another. They
get this part of their character from having so much desire.[11]

## Markets

Whereas the association of town with *tamaa* was a product of colonial
and postcolonial experience, local disposition toward the market was
more complex. The productive energies expended by women in the
market have long reverberated with subversive reproductive potentialities, and markets challenged male surveillance and the control over
female mobility that was implied in the patriarchal relations and closeness of the *kihamba*.[12] In these markets, which are among the oldest in
East Africa (Koponen 1988), women developed independent forms of
social organization and techniques of self-policing; markets also served
as a safety net in times of extreme need and as a source for personal
accumulation of money through diligence and entrepreneurship.[13] As
contested loci of control over women's work and mobility, markets
produced enduring tensions that became reinvigorated as the numbers
of petty traders grew during the 1980s.

The association of markets with female agency seems always to have
threatened aspects of Chagga patriarchy and patriliny epitomized by
the *kihamba*. In the nineteenth century, markets that supplied caravans
offered women the chance to have casual relations, if they so desired,
with men who would not stay long enough to raise suspicions.[14] A
widowed woman who had not been remarried into a leviratical union
might seek to become pregnant as a way of acquiring exclusive control over a child. The woman might suppress inquiry into the identity
of the child's father by stating that "it was a blessing brought to me

from the market" (Gutmann 1926:196).[15] Indeed, the markets were so strongly marked as female space that even uninitiated boys who were not yet fully incorporated into gender hierarchies were discouraged from going there. Male initiation lessons reinforced the idea that the market provided women with a tool for subverting men; they included frequent reminders specifically not to divulge secrets there (Fosbrooke 1952:101). The enduring alternative formulation of reproductive capacity suggested by the productive space of the market was also inscribed in sexuality and in the physical bodies of women. In the 1990s in Mbokomu it was said that one remedy for infertility was for a couple to have sexual intercourse in the market at night. In addition, *dawa*[16] made from the flesh excised during the initiation of a woman was thought to bring good business in the market.[17]

In the 1990s, conflicts between men and women over going to marketplaces were a common source of antagonism and domestic violence. These battles were usually prompted by the distrust and jealousy *(wivu)* of husbands and played upon their fears of losing control over the productive and reproductive mobility of women (see Silberschmidt 1992). In at least two cases recorded from 1991–92, men attempted to disfigure their wives in order to assert their dominance and dissuade potential seducers.[18] In his analysis of the association of AIDS with female mobility and commercial activities (including sex work) among Haya, Weiss observes that in "a patrifocal culture, the mobility of women is essential to social reproduction. Marriage is constituted by women's movement between the focal sites of agnatically held households. Moreover, this mobility is not simply women being moved by men. . . . Rather, there is coordinated control of the complementary relation between women's mobility and men's fixity" (1993:32). In Kilimanjaro, the market and the female society that flourished there did so within a context that retained such cultural values, even as the social conditions and interdependent hierarchies surrounding marriage had completely changed since the days of the *kihamba* regime.

One friend recalled her parents' marital conflict and the role that the market played in it: "I look at my parent's marriage. They are miserable. . . . Since 1976 my parents have lived separately. Because they are Catholic, they are not allowed to break the marriage, but they would if they could. All they do is fight. They have a case coming to court soon, in fact. They never loved each other, and they were fighting every day. . . . All of their fighting started because he didn't want her to leave the house at all. He didn't want her to go to the market. He thought men would start to look at her—desire her *(-mtamaani)*. It was necessary, though, for my mother to rely on herself. She did this partly through going to the market anyway and partly through her children who now provide her with what she needs."[19]

The market to which the woman referred is located at Kiboriloni, and in the early 1990s, it had become the largest weekly market in Kilimanjaro region. Kiboriloni, a ward of Moshi town with a population of about 4,500, lies just off the Moshi–Dar es Salaam road. Twice a week the area flooded with buyers and sellers of used clothing, printed cloth, foodstuffs, and numerous commodities and tools. On two additional days the market was open for the sale of used clothing, or *mitumba*. Kiboriloni was once located high on the mountain and moved to its present location in the 1940s—a history of place that mirrors that of the people who trade there. The market was one stop on a weekly circuit that took both men and women through the year. On market days, the trade sprawled along the roads and wound its way behind a cluster of butcher shops, bars, guest houses, stores, and private residences to a large open area that was once sufficient to contain it. The transience of Kiboriloni market was uniquely captured by the words on the bright yellow plastic bags that were sometimes sold there. The bags, which advertised the duty-free services at a European airport, were printed with the slogan "Buy and Fly." In the late 1980s and early 1990s, the weekly cycle for many men and women in the informal sector started with crossing into Kenya in order to smuggle cooking oil, soap, cosmetics, and molded plastic dishes and shoes back across the border. Some men traveled from Moshi to Dar to sell bananas, buy used clothes, and then return to sell the clothes. Women were heavily involved in the used clothing trade, as well as in the sale of *khanga* and *vitenge* (singular: *kitenge*, a printed cloth usually sold in two pieces and worn by women), which they obtained from Tanga, Arusha, Kenya, Dar es Salaam, or local wholesalers. Others, both men and women, were selling locally made tin lamps, rope, spices, as well as bananas, maize, millet, meat, and other staple foods. The whole market was ringed by small restaurants, bars, butcher shops, and guest houses.

The cultural ambivalence toward markets figured in local consciousness about AIDS in a number of ways. Most important, the market represented a near inversion of idealized forms of social reproduction: the inculcation of good *tabia*, the direction of sexuality toward reproduction, and the channeling of desire into valorized productive pursuits. One young man who lived in Kiboriloni, a civil servant in his early twenties who claimed to be a devout Lutheran, seemed to cling to what he called "the Christian life" like a shield against the temptations of the market.

> [Does Kiboriloni have a bad reputation?] It has a good reputation for business. But its bad reputation is as a place of depravity [*uhuni*]. There are drunks, dope smokers, moonshine makers—it's a hub for all kinds of dirty things. But any place with a lot of money floating around will be like this. Any place where there are a lot of people mixing from all over—where people stay who come from various ethnic groups you get all this. It's the money that causes the *uhuni*. I could just take a girl aside and start drinking with her, spending money. . . .[20]

Town and the markets were spatial idioms for the new disease that must be seen not just in terms of "upward" social mobility and a taste for new lifestyles and things but also in terms of the trends in social reproduction and geographic mobility at the historical moment during which the epidemic began. These trends were largely, though not exclusively, stamped with the discursive mark of the declining authority of Chagga manhood and the precocity of young Chagga women. The interpretations given to the perceived shifts in the social distribution and contexts of fertility illustrate how the complexities of demographic process have been simplified in popular consciousness and enrolled in a cultural critique of youth and gender.

### Spatial Idioms for Sex and a New Disease

The language surrounding sexuality among young people in the 1990s reflected the jumbled experiences of Tanzanians as they cobbled together their adult lives in the morally contested spaces of town and market. City streets and marketplaces such as Kiboriloni enriched the street talk about sex among young people. Young men increasingly learned about sexuality through their day-to-day experiences in cities, schools, factories, or the marketplace. Girls, meanwhile, were learning about sex through a combination of personal experience and an apprenticeship system in which their instructors tended to be older female schoolmates who emphasized sexual technique rather than marital responsibility, as their aunts once did. In this atmosphere, many modern institutions such as schools that once held the promise of aiding Chagga in reconfiguring social reproduction seemed to fall into disrepute. One married woman from Mbokomu told how young girls learn about sex: "Today, the girls are taught how to 'play the hips.'

The boys love it, but if you do it in the village, they will call you a prostitute. Now girls teach it to each other at school. When they learn it, the 'teacher' stands behind the girl who is learning and moves her hips for her. Then they switch, until the girl who is learning gets the hang of it. They call it 'going to class.'"[21]

Among young men in Moshi and the rural wards of Mbokomu, the wordplay used to discuss women, sex, and relationships drew on technology, the city, and market life—much of it incorporating English cognates. The aesthetics of this slang were a hodge-podge of images. In addition to using English words for sexual relationships such as "boyfriend" and "girlfriend" (often in preference to the Kiswahili *rafiki*), young people made the noun "sex" into a verb--*sexi*.[22] Common words for orgasm were the English words "trip" and "piss."[23] Should a young man notice a companion turn his head to look at a woman, he might say, "You've got a neck like a fan and eyes like light bulbs," mixing Kiswahili and English.[24] Some men explicitly evoked the marketplace when discussing the transactional aspects of sex: taking a man's semen was said to be "a woman's part of the bargain." In this context, using a condom was "like getting cheated since the man spends his money to create the atmosphere in which a sexual encounter can occur."[25] A taxi driver described a sexy woman by saying that she must have "legs like beer bottles"; "legs like soda bottles," he thought, were too thin. A common euphemism for vagina was "machine," and *kusaga* (literally "to grind") described sexual intercourse. The taxi driver also conjured up conceptual linkages between desire, money, and sex when he said that, "if you don't please a woman sexually, she'll insult you: 'What kind of man is this?! He's free! I didn't spend a thing! He's not worth anything.'"[26]

Euphemisms for AIDS, STDs, and condoms were also technologized and commodified. AIDS was called *umeme* (electricity), and genital herpes was called by the name of the soft drink "7-Up" (because the lesions disappear after a seven days; "it's up"). Condoms were likened to bullet-proof vests or referred to by the trade name of a puncture-preventing sealant for motor vehicle tires, Oko. "Use Oko!" went the radio ad, "Don't get a puncture!" The metaphorical use of this advertising jargon was straightforward: use a condom, and don't get AIDS. What was significant in this case was that the part of the popular imagination that seized upon such fragments of text and turned them into widely used street talk fixed upon a product that signified both mobility and risk. Yet behind all these ironies and inversions of meaning lay a shadowy conceptual link between productive and sexual action.

AIDS was a disorder that could disrupt the connection to a vestigial way of life with seeming caprice; "Getting AIDS," went a wry double-entendre, "is like breaking your shaft in the *shamba*." The *shamba* (field) in this case is no longer that space where the productive labors of men and women give material sustenance, but the metaphorical "field of love" in which desire was sown and deadly disease harvested.

The wordplay involved in likening AIDS to breaking the shaft of one's hoe, to a puncture, or to an accident at work (as another saying went) placed contradiction at the center of popular understandings of the causes of the disease. AIDS was simultaneously a category of random misfortune (a puncture) and the outcome of one's choice of "*shamba*," what "work" one chose to perform there, and what "techno-logical prevention measures" one took when "on the road." In Haiti, as Farmer (1992) has shown, several explanatory frameworks about the causes of AIDS co-existed. In popular consciousness, they were linked by the idiom of AIDS having been "sent" as either a part of a First World conspiracy against the Haitian peasantry or as a form of sorcery in the struggles of Haitian against Haitian in the context of the crushing poverty of village life. In Kilimanjaro and elsewhere in Africa, how-ever, no such linking idiom existed. In Rakai, Uganda (once seen as the epicenter of Africa's AIDS epidemic), as in Moshi, few informants were troubled by the sense that AIDS was both a matter of misfortune and a matter of personal culpability. AIDS was related simultaneously to the idea of a new and deadly pathogen and to themes of jealousy, ill fortune, personal culpability, and witchcraft (Barnett and Blaikie 1992:43).

### "AIDS Is an Accident at Work" (*Ukimwi Ni Ajali Kazini*)

The concepts of *tabia* and *tamaa* and their power in mediating interper-sonal relationships were not confined to the judgment of actions in the context of male-female seductions, flirtations, or sexual relations. *Tabia* and *tamaa* were concepts that explicitly reflected the interconnections between personal resources, production, and reproduction, between energy, work, and sex. As one young pull-cart operator said, "I am working hard, and so I don't really think about *tamaa*. Work tires you out. If it tires you out, you can't have *tamaa*. You also can't have *tamaa* if you don't have any work—you can't have *tamaa* until you have some money. What I desire now is my nice house, my nice car, my TV satel-lite dish. And I want a wife. I still really want these things, but I have no idea if I will ever get them."[27]

Good work was the satisfaction of desire. The salubrious effects of good work on the person were thought be protective against the temptations of excessive *tamaa*. Work was an activity that not only provided the means of survival, but it also built good character by requiring the maximum expenditure of physical and mental energy in the most historically valorized mode of production. In answer to questions about how "good work" is related to intelligence, a truck driver from Old Moshi explained that an individual uses an in-born faculty of intelligence to discern the moral value inherent in certain forms of labor—such as farming: "When someone is born, he is born with a certain intelligence in the brain. Whether or not someone goes to school—whether or not they study—that intelligence can take them far. We say this is *akili*. Your *tabia* comes partly from your *akili*. A child learns—sees various things—someone farming, for example. If a child sees that and comprehends the significance of farming, that's *akili*. *Akili* is how the brain works to understand the importance of work that is done with the hands—work that brings the necessities of life to the one who performs it."[28]

The notion that an activity such as farming would bring about an appropriate state of exhaustion in young men was based only partly on the idea that such work would literally make them too tired to engage in risky actions. At a deeper level, a state of tiredness or exhaustion (*-choka*) from good work implied that both the body and the mind had been exercised in approved forms of labor requiring intelligence and strength. The exhaustion engendered by good work brought "the necessities of life," and to be tired in this way was to have expended one's energy on the kinds of activities that built good *tabia*. The tiredness of good work also implied a moral commitment to the spatiality of preferred forms of productive and reproductive social relations, as men would be too tired to "wander around." Not all forms of exhaustion were protective; only tiredness arising from good work left an individual with no excesses of *tamaa*. During an AIDS education speech to secondary school girls (many of whom were in their late teens or early twenties and presumably sexually active), the presenter stated that a vigorous sex life (implied by the use of modern contraception) would result in a state of exhaustion that would destroy the capacity of the girls for the "proper" labors of school work: "Pills—leave them! You can destroy your ability to have children. The injection, and the rest of it—leave it! Teach yourself how to say 'no.' The pill works by hormones, and the only ones who use these pills are the ones who have the character of sleeping with guys. They have all sorts of side effects. They make you nauseated. You can get all the symptoms of being pregnant. They tire you out. You can't work, you can't study . . . all because you have said 'yes.' "[29]

In order to explore the moral hierarchy of different kinds of occupations in depth, I employed a modified pile-sort technique (see Bernard 1988:234–37), in which different occupational categories were written on index cards. Informants were asked to sort the cards into four piles: the "best" jobs (defined as those that bring a good income and high status), jobs at which one could earn a living and enjoy respectability, jobs that do not pay well and do not carry much status, and jobs that bring a poor standard of living in all regards. Those who participated in this exercise generally found it easy to rank the jobs.[30] While there was little unanimity on the best kinds of work, three jobs were at the bottom of almost every one's list: small businessman/market woman, bar worker, and guest-house worker. Other forms of nonagricultural manual labor such as factory worker were also frequently near the bottom of participants' lists.

Conceptually, business (biashara) was virtually the antithesis of work—a few steps up from thievery. One informant, a school teacher from Old Moshi, described her brother by stating flatly, "He doesn't work; he just does business" (Hafanyi kazi; anafanya biashara, tu).[31] This conceptual opposition existed partly because business "doesn't tire the body or the mentality—it's the easier thing to do. The hoe and the shamba—now that's honest work."[32] Farming, the quintessence of work, implied a stationary existence; farms don't move and farmers would be too tired to "wander around" at the end of the day. Business, on the other hand, implied travel, transience, and the importation of commodities—the root of all desire. One clue to the close and widely shared symbolic association between work and sex is in the ironic double meaning of the Kiswahili word kazi. Kazi literally means "work" but is also a euphemism for sexual intercourse—a form of work that produced a variant of exhaustion with its own effects. Young people often played upon these layers of meaning in the concept of work with a favorite slogan of the early AIDS era, "AIDS is an accident at work." The irony turned not only upon the pun but also upon the fact that the conditions most associated with risky sex (i.e., business) were a mere parody of "work" in the local schema.

## "AIDS Is Business" (Ukimwi Ni Biashara)
## Wahuni: AIDS and the Pathology of Lifestyle

If work implied fixity, dependability, and good tabia, the whole complex of activities emerging in the informal sector implied nearly the opposite. This was encapsulated in the particular scorn reserved for characters such as businessmen and bank tellers, who were thought to be in constant contact with money. The generation of meaning in the AIDS epidemic in northern Kilimanjaro was not only a lamentation over the slow loss of men and their potential for cultural reproduction; it was a commentary on the very moral character of community. In many contexts (often in AIDS prevention and education speeches) the bodies of youth were represented as being clothed improperly, fed improperly, absent improperly, sexually active improperly, fertile improperly, and laboring improperly. This cultural vilification was facilitated by the melding of an available cultural category of person, the *mhuni*, with the devalued bodies of young men and women. The Kiswahili word *mhuni* (plural: *wahuni*) has long been used to refer to a single man, often living on his own, and has had the connotation of "one who wanders about for not good purpose . . . a rebel . . . profligate" (Johnson 1939:137–38). In the age of AIDS, the term was applied to young men and young women and was reinvested with a damning force.

The reinvention of the *mhuni* pathologized the changing character of adulthood in Kilimanjaro. As long as the rural population in Kilimanjaro could afford the costs of social reproduction, the dislocation of productive manhood was culturally tolerated—if not celebrated. Such arrangements began to look altogether less tenable, however, as options in the formal economy shrank, upward mobility afforded by education disappeared, the returns on one's productive efforts weakened, and family relations already strained to great geographic lengths were wrenched by diminished remittances. In light of AIDS, however, stories and images of sexual chaos of *wahuni* abounded in local dialogue about young adulthood and were paralleled by notions of random and nomadic lifestyles. An association between unbridled sexual desire and a lack of fixity within controllable geographic and social landscapes bolstered the personification and embodiment of AIDS in youth. Kilimanjaro's variant moral demographies were central rhetorical devices in diatribes against youth and in explanations of how they came to be so much at risk in the epidemic. The *mhuni* became a sort of late twentieth-century East African rake, emblematic of the pathology of personhood associated with cities, markets, travel, and business. Those who contracted the virus, in fact, were called *"wagonjwa wahuni"* (the *wahuni* sick ones) by a participant in an AIDS seminar.[33]

*Wahuni* were the absolute antithesis of proper Chagga young men and women. They were sometimes called by the epithet *bo'n-town* (i.e., "born-in-town"), which even more clearly asserted the notion that young people came entirely from urban roots and had no connection to the mountain. The typical female *mhuni* was a bank teller. The typical male *mhuni* was a small businessman operating in the markets. A voracious desire for sex, money, or, preferably, both at the same time was emblematic of the insidious *tabia* of the *mhuni. Wahuni,* it was said, were after the easy life; what they wanted, they didn't want to work for. Bank tellers were said to riffle through account files seeking the wealthiest customers to seduce. Male market sellers were reputed to give discounts on their wares to female customers in exchange for so-called "express" service at the numerous market guest houses.

Young adults themselves recognized and responded to the idea of the *mhuni* with a mixture of contempt and a modicum of empathy. They often explained how they struggled to survive as the cost of living soared and opportunities shrank. Education, which once led to status occupations, was no longer seen as an advantage in the job market. Around Kiboriloni, those who left school early (or attended only on nonmarket days) might be seen to be getting the jump on their peers, many of whom would inevitably later end up with a gunny sack spread out on a small patch of ground in the market, competing with former schoolmates to sell identical goods. Many young businessmen talked dreamily of getting involved in the tourist trade, becoming a driver or car mechanic, or striking it rich in the tanzanite mines of Arusha. The predicament of such young men was understood by young and old alike. Yet many youth were treated by and treated one another unsympathetically, their dreams seen as wildly impractical, their energy wasted on unprofitable business ventures, local beer, and taking their pleasure with young women who were seeking their own tenuous toehold on security through offspring and the possibilities for marriage that their apparently precocious fertility once seemed to offer.

Twenty-seven-year-old Rose was living with her parents in the Majengo section of Moshi. She was not married, had no children, and had just finished a computer course in Arusha. Rose was looking for work and hoping that her brother would be able to offer her something in his business in Dar es Salaam. I met Rose while conducting a household survey with my research assistant, Gertrude; Rose was visiting with one of the survey respondents when we paid a call. Before our trip to Majengo, I had been discussing with Gertrude how to go about interviewing on the topic of *wahuni*. I took one look at Rose and asked her for an interview. Rose was dressed in what seemed to me almost a parody of *mhuni* style. Her hair was braided "Rasta-style," with two-tone extenders, and bound with a fancy, brightly colored head wrap. Her face was heavily made-up, complete with gold lipstick to match her gold nail polish on the fingers of the right hand only. She wore a loose-fitting man's dress shirt unbuttoned halfway, tight-fitting blue jeans, and foam rubber thongs, with gold polish on her toenails. Rose wore gold filigree earrings, a "disco chain" (a gold necklace), and gold rings on two fingers of her right hand.

When the survey was completed and I interviewed Rose, I was surprised by what she said. Instead of a narrative along the lines of "I was a teenage *mhuni*," Rose launched into something of a diatribe against *mhuni* ways and the excesses of her peers.

> [Where does *uhuni* come from?] Young people today like to *starehe* more than doing work. They want to live in a way that they haven't struggled to get. The easy life. A *kijana* sees a girl, thinks she's cute, and he just wants to enjoy. This kind of stuff brings *uhuni*. [Can you tell if someone is an *mhuni*?] You know if a woman is involved in this lifestyle if she doesn't have work, but she still is a smart dresser. Where did she get the money from? Men. She is a prostitute; an *mhuni*. She does it almost like a kind of work.
>
> [Do *wahuni* have a lot of sexual desire?] Yes. Like bank workers. They work; they get a salary of the usual level, but when they get the chance, they go through the accounts to see who has a lot of money. When he comes into the bank, they fight each other to serve him. They flirt with him. It's all of this wanting a better life than you can afford. Men today don't see the future. Whatever he has today, he uses it. He wants everyone to know that he has money. He *starehe*s. Ladies see money, and they get confused, because that's what they're after. Life here in Moshi is after money. This is not the original Chagga *tabia*; it's because of economic conditions. If you have work, you're not left with enough time to make *uhuni*. When you come home you're tired.
>
> [Are there *wahuni* on the mountain as well, or just here in town?] *Wahuni* are much more common here in the city than on the mountain. They look just like everyone else, but they have no respect, no shame, and no sensitivity. If they have AIDS, they want everyone to get it. [Do you know anyone you think fits the description of an *mhuni*?] I know one girl—three of her boyfriends have already died. She's still got good health, and she's going around infecting people. These *wahuni*s, whether male or female like to fuck [-*tomba*] more than other people. They also stick to their own kind; if they go outside their own group, there's nothing to talk about. [Where do you find *wahuni* in the city?] The disco is a nice place to find them. Like the bank tellers. Uch. They're such *wahuni* they even try to pick up the husbands of women who have just died [she implies that these hypothetical women have died of AIDS],

or they won't even wait till she is dead—they just go for the husband. The problem here is that if they just go with this husband, they cause him to forget his home completely. This is terrible. And these guys, you know the way they think, "The way that woman dresses . . . now how does she look naked?" These are totally usual ideas for men.

[How do *wahuni* handle money?] Instead of using it for their own futures, they just use it thoughtlessly. I don't understand why they don't think of the future. If a person inherits some wealth, for example, he is totally defeated in organizing anything with it. The next time you turn around the money is finished. People just forget themselves. They have the thoughts of children, not of adults. [What about women who become *wahuni*?] People are very jealous of a beautiful woman. They think she wants to show everyone how fine she is. To be beautiful is easy and dangerous. You can get sucked up into the mob psychology with the *wahuni*. The *wahuni* are self-loving, boastful, and vain. They're the ones who wear "*skoonas*" [i.e., schooners]—you know, those shoes where the women sail along on high heels, and each shoe goes "ka-klack, ka-klack, ka-klack," and they draw everyone's attention. The mob psychology works on them because if you don't fall in line, they call you *mshamba* [a "hick"]. They get so annoyed if you are among them and just act like a normal person. I'll tell you one thing, though: If I got stuck working for the government, I'd be *mhuni* for sure. The salaries are just too low.[34]

The emergence, reproduction, and proliferation of these images of miscreant youth are microexamples of the sort of "modular cultural artefacts" that Anderson (1983:4) applied to the creation of concepts of nations and nationalism: "The creation of these artefacts . . . was the complex 'crossing' of discrete historical forces. . . . once created, they became 'modular,' capable of being transplanted, with varying degrees of self-consciousness, to a great variety of social terrains, to merge and be merged with a correspondingly wide variety of political and ideological constellations." The *mhuni* became a hegemonic, dominant ideological representation to which everyone could relate and with which none would identify, the "enormous range of [its] applicability . . . a direct consequence of [its] simplicity" (Moore 1996:196).

In the name of cultural realism, to paraphrase Legge (1997:13), social actors in Kilimanjaro switched the villainous stereotype of the *mhuni* for the truth of each economically disenfranchised man and woman and so generated a folk epidemiology in which all could participate. The *mhuni* was not so much an invention of structurally favored elites in a classic struggle of elders and juniors, but a malleable, embodied sign that became part of taken-for-granted notions of young people.

In nearly eighteen months of fieldwork no one ever suggested that *wa-huni* did not exist or that they were somehow "invented" in order to stereotype members of a disaffected or disenfranchised generation. Rather the *mhuni* became an elastic category that could be stretched to fit any particular situation. Within the bodies and personae of youth, the reconfiguration of the *mhuni* represented the intersection of epidemic disease and demographic momentum, epidemiologic indices of risk and pathology, demographic narratives of the attenuated demise of cultural integrity with its "imagined" ideal of the *kihamba* regime, and local histories of sexuality, desire, and development. The *mhuni* also allowed people in Kilimanjaro to engage in an easy denial of personal risk: "If AIDS is a disease of *wahuni*, and I am not *mhuni*, I am not at risk." Elsewhere in Africa where the epidemic had already become much more severe, personifications of AIDS reflected more bitter sentiments. In Rakai, by contrast, AIDS was referred to as *mubbi*, "the robber," for it robbed people of their full adult lives, of a sense of security and trust in their partners. It robbed families of their ability to perpetuate themselves, the elderly of their expectation that they would be cared for in old age, children of their parents, and families of their resources (Barnett and Blaikie 1992:52).

## Beer Bellies and Big Bottoms: The Cultural Anatomy of Desire and Risk

Although Rose suggested that *wahuni* "look like anyone else," there was a distinct iconography of *mhuni* anatomy that spoke to the physical manifestations of their excesses. The stigmatization of women as "vectors" for STDs, including AIDS, has been well documented in many settings (see, e.g., Brandt 1987). It is important to note, however, that in the cultural signification of AIDS in Kilimanjaro, men were vilified as much as women—if not more so. The *kitambi* (a man's beer belly) and the "*wowowo*" (a slang word for a woman's large buttocks) were often exploited as symbols of insatiable desire for consumption. *Wo-wowo* was a nonsense term understood throughout Tanzania because of an advertisement for a night club in Dar es Salaam that appeared regularly in national newspapers. The illustration accompanying the advertisement depicted a small, balding man who has been knocked nearly unconscious in a collision with the enormous rear end of a woman in high heels and a tight disco outfit. While the woman continues to dance with oblivious abandon, the man sits on the floor, clutching his head, his eyeglasses askew. Above him, and literally behind the back(side) of the female dancer appears the snickering word *"wowowo."* The *kitambi* and the *wowowo* became standard accouterments of images of *wahuni.* They were iconic of the disordered space between the bodies of men and women revealed in diseases of development such as AIDS.

In 1993, KIWAKKUKI sponsored an AIDS-education drama competition in Moshi. The participants included women's groups, church youth groups, government and private secondary schools, and a teacher's training college. In nearly every play or play-poem *(ngonjera)* performed, a businessman with a *kitambi* or a high-heeled woman with a *wowowo* represented the malevolent presence of HIV in the story line. Eventually, evoking the symbolism of the syndrome, the *kitambi*s and *wowowo*s withered away with the health, wealth, beauty, and the sanity of the victim—AIDS signified the simultaneous, slow negation of the body and the person.[35] In one of the play-poems a businessman with a *kitambi* wooed successive partners one after the other at his favorite bar. The businessman contracted a different STD from each woman. Each time he fell ill, he begged his muse, "Pesa" ("money"), to help him recover.

Finally, the businessman fell ill with a disease that wasted his *kitambi*—a sight from which Pesa fled in horror. As the businessman staggered about the stage with a pale powdered face and clothes that had magically become tattered and too large for his wasted frame (denoting his descent into poverty and madness), the play-poem concluded with a song that admonished *"UKIMWI ni tamaani! UKIMWI ni zinaa! UKIMWI ni uhuni!"* (AIDS is to desire! AIDS is promiscuity! AIDS is a profligate lifestyle!).[36] In another performance, set in an office, an affair quickly developed between a secretary and her new boss. Sakina, the secretary, had a *wowowo* that her boss made a point of staring at wide-eyed for the benefit of the audience—who obliged with uproarious laughter. The boss, who began the play with a hefty middle, gradually withered away until his wife commented that "even your *kitambi* is disappearing."

## Signifying Risk in AIDS Control Messages

Several years elapsed between the time HIV was identified in Kilimanjaro and the implementation of programs by AIDS service and education organizations, but by the early 1990s a variety of anti-AIDS efforts were under way.[37] The largest and best funded was the education component of the Tanzanian/Norway AIDS Project (MUTAN), funded by

Norwegian government aid. The Lutheran and Catholic dioceses also had AIDS education programs, as did KIWAKKUKI. These addressed different audiences and had different approaches to prevention education, yet commonalities existed among them in the way they signified AIDS and risk. All of them, for example, addressed themselves to young people and to women left behind by migrant husbands. In doing so, the AIDS education speeches they presented combined professional and popular epidemiologies of AIDS that were laced with what Seidel has termed the "competing discourses" of AIDS in Africa (Seidel 1993). In Kilimanjaro, AIDS educators have communicated with audiences by mixing medical information with images of misallocated energy, desire, business, and the personage of the *mhuni*. If the examples of AIDS education recounted here seem overdrawn, it is in the interest of an account of AIDS education as it was practiced in certain contexts rather than as it was theorized about by donors, consultants, and critics. This account is not an evaluation of the effectiveness of AIDS education, nor is it a statement about the skills of particular educators; the point is to explore the layers of meaning in the practice of AIDS prevention.

A "medico-moral discourse" in which monocausal epidemiological notions of risk have, inevitably, conveyed value judgments about "risk groups" (Seidel 1993:176–78) was a feature of most HIV prevention in the region and encoded powerful critiques of the failure of youth to exhibit good moral character. In the same speech to secondary school girls in which she warned them against contraception, a MUTAN educator incorporated the image of the *mhuni* as an unspoken referent in her discussion of risk, desire, and businessmen in the marketplace. The goods that the hawkers purveyed in the markets were presented as tokens of infected desire and temptation, the tainted icons of illicit wealth. Only the *tabia*-enhancing effects of hard work, the students were told, could save them from the guile of young men and the fatal allure of their wares.

> Why do girls have the *tabia* of going with young men? It's jealousy [*wivu*]. Jealousy of nice clothes. The clothes are there in Kiboriloni, but how do we get the money? We deceive our parents. We look at the guest houses for lorry drivers who have a lot of money. If you are wicked, you can get any idea at all into your head, and you won't succeed in school.[38]
>     It's the markets. The market of Himo, the market of Kiboriloni. If you go there, your entire life as a woman will be crippled. You'll have problems for the rest of your life, even if you don't get AIDS. . . . Kiboriloni is practically in town . . . it's not far away. . . . You are

good girls, but there in Kiboriloni, there are moccasins. Moccasins deceive. Moccasins will fail you. Moccasins will bring trouble— the same with watches, the same with sandals.

You must change your *tabia.* You must understand. Not far from here there is a place called the Countryside Inn. [The students laugh.] Many students go there. The men drive up in their cars with tinted windows. . . . Many girls who get pregnant get abortions. They become infertile.

What should we do to change *tabia?* From morning to night you put in a hard day of work.[39]

The audience regarded the presenter's speech, which also included exhortations for the young women to eschew oral contraceptives, as a slightly embarrassing display of demagoguery more for the benefit of the school headmistress seated in the corner of the room than for the students, whose needs for practical information and support were left unaddressed.

Priests and ministers also addressed AIDS in sermons and speeches both in- and outside church. In 1991, the workers of KCMC made one of the hospital's pastors their guest of honor at activities to mark WHO's World AIDS Day. In his remarks, he equated cultural loss with vulnerability to AIDS and evoked "disco" to signify a polyglot culture of bad *tabia.*

This doctor believes in his religion more than he believes in condoms! Don't break this machine of society that God has given us. Don't welcome this unwanted guest. We have a mixture of cultures now. We have thrown out the teachings of the elders. We must return to our culture, our traditions, and to God. Do they have trouble with AIDS in India? China? No! Why? Because they have a strong religion and a strong culture.

We must tell our youth that "if you do not change your ways, you will die of AIDS, and we will die of broken hearts. God will forgive you tomorrow if you leave aside bad *tabia.*" They must leave the discos behind. Disco. It's a European thing. Why do we need such noise?[40]

In 1992, KIWAKKUKI held a three-day training session for members who had volunteered to serve as home visitors to people with AIDS. The training was funded by MUTAN and was run with the assistance of AIDS counselors from the regional hospital. The closing speech was given by a Lutheran pastor and exemplified "medico-moral discourse." The following extract from his speech contains a dense and highly political interweaving of biomedical knowledge, Christian morality, and

a critique of modern locations of moral value in productive and reproductive relations.

> Some time ago I was one of a group of pastors who went to Kagera,
> where AIDS started out in Tanzania. We traveled through some
> of the countryside there—and it is truly astounding. Houses are
> closed up; the border area with Uganda is empty. . . . We went to
> the RMO [Regional Medical Officer], asked to visit some of the
> afflicted on the wards, but when we went in we were told we
> should stay far away from them. That they are "very dangerous."
> Those days the word was to separate the sick—to fear the bed-
> clothes, the saliva, even their breath.
>
> Today we realize that the problem is not with those dying in
> their beds; it's with those sick ones who are still moving around.
> AIDS is spread by promiscuity and adultery [zinaa na uasherati],
> not by breathing, saliva, or mosquitoes. Promiscuity, adultery, and
> homosexuality/anal intercourse [ulawiti]. Men who want women
> along the road. Medical science has proved beyond a shadow of
> a doubt that he who does not lead a Christian life will die. His
> family will die. His house [clan] will die. Medical science has
> shown us that there is no reason to abandon the bedridden. We
> must make them comfortable, be sensitive towards them. We can-
> not blame the sick; who knows how they got their AIDS? You
> women are the ones in danger. I say this with great bitterness. Your
> man comes home with a kilo of pork and AIDS. "Oh," he says,
> "I'm so sorry!" How should we help her, this mother of children?
> It's a problem. Condoms? Condoms can't be relied upon. Your
> work is enormous and difficult. Women are in great danger. What
> way is there to look after the woman whose man wants fresh pas-
> tures? Go to Kiboriloni to see how people live. See this man with
> his kitambi. He doesn't have AIDS yet, maybe, but go to Kibori-
> loni—it's not far from here.[41]

This speech, delivered in the rhetorical style of a sermon, was an
eloquent act of signification. Take, for example, the final few lines
quoted above, "Go to Kiboriloni to see how people live. See this man
with his kitambi. He doesn't have AIDS yet, maybe, but go to Kiboriloni—it's not far from here." This sequence of statements makes sense
because of the tactical and almost spontaneous use of signs (the market,
men's embodied excesses, AIDS, and "here"—a church-run facility) in
which the pastor also incorporated himself and his listeners as signs
(by emphasizing the proximity of speaker and audience to the locus
of epidemic contagion). From my perspective, the speech epitomized
the symbolic life of AIDS as a cultural critique of development and
young adulthood; for the audience it was compelling and resonated
with meaning and experience. Most of the women with whom I dis-

cussed the speech thought it was a fine way to close the home-care seminar.

To be sure, not all formal AIDS education contained such overdrawn caricature of risk and contagion. In fact, more interactive formats often highlighted the fact that many community members perceived AIDS to be a result of hard times and social change, for which young people could hardly be held accountable. Between 1991 and 1993 the bulk of the formal AIDS education work conducted by both the Lutheran and Catholic dioceses was directed by expatriate women. In the Lutheran diocese, the director of the health education program launched a series of day-long seminars for parishioners in many urban and rural locations. In these seminars, the image of the *mhuni* was seldom invoked. In addition to information about modes of transmission and statistics about the state of the epidemic in Kilimanjaro, the presenter focused on compassionate treatment of those with the disease. In order to generate discussion about this topic, the facilitator often asked members of the audience to perform an improvisational skit based on the premise that a young woman had acquired AIDS as a result of her desire for a pair of moccasins. As we have seen, her assumed use of sex to get the shoes was a concise piece of a cultural etiology to which the entire audience could relate.

The skit was specifically designed to engage the observers in an interpretive exercise. The audience was asked to comment upon the actions of the performer portraying the girl's mother, who responded to her daughter's condition with suspicion, fear, and shame. The discussion generated by the skit often revolved around a now familiar set of themes and returned to the premise of the skit—that the young woman was infected in town through her desire for symbols of a certain kind of lifestyle. The representational medium of this skit allowed significations that were sympathetic to the plight of young people to emerge. After one performance, an older man stood and offered an account of local conditions of risk in which culture, development, and poverty—not itinerant businessmen of bad moral character with excesses of *ta-maa*—were seen as problematic: "The problem is that today it's difficult to find work. This young girl wanted a new pair of shoes. This isn't bad. The problem is that we cannot find work, and it's hard to return to a way of life that is past—cutting leaves for the cows [i.e., a *kihamba*-based life]. The youth see houses with cars and telephones. . . . But the conditions of poverty are what life is now. We must help the youth to realize the life that *they* see is good. Bridewealth, for example, must be lowered or abolished altogether. Young men are still unmarried at the age of thirty and thirty-five. They cannot afford the bridewealth,[42] and so begin to visit loose women."[43]

## Do as I Say, Not as I Do: Sign Users as Signs in AIDS Prevention

The saying "AIDS is business" is a double-entendre; it derived half of its meaning from the cultural associations I have just outlined and half from another way in which AIDS represented a disease of disordered development. As Lyttleton observed in his study of AIDS control in rural Thailand, many programs employed a top-down model of information dissemination that replicated the structure of many previous development programs (1996:25). MUTAN was largely based on a "project" model, and its effectiveness was mediated partly by how audiences assessed MUTAN against their previous experience of development projects in general. Although messages about AIDS succeeded in conveying potentially life-saving information to most of the adult population of Kilimanjaro, there were many reasons why the distribution channels for these messages were suspect.

For many young people, development projects were frequently seen as ephemeral and ineffectual additions to the local landscape and as cash cows for a handful of local elites.[44] With its new cars, videos, computers, and plum salaries, MUTAN often appeared to fit this mold, hence the cynical critique "AIDS is business" was often uttered in reference to it. Intoned by priests and AIDS educators, this phrase signified the pathology of small business life. It had quite another meaning when uttered by a young kiosk-operator upon catching sight of a regional official transporting bags of maize in the back of a MUTAN Land Cruiser for his profitable trade in Kiboriloni. The widespread sentiment among young people was that the members of the formal health-care sector who found employment as AIDS educators and counselors were primarily motivated by the topping up of their salaries and other benefits rather than a strong commitment to AIDS prevention or the care of the AIDS ill. Even when MUTAN was aware of these impediments and went to extraordinary lengths to allay the community distrust generated by medical research on sexual health, the obstacles could not always be overcome (Klouman et al. 1995:208–9). For their own part, the nurses and medical assistants who made up the bulk of the Tanzanian project staff felt grateful for and entitled to the financial boost to their meager public-service salaries that came from employment by the project. In Tanzania, it has been conventional practice for aid projects to pay local staff salary top-ups and allowances (posho) for attending meetings and workshops. These allowances often amounted to substantially more than the government salaries the employees received, which, in the early 1990s, were in the range of $20 to $40 per month.

Regardless of the reasonableness of assembling a decent wage through working for foreign aid projects, the credibility of many Tanzanian health-care workers involved in AIDS work was further hampered by the experiences that many young people had of reproductive health services based in the government health system. Those who preached concern for the sexual health of the public came from among the same class of individuals who provided illegal abortions and extorted money from young people to treat their STDs or even to write letters of reference to the zonal hospital for treatment.[45] As one Tanzanian sociologist put it, owing to declining funds and shortages of drugs in the 1980s, the national health-care system (in addition to the "system" more widely conceived) came to operate on the basis "not of technical know-*how*, but of technical know-*whom*" (Lugala 1994). For the relatively small proportion of Kilimanjaro's youth who came into contact with AIDS educators (Setel and Kessy 1992), this fact militated against health-care workers serving as credible or sincere models of behavior and attitudinal change, or even as genuine in their concern for sharing AIDS education. The Tanzanians involved in AIDS work were clearly seen as privileged and elite among a local class of workers who already had power and status (see Setel 1997). Within the hospital itself, money available for AIDS-related activities had a serious effect on work relations between MUTAN employees and co-workers.[46]

Furthermore, the persons employed by MUTAN educators, along with the agents of every other institution and organization that engaged in AIDS education in Kilimanjaro, occupied structural positions in relation to their audiences that had a profound, unspoken effect on the outcome of their encounters. Structural relations affected how audiences were defined, which issues were emphasized, which were left out or avoided (condoms, for example, were often excluded from these talks), and what moral messages were conveyed as subtexts to educational information. In this way, the fact that sign users became signs in their own acts of signification often worked against effective communication. Structural inequalities were reinforced, for example, by the obvious disdain shown toward a group of guest-house workers at an AIDS seminar led by the regional AIDS coordinator and the regional AIDS counselor. The counselor was from an elite family with a conservative Lutheran background. During her colleague's presentation the AIDS counselor sat to the side, pointedly ignoring the proceedings and leafing noisily through a *Newsweek* magazine. When she stood to present, she directly confronted the guest-house owners, stating, "One of the taxi drivers in our other seminar said that guest houses spread promiscuity—that each room comes with its own woman." The owners objected, to which the counselor answered, "Well, that's as may be, but how can guest house owners help us?" The content and tone of her response indicated that she expected that the guest-house owners were meant to help the AIDS educators rather than the other way around, and that she was deeply skeptical that such assistance lay within the realm of possibility.[47]

The credibility of the church as a source of compelling prevention also became strained for some young people. In the border market of Himo, Catholic priests were called *padri tundu*, "mischievous priests," and certain children there were rumored to be the evidence of their misdeeds. I asked my friend the Moshi carpenter whether he felt the church was a credible source of AIDS education. In reply he stated:

> Twenty-five years ago the church was very concerned about social development. The whole leadership had a big commitment to develop society. They had networks of kindergartens, primary and secondary schools, dispensaries and hospitals. They had all kinds of locations at which they would provide services. . . . At a village level, people were committed. The priests and ministers were well educated and understood things better than the local folks. Thus when they saw that so-and-so was having psychological problems, they could help him. . . . It has now gotten to the point where the commitment of the clergy and church has been lost. . . . This has been caused by hard economic conditions. Priests concern themselves with their personal wealth. There was a spiritual commitment among them, but now they just go to work and wait for their salaries. . . . No one is helping the people. No one is thinking about the problems. Their work is to serve, but they just don't do it.[48]

## Everyday Significations of AIDS and Prevention

People in Kilimanjaro were aware of AIDS and, when they could or were motivated enough, responded to the epidemic in their own ways. These responses were not always ideal from a prevention standpoint, but nearly everyone interviewed during the course of fieldwork stated that they had altered the kinds and qualities of the relationships in which they engaged, and placed a new emphasis on "faithfulness" *(uaminifu)* in marriage and relationships. Some had adopted measures that they believed to be protective, like selecting only "clean" partners or using condoms consistently with *starehe* partners. Others attempted to appropriate some of the power of the medical vision of AIDS by devising a self-test in which they scratched themselves with a sharp object and then observed how the wound healed.[49] Much has been made of the gallows humor of young men, of fatalistic slogans such as "AIDS is an accident at work," and of wordplay with the acronym "AIDS" such as "A*cha* I*niue*, D*ogodogo* S*iachi*" (Just let it kill me, I'm not leaving young girls alone). Yet one should not mistake such discourse for behavior. Studies from elsewhere in East Africa (Mukiza-Gapere and Ntozi, n.d.) support the protestations of young people in Kilimanjaro that AIDS had "changed their way of life" and their sexual behavior. Most informants in Kilimanjaro were adamant that AIDS had changed behavior. One man, a carpenter in his thirties living in Moshi, spoke for many when he told me:

> You don't see so many men with women in places of entertainment now. Previously, if you went to a bar, 90 percent of the men would be with girlfriends. But now you will only find the men there. A lot of people say it's because the price of beer has gone up so much, but really it's because of AIDS. If you find a pair, it will be a long-time girlfriend or a special friend.
>
> AIDS has ruined their way of life. The greatest entertainment here is sex. Our way of life has been very seriously affected. Even with one girl there is not much fun. You need to have several to have a good time. Change means risk. Life has become very miserable.[50]

Yet while many people acknowledged it as a present threat, AIDS remained an ambiguous entity, obscured by rhetoric and clouded by contradictions. In his short story entitled "Death from AIDS," Clement Merinyo represents the daily lives of young men in the shadow of the epidemic as filled with uncertainty, scepticism and denial.

> AIDS was a topic of conversation of the young businessmen when they got drunk.
>
> "Don't get used to AIDS my friend," a person would be told with portent when one of the bar maids showed signs of wanting him.
>
> "AIDS! You can even get it from needles at the hospital, man," the taunted man would say, defending himself. "You want me to abstain from eating roasted meat because I'm afraid of AIDS?" In their circle they called women "the roasted meat you eat when you drink beer."
>
> "Hey, isn't AIDS just like an accident?" another would say, doubtlessly defending and guarding his *tamaa*. "If it has been writ-

ten that you will die from AIDS, you will die from AIDS, no matter
what you do. Even the priests in Europe, I hear, are dying from
AIDS." . . .

"Don't you care about your life?" he would be thrown the question, "why do you . . . ?"

"Why do doctors smoke cigars and drink booze? . . . Those who
themselves warn about the sickness and damaging effects of these
practices! I can do without your meaningless stubbornness, man!"
(Merinyo 1988:35–36; my translation)

Such scenarios rang true to the impression given by many informants.
Most, however, had stories to tell of their own moments of realization
of vulnerability. For some it came with the death of a close friend or
family member; for others it came in a flash of recognition when the
idea of taking a *starehe* partner suddenly lost its appeal.

Audience interpretation of AIDS education was thus based upon
more than its narrative content or its moral subtexts. The ostensibly
context-free sex of the AIDS education flip chart or prevention seminar
(see Dixon-Mueller 1993; Ahlberg 1994:225) was viewed by young people in the context of their social relations. The meaning of prevention
work derived from the fact that the persons who engaged in it themselves operated as embodied signs; the AIDS educators' tactical use
of signs of moral turpitude was undercut by a host of nondiscursive
significations that inhered in their status as health workers and their
participation in a form of project-based intervention that many young
people viewed with great cynicism. As such, AIDS educators were
not in control of their own signification and generated meanings independent of the prevention messages they uttered. This is not to say
that educational messages had no meaning in and of themselves, but
that they did not have a meaning independent of the institutional
pragmatics through which they were manifest. In this context I follow
Rochberg-Halton in using "pragmatics" to mean the layered relationships between signs and their users, in which the users and their behaviors are also signs and in which use can only be understood within
the cultural context of ongoing inquiry, or signification (Rochberg-
Halton 1986:4).

The pragmatics of AIDS education were manifest in multivocal and
multilocal semiotic events throughout Kilimanjaro, a semiotic that was
in equal measure semantic and somatic, and encompassed by demographic, economic, and epidemiologic circumstance. This signification
happened with spontaneity and immediacy through the use-signs of
body and language. Institutional and noninstitutional interests converged and diverged in seemingly unpredictable ways and in countless

THE "ACQUIRED INCOME DEFICIENCY SYNDROME"      181

social situations: in hospitals and homes, in blood labs and churches, over the graves of the dead for the benefit of the living, between patients and practitioners, between educators and audiences, between priests and parishioners, and between researchers and researched. For recipients of AIDS control messages, a series of seamless, interdependent interpretive acts made up the experience of prevention education. No one came to this encounter a tabula rasa; even if members of the audience had no prior knowledge or expectations about AIDS and risk (and very few did), they all had a structural position in terms of gender, age, and social standing that served as an embodied vantage point from which all other acts of signification were viewed. These structural relationships between AIDS service providers and their intended audiences greatly influenced communication. As audiences experienced representations of themselves as persons at risk, some found self-recognition. For others, there were too many dissonances between the images of themselves-at-risk and the very physical presence of pastors, nurses, and physicians as corporeal agents of meaningful action. These dissonances began with practices as mundane as educators' arriving at an event chauffeured in shiny new Land Cruisers and unloading video screens, generators, and public address systems. Not a word of AIDS education needed to be uttered for a powerful and inevitable set of associations to exist over and above the issues raised in the semantics of an AIDS information campaign.

The cultural signification of AIDS in Kilimanjaro was distinct from the epidemiologically "proven" presence of the disease (to which we shall now turn), but no less steeped in a process of interpreting conflicting and ambiguous signs of the disease. In Kilimanjaro, as elsewhere in Africa (Romero-Daza 1993), public health education moved in advance of the epidemic, leading to high levels of knowledge in relatively low prevalence areas. Even where widespread awareness of AIDS occurred in the context of high prevalence, such as parts of Uganda, the language used to describe the shared experience of the epidemic often served to heighten the numerous ambiguities surrounding the disease, allowing people the option actively to "not know" about it (Obbo 1991:85). Yet, paradoxically, such "not knowing" was a form of knowing all the same (see Last 1992). In Kilimanjaro, the balance between knowing and not knowing about AIDS was struck in myriad ways. Often it had to do with the legitimacy that young adults and older elites attributed to various sources of knowledge, some of which were shot through with symbolic tensions that undermined the transfer of information. The institutional authority of AIDS educators from the formal health-care sector and religious figures did not translate into a ready platform from which to communicate about the epidemic. The AIDS epidemic in Kilimanjaro acquired its meaning from an amalgam of local moral demographies and the models of personhood that fit within them, disparate and often conflicting pieces of information about HIV and risk, and whatever direct experience individuals had with this ambiguous new disease.

## CHAPTER 6

An Epidemic of Clarity, a Disease of Confusion:
Professional and Popular Epidemiologies
of AIDS

### Significations of AIDS and the Bodies of Young Adults

In previous chapters I illustrated several of the major paradoxes and
contradictions posed by AIDS in Kilimanjaro: that contemporary sexual ideologies have been based upon the nostalgic referent of an unsustainable demographic regime; that modernity was seen as the salvation
of the Chagga and in light of AIDS has been recast as their curse; that
sexual culture in Kilimanjaro, spoken of in terms of randomness, has
in fact been organized; and that vulnerability to HIV was born of demographic and economic necessity and yet has been attributed to excesses
of bad character and desire among the young. In this chapter, I shall
examine one more layer of contradiction in this inscrutable plague: that
of expectation and experience. Although the first AIDS case had been
diagnosed in the region in 1984, until two prominent men in Moshi
died of the disease several years later, few believed it had arrived in
Kilimanjaro. Even then, it was not until 1988 that a majority of respondents to a household survey conducted in Moshi recognized AIDS as
present in Kilimanjaro (Setel and Kessy 1992). The local histories of
AIDS, as they were recounted by doctors, villagers, townspeople, and
epidemiologists, were layered with expectations, conjectures, and pre-
sumptions, many of which centered on stereotypes of *wahuni* and an
urban disease model. As diverse sets of actors came to grips with the
idea of AIDS in Kilimanjaro, they wove together expectations about
the epidemic from numerous sources. The precise language of clinical
practice and epidemiology, however, stood in stark contrast to the ambiguities and silences surrounding the lived experience of the disease.
Over time, an inchoate and varied cultural discourse about development and cultural dislocation was spun into a web of basic, taken-for-
granted home truths in both professional and nonprofessional epi-

demiologies of AIDS. Because expectant knowledge of the epidemic preceded lived experience with it, the popular epidemiology of AIDS in northern Tanzania differed from its identification and investigation in some other African locales and paralleled it elsewhere. In places such as Kagera, Kinshasa, and Kampala, medical research and public information campaigns *followed* an awareness that a new disease had stricken many young adults, while in Lesotho knowledge moved *in advance* of high rates of disease (Romero-Daza 1993).

This period of the AIDS epidemic in Kilimanjaro was as much about constructing local knowledge about HIV as it was about managing its ambiguities. In coming to grips with the idea of HIV, epidemiologists and laypeople all created representations of the disease, used these representations to generate new ones, and so built up a layered portrait of the natural history of the epidemic. Certain meanings central to AIDS, such as those related to *tabia* and *tamaa,* were unshakably embedded in what people in Kilimanjaro understood being human to be. Other meanings, including those attached to the moral demographies of Kilimanjaro and the popular and professional narratives of the epidemic, were more explicit in the public debate. While no one challenged the notion that promiscuous sex was a feature of excessive desire and bad *tabia,* young people in Kilimanjaro, as elsewhere in Tanzania (Muhondwa 1991), did express skepticism about epidemiologic narratives of AIDS and risk. They doubted the credibility of some of the sources of knowledge and pointed out lacunae in the "science" of AIDS. For example, individuals who were assumed to be vulnerable to infection seemed to go unscathed, while others, who did not conform to their expectations of risk, perished. There were gaps between the expectations that they had of the epidemic based on the advanced warnings they had received and the experience of the disease as it began to emerge among them.

Before they became part of the symbolic discourse of the AIDS epidemic, men and women—as embodied signs of adult personhood—experienced dislocations and relocations that shook them free of cultural and social conditions in which qualities of personal action could be readily slotted into a shared system of meaning and belief. In the way they bore children, made love, moved, became ill and died, their bodies came to betoken disordered development. Over a number of years, epidemiologists quantified and located the whereabouts of AIDS in Kilimanjaro. This local, geographic quest for the virus required using the bodies of young Tanzanians as starting points for the application of various scientific methods and technologies. Clinical case definitions, HIV blood tests, and case control studies were brought to bear upon patients in hospitals and upon blood samples taken from occupational and demographic subgroups of the Kilimanjaro population. These professional activities thereby accomplished the epidemiologic goal of locating HIV in terms of person, place, and time. The cultural process of coming to terms with this new disease was also based upon information contained in the bodies of adult men and women. However, the nature of that information and the interpretive undertaking were somewhat different. The cultural generation of meaning required no formal education, no capital-intensive technology. It required nothing other than an ability to engage in collective creative thought about a disease that remained a chimerical presence for most, long after scientific authorities had announced its epidemiologic arrival.

Epidemiologic inquiry entails the generation of inferences about causes and conditions associated with the presence and absence of disease. These inferences are based upon the visualization, manipulation, and interpretation of clues to the whereabouts of somatic disorder—an inquiry that depends upon the interpretation and enumeration of physical signs of AIDS in aggregates (samples, cohorts, and cases) of individual bodies, both sick and healthy. It should be noted that by "signs of AIDS" I do not mean *symbols* of AIDS, or metaphoric, textual, inscribed representations of AIDS, but "signs" in the real, immutable, corporeal, and clinical sense: the presentation of certain clinical conditions, the darkened bands of a Western-blot test strip which indexes the presence or absence of constituent proteins of HIV in blood samples, and the relative HIV prevalence rates among pregnant women and blood donors (see, e.g., Good 1994:71–76). In the early 1990s there was a rumor in Moshi that a physician at KCMC could diagnose AIDS by simply looking at a person. On one hand this rumor can be seen as a naive belief in the divinatory powers of biomedicine; on the other hand it represented a popular realization that medicine, in its own terms, was indeed capable of signifying the presence or absence of disorder on the basis of the visualization of signs.

As epidemiologists began to sketch the presence and prevalence of AIDS in Kilimanjaro, the economically and demographically circumscribed bodies of young people were a starting point for another kind of search—a cultural pursuit of meanings for this emergent disease category. Unlike the clinical and epidemiologic inquiry, the cultural quest for comprehension was not based primarily upon inferences built upon indexical and clinical signs such as blood test results or swollen lymph glands; it was constructed mainly from the manipulation and interpretation of a different, though no less real, set of signs. These included stories, rumors, and health education messages about AIDS; the lack of fixity of young people; their moral character as revealed through their purposeful actions; their habits of consumption; and, for those who were affected by the disease, the symbolism of their wasted and weakened bodies.

Because both the medical and cultural searches converged upon the same set of objects (i.e., the bodies of adult men and women that contained an unprecedented capacity for disorder), they could not help informing one another. As Good points out, "Medicine, as a form of activity, joins the material to the moral domain" (1994:70). One set of objects, then, was capable of producing signs with different ontologies, ontologies that depended in large part upon the interpretative techniques of whoever was engaged in using those signs (and thereby producing new ones). These signs all pointed back to an apparently common origin—the disordered and dislocated bodies of young people. These bodies, then, became "material-semiotic generative nodes" (Haraway 1991:208) circumscribed by history and demography. Stated slightly differently, because both cultural and medical knowledge of AIDS was based upon the bodies of youth, epidemiologic representations of the disease could not help serving as cultural evaluations about the nature of young adult life-styles. Simultaneously, the popular inquiry into the epidemic incorporated certain elements of scientific epidemiology, studding the cultural signification of AIDS with bits and pieces of medical knowledge about the disease. In this sense, cultural knowledge and medical knowledge converged and at times became indistinguishable from each other. This proximity of inquirers and the contiguity of their inquiries meant that there were many occasions on which science *was* culture (see Haraway 1991). In practical terms, there was perilously little difference in meaning between a priest's claim to AIDS counselors that medicine had scientifically proved that leading a Christian life was the only way to prevent death from AIDS[1] and an AIDS researcher's decree to fellow scientists that the epidemic would "kill everyone in Kilimanjaro with a certain lifestyle and leave the rest of us alone."[2] This sort of syncretism has also been observed in Ivory Coast (Caprara et al. 1993:1233) and Uganda. In Rakai, as in Kilimanjaro, an "understanding of the scientifically established chain of causation is then used as the foundation for a moral evaluation [of people with AIDS] based on their disregard of traditional family and communal values" (Barnett and Blaikie 1992:49).

Three cases of people who suffered from AIDS are presented at the end of this chapter. Their life stories point to the confusions and quandaries of those who actually confronted the disease in the early 1990s. With the oracular power of the X-ray, epidemiologic estimates of seroprevalence based on blood tests laid bare the scope of the HIV epidemic in the Chagga social body. Yet like the X-ray, these statistical snapshots removed all traces of the individual identities in whose blood the portrait of the epidemic was drawn with such seeming clarity. In the early 1990s there was as yet no culturally tangible frame of reference for the disease, no common folk epidemiology based on experience. What common cultural images and themes did exist were based more heavily upon expectation—not because AIDS was absent, but because by its very nature it was gradual, nebulous, and invisible to many people. Cultural expectations about disease and the diseased gave rise to a recapitulation of images of social and biological pathology in the personage of the *mhuni.* This personage served as an icon of contagion and thus allowed AIDS to betoken the embodiment of diseased development and cultural dislocation. The *mhuni,* like the *kijana* in "Hey, Listen!" was culturally substituted for the dogged ambiguities of actual experience and the characteristics of the real individuals who began to sicken and die from AIDS. In the skits discussed in the previous chapter, there was never a doubt about the progression of the narrative or about which characters had the virus. Every *mhuni* fell ill with AIDS and exhibited every gross sign and symptom thought to be associated with symptomatic disease, including fever, drastic weight loss, and dementia. In this respect, the KIWAKKUKI drama competition epitomized the way in which most public discourse about AIDS concerned shared expectations of the epidemic, not a collective experience of the disease.

## The Power and Appeal of Biomedicine in the Colonial Era

The synergy between popular and professional epidemiologies of AIDS in Kilimanjaro had its roots in a Chagga enthusiasm for Western medicine that paralleled the local commitment to churches and schools. Since shortly after its arrival, Western medicine has had an authoritative voice in local experience. Medicine—whether Western or African—has always been an instrument of social and cultural power through its capacity to define, act upon (and in), and claim authority over bodies, and thus over the persons residing therein (e.g., Comaroff 1993; Feierman 1985; Lyons 1992; Turner 1984; Vaughan 1991). In sub-Saharan Africa, colonial medicine was strategically positioned to act upon sectors of the population, including women, urban laboring populations, rural agricultural workers, migrant labor, and Christian converts (Curtin 1985; Hunt 1992; Packard 1989; Ranger 1981; Turshen 1984). To varying extents, biomedicine was aimed at all of these populations in Kilimanjaro during the twentieth century. At the same time, however, Chagga domesticated medicine in their own way. They engaged with Western medical epistemology in a critique of the *kihamba* regime, they enrolled medicine in the construction of new and "modern" adult identities, they went to clinics in droves, and they sought personal advancement through health as a profession.

Before the arrival of Western medicine, Chagga handled disease and personal disorder through a variety of techniques. Models of disease etiology, and explanations for injury and death, were similar to those found elsewhere in East and Central Africa. Disease, as a category of misfortune, was often held to be a somatic manifestation of social distress and indicated the malevolent agency of witches, transgressions against the ancestors, or the consequence of curses and maledictions sent by an antagonist. Witchcraft, sorcery, and curses were the most pronounced ways in which social inequalities and opprobrious human agency figured in the cause of disease and misfortune.[3] Chagga countered curses, witchcraft, and other illnesses with widely known herbal remedies or through recourse to healers, or *waganga* (singular: *mganga*), often from outside groups.[4] Among Chagga, the different types of medical experts include diviners, herbalists, midwives, and surgical (circumcision) specialists. Although recognized and revered, *waganga* have not been accorded particularly great political or religious status. They could be either male or female and were often selected by their parents to receive training; some acquired the power to divine through dreams or visions.[5] In addition to forms of healing indigenous to northern Tanzania, Islamic healing, which may have entered the mountain system with the arrival of coastal caravans, has become an important part of the medical pluralism of Kilimanjaro.

Biomedicine made a popular debut in Kilimanjaro in the late nineteenth century. Johnston (1886), for example, was sought out for medical attention in the 1880s, and clinical medicine had its first sustained presence on the mountain when German doctors arrived in 1889. Once established on the mountain in the 1890s, biomedicine made the Chagga objects of research, treatment, and policy. Through a familiar colonial rhetoric of differentiation and distinction, medical practice served to reify a view of traditional ways of life as primitive and unhealthy. This set the stage for practitioners of public health and hygiene to extend to Chagga the civilizing project of transforming Africans into a colonial image of healthy human beings. Through the same kind of "education of the senses" that was at work among Europeans at the end of the nineteenth century (Gay 1984; Haley 1978), the early medical missionaries read passive African bodies for signs of ill health in a broader project of evaluating African persons and cultures (Comaroff 1993; Setel 1991a; Vaughan 1991). Colonial authorities attempted to entice Africans into this "training for civilization" through promoting the active use of their bodies as well. In 1931, for example, football matches were organized in Kilimanjaro by the sanitary superintendent "in order to inculcate in the younger generation the love of healthy sport" (Bailey 1931:4). From the colonial perspective, medical research and treatment were primarily useful for maintaining a healthy labor force. Research tended to focus on the diseases most debilitating to productive labor; malaria, tuberculosis, and sleeping sickness were all the subjects of major medical research in Kilimanjaro in the twentieth century. Early health campaigns in the area included the production of lymph at Moshi hospital, the vaccination of thousands against smallpox in 1908, and the treatment of yaws. Reproduction was also an early concern; obstetric services were among the first specialist services offered to Chagga in the 1920s.

Tuberculosis prompted significant attention to African ways of life on the part of the colonial health sector in Kilimanjaro, a concern reinvigorated in the age of AIDS by the common association between HIV and tuberculosis infection. While the link between tuberculosis and a medical critique of African ways of life was more acutely articulated in places such as South African mines (Packard 1989), in Kilimanjaro it surfaced in connection with the unhealthiness of a growing population. Tuberculosis was said to be particularly common on the southern slopes because of the climate and the crowded living conditions (Clyde 1962:119). In 1930, more than 13,000 Africans in the Northern Province were tuberculin tested, revealing an incidence of eleven cases per thousand in parts of Kilimanjaro (Tanganyika Health Division 1963). In order to confirm infectious cases, the research director, Dr. Wilcocks, found it necessary to solicit the participation of residents of rural areas through the use of a portable X-ray: "He took the [X-ray] films with a portable machine in which the power was derived from a generator spun by the jacked-up rear wheel of his car, a current of 220 volts being developed. The tube was supported by a telescopic tripod placed above the chest of the patient, who as often as not lay in the grass by the side of the road. Even thirty years later the fear of witchcraft makes people in some districts reluctant to part with a drop of blood for a simple examination; Wilcocks must have been unusually persuasive to get his subjects to lie down under so imposing an apparatus as his portable X-ray" (Clyde 1962:120).

In this assessment, Clyde was obviously unable to appreciate that Africans might have had a culturally informed set of sensibilities about various bodily substances; it was probably fortunate for Dr. Wilcocks's research that he did not need stool samples from adult men. Nevertheless, the apparent compliance evinced by Chagga in the face of this particular colonial apparatus may attest more to an openness on their part to rethinking their embodied relationship to a rapidly changing social order than to the persuasiveness of the physician. Their eager uptake of medicine illustrates the zeal with which Chagga adopted new practices related to their bodies and consciously engaged in altering the cultural meaning of health and illness.

Many Chagga needed little or no persuasion at all to engage with biomedicine; they fairly flocked to clinics for treatment. That medical services were not only acceptable but also in demand is evident from the rapid growth of the sector in Kilimanjaro. Chagga readily accepted Western medicine, eventually making Moshi hospital (arguably) the busiest and largest in the Tanganyika Territory. The hospital in Moshi opened to paying African patients in 1922 after the district commissioner persuaded a group of chiefs to build the native wards at their own expense (Clyde 1962:115). An operating theater and office were added to the facility soon after. Outside Moshi, hospitals were established at Kilema and Machame early in the century. These facilities were ringed by four or five dispensaries. On the mountainside, European patent medicines were successfully sold in coffee co-operative stores from 1935 onward—over the objection of Lutheran missionaries, who had, until then, enjoyed a profitable monopoly over the products (TNA J.1.11841).

Meanwhile, inpatient and outpatient medical services were in demand at government and mission installations. Maternity services became available in the early 1920s and, as in Central Africa, they served the goal of "training African mothers for civilization" (Hunt 1992).[6] Chagga were heavy users of the Moshi hospital despite having to suffer appalling conditions, having to pay for treatment, and having to cook for inpatients.[7] By 1952 the hospital was inundated with African patients. Year after year, Medical Department Annual Reports ranked the hospital as one of the territory's busiest, stating that it suffered from continual overcrowding. In 1956, it had also become one of Tanganyika's biggest health installations, requiring an ancillary health infrastructure on the scale of that of Dar es Salaam—a city many times the size of Moshi.[8] In the late 1960s, the mountain and town were served by six hospitals, including a zonal referral hospital (KCMC) and a latticework of health stations and dispensaries operated by Catholic and Lutheran churches, and other private concerns. By this time, Mawenzi (the renamed Moshi hospital) alone saw more than more than 267,000 outpatients annually (Figure 6.1).

Given such active participation on the part of the local population, it is not difficult to see how biomedicine became important in the representational politics of development and social change in Kilimanjaro. Medicine aided a basic re-vision of ideas connecting persons, bodies, and culture in the mountain system. This process took the form of a critique of traditional mountainside life and was furthered by medicine's modern aura, the appeal of its clinical efficacy, and the fact that Chagga were as eager to become medical practitioners as medical subjects. In the 1930s, sanitary policy was used as a vehicle for directing a mixture of medical, moral, and educational criticism at local culture—first by Europeans and then by Chagga themselves. From the 1930s onward, the power of biomedicine as a symbolic system was exploited by people in Kilimanjaro in a new, medicalized language for describing their own social world to themselves. Through their partici-

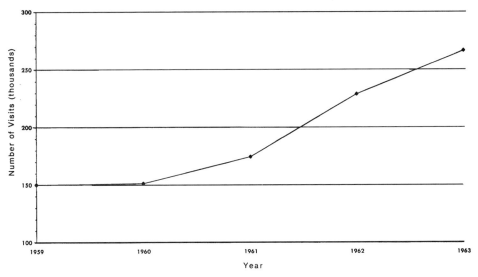

Figure 6.1. Outpatient visits to Mawenzi Hospital, 1959–63. (Source: Tanganyika Medical Department 1959–63)

pation in preventive health campaigns, disease control, obstetric services, and nutritional and sanitation surveillance, they became part of
an institutionalized mode of representing distinction and differentiation that turned in upon their own social body.

The power of biomedicine as both a representational device and an
instrument of direct social control became evident in a number of are-
nas. Perhaps the clearest example in the archival record is to be found
in documents relating to the recruitment of African District Sanitary
Inspectors (ADSIs) during the 1930s. The ADSIs represented a subtle
and hegemonic exercise of medical power in the re-vision of "tribal
life" and in the creation of social knowledge about unhealthy practices
in the Chagga social body on the mountainside. Such medical construc-
tions of "cultural predisposition" to disease among Africans were a
feature of colonial medical practice throughout British-held Africa
(Vaughan 1991:46).[9] These inspectors were engaged in the surveillance
of their home communities, simultaneously carrying colonial policy
into the *vihamba* and carrying out the visualized signs to back up the
disparagement of Chagga ways of life. During a series of visits to
ADSIs working in the *kihamba* zone, the sanitary superintendent, B. T.
Bailey, marshaled facts and figures for a medical diatribe against
Chagga not under the influence of missionaries. Traditional banana-
fiber or grass-thatched huts were unsatisfactory, while "many mission
converts under the supervision of their teachers build much better
dwellings of stone or sun-dried brick, which are adequately lighted
and ventilated" (Bailey 1931:2). Likewise, the bodies of nonmission
Chagga were "filthy for the greater part of the year. . . . The mission
converts generally present a better appearance" (1931:4). Ultimately,
Bailey targeted almost everything that was customary to *kihamba* life:
burial customs, the habit of men defecating in the banana groves, traditional building materials and techniques, water-conservation methods,
modes of dress, methods of distributing and cooking meat, and child-
rearing practices all were designated for a sanitizing encounter with
the hygienic enterprise of ADSIs and the health department.

"Propaganda," as the medical department called their health education efforts, was an important technique in this covert struggle over
reconstructing Chagga persons and instilling in them a modern, West-
ernized sense of embodiment. Political leaders, churchgoers, and students participated in this project by distributing handbills encouraging
vaccination and other "healthy" habits. Disney films about hookworm
and malaria transmission were shown to several audiences, and in the
1950s, a large pilot health-education project was mounted near Mwika

that used slides, photographs, posters, and seminars—not dissimilar in form to multimedia AIDS prevention efforts launched forty years later. Chagga leaders were enrolled in support of the formal health-care sector. District leaders willingly enlisted to report cases of infectious disease, including anthrax, smallpox, and pertussis from all over the mountain. Through the judicial power that they retained under the British, *mangis* enforced public health codes and collected fines levied on butchers for selling rotten meat traced to them in cases of food poisoning.

A further dimension of medicine's transformative effects in Kilimanjaro lay in its ability to go beyond merely representing the disorder and unhealthiness of tradition and toward promoting the active construction of new subjectivities. Medicine and its agents, both European and African, worked to encourage the internalization of an ideology of what modern and healthy Africans were meant to do: how they were meant to work, dress, house themselves, and feed their children. This ideology was taken up by urban residents, who showed a predilection for assimilating new, medicalized ethics of parenthood. A South African ethnographer visiting Moshi noted the growing popularity of bottle feeding: "For their babies, they even take graduated bottles of European manufacture for the milk which they give their children, because they can read from these bottles the amount of milk consumed" (Lehmann 1941:341). Whereas Vaughan (1991) has found that Africans were rarely anything but the objects of the medical enterprise in Africa, one set of arrangements between a hospital, a school, and Moshi social clubs is particularly illustrative of how biomedicine worked hand in glove with other colonial institutions in an effort to instill in Chagga a new self-consciousness, to reeducate their native sensibilities. In 1949, at the Kibong'oto Tuberculosis Hospital and Sanatorium, the salubrious effects of "occupational therapy" (read: "industrial-style labor") and medical attention represented a concern for effecting not just a physical cure, but a transformation in the consciousness of patients. These activities constituted an orchestrated effort to foster new subjectivities among Africans through the medium of their bodies.

> Weaving was started in January after the purchase of one large thirty-six-inch loom and a number of smaller looms, which were supposed to be bed looms, but they could only be used by a small number of patients as the vast majority were too ill to take advantage of them. The knitting of scarves and pullovers was continued by male and female African patients, who were paid a percentage of the profits arising from their sale as a reward for their labour.

By the end of the year, a gross profit of 1,400/- had been made on articles woven and knitted. Two contracts with Machame Girls' School for uniforms, underwear and bedding were fulfilled. Tin work was continued, but scrap tin was difficult to obtain, and all that the workers were able to gain was a little pocket money. Towards the close of the year, leather work was started, being developed through patients who had been cobblers, and this is gaining in popularity. . . . The hospital is greatly indebted to the staff and children of Machame Girls' School who arranged a fete to raise money to assist in the work of occupational therapy, and to the Moshi branch of the Women's Service League who organized a garden party also in aid of the hospital, whilst special gifts of sweets, cigarettes and food were presented to the patients at Christmas by the Red Cross Society. (Tanganyika Territory Medical Department 1949:15–16)

Chagga were not just willing consumers of and participants in the practice of medicine in the Tanganyika Territory, they also wanted to become its agents. From the late 1920s onward, Chagga sought employment in health care. Nearly every recorded request for an increase in Western medical services was accompanied by an equally explicit appeal for employment of young people in the health sector. Through the demand for services and the demand for jobs, different sectors of society effectively appropriated elements of biomedicine to their own ends— at the same time that it was engaged in transforming them. Local health workers from Kilimanjaro first acquired medical training in large numbers in 1927 at the hospital in Kibong'oto, where they were taught to perform collapsed-lung therapy for tuberculosis treatment (Clyde 1962). From then on, there were a number of occupational categories in the health sector that appealed to more and more young people. In the 1930s, *mangis* requested training for their subjects as sanitary inspectors in order to "help raise people up to a civilized condition" (TNA 5.312), and schoolchildren went so far as to write letters to the district commissioner begging for "the opportunity to study Public Health work" (TNA 5.312).

In the biomedical encounter with Africa, local medical practice has often been described by public health practitioners as being firmly, even maddeningly entrenched—as an obstacle to development. As Schoepf has noted, the effect of this perception in international health practice has been the position that "culture is viewed as an obstacle to change. . . . Simplifications of cultural phenomena [have served] to cast blame upon peoples who are perceived as 'different' for the failures of medical knowledge or health care delivery systems" (1992:356). Chagga leaders were impatient to avail themselves of modern services and seemed at a loss without the facilities and the jobs their presence would entail. Those who might reasonably have been expected to be among the most culturally conservative were in fact in the vanguard of pushing for change. *Mangi* Marealle wrote in the 1940s that since the departure of a government sanitary inspector from Marangu, "the filth has overtaken us and the latrines are not made clean. Other places aren't built in such a way as to avoid stomach diseases . . . that person or someone else to do that work should be returned to us" (TNA 5.312). As they did in the case of education and the establishment of schools (Lawuo 1980:85), Chagga formed pressure groups to lobby simultaneously for health services and for employment. The *mangi*s appealed for the construction of a training facility for medical auxiliaries in Kilimanjaro, complaining that the school in Mwanza on the shores of Lake Victoria was too far away and that its lowland location was too unhealthy for Chagga youth. Strikingly, leaders even went so far as to foretell the stagnation of development unless more curative services were provided by a professional class of Chagga to other Chagga:

> *Medical Attention.* We need more attention to combat the many diseases which are now spreading; more government hospitals and dispensaries should therefore be built. It is true that there are some Mission hospitals, but these are not in any way enough. . . . There might be a question of staff: at the moment we have many of our boys in military medical corps, who, when demobilised, will be found very useful in this direction. The Native Treasury could be enabled by financial assistance from the government in erecting and staffing these dispensaries. . . . Many Chagga youngsters are willing to get trained as nursing orderlies and dressers, and those of a higher standard still as medical auxiliaries. . . . Progress cannot be expected of a people with unhealthy bodies. (TNA J.1.11841, letter from Chagga Chiefs to Provincial Commissioner, 26 Jan. 1946)

Overall, however, employment in government medical services in rural areas was only open to a lucky few. From 1960 to 1965, of an estimated 2,666 Africans employed in education, health, administration, and agricultural extension work, roughly 180 had jobs in the health sector, while the vast majority (2,380) worked in education (estimates based on Moore 1986:136). Regardless of the small actual number of practitioners, it was clear that medicine was a high-profile institution that offered some hope of accommodating a few of the youth who required new kinds of productive adult lives.

As should be clear, this increasingly medicalized outlook not only represented an alternative and modern approach to matters of ill health and hygiene, but it was also intimately connected with what local actors perceived to be their push toward development and civilization. As agents of biomedicine, young, salaried health workers felt themselves to be in the forefront of this charge. This attitude was part of the colonial medical service from at least the 1930s, as can be seen from the comments of health workers such as the native sanitary orderly who, while investigating typhoid in Moshi, commented that "the Chaggas are living unsanitarily. I taught them what to do on their premises" (TNA 5.12.5). Some years later, rural health auxiliaries elsewhere in Tanzania looked forward to the task of "educating all the people in rural areas to know what is good for their future and what is not," and "to direct them on how they would perform their life" (van Etten 1976: 121). The zenith of local linkages between medicine and development under colonialism was probably the establishment of the Chagga Medical Executive Committee in 1950. The committee consisted of a chief, an African physician, and the district commissioner. Again, the goals were to provide both more medical services and more jobs for Chagga.[10] Local dispensary staff wrote to the colonial government on behalf of the proposed committee and extolled the notion of Chagga control over preventive and curative services for sexually transmitted diseases. The committee "will be a great step towards civilization and progress," one dispensary worker stated (TNA 5.12.12, undated letter from Roderick Ndefungio).

Thus, in the colonial era, medicine operated within Chagga culture on a number of discrete yet interconnected levels. First, it was part of the colonial package of church, school, and clinic that Chagga readily took to. In doing so, Chagga took on board biomedical assessments of the healthiness and unhealthiness of *kihamba* life, and made a "cultural commitment"—to borrow Moore's term—to altering perceptions of health and bodily order. States of health, in turn, were increasingly thought to reflect levels of development, thereby giving medical practitioners, both African and European, special authority and status in this development-oriented population. Despite the contradictions noted in the previous chapter, medicine has retained an authoritative voice in cultural dialogues about social change. The emergence of a category of illness called "diseases of development" *(magonjwa ya maendeleo)* attests to this. This domain of disorder included AIDS, smoking, diabetes, obesity, alcoholism, and hypertension. A booklet about the subject, entitled *Magonjwa ya Maendeleo* (Mpensela 1990), was readily available at newsstands in Moshi. The booklet was festooned with images of *kitambi*-weighted businessmen. This iconic image of questionable *tabia* and *tamaa* became linked to a whole category of diseases associated with the negative effects of development, not just AIDS.

## Epidemiologic Rumors and Experiential Facts
### The Urban Disease Model

The scientific epidemiology of AIDS in East Africa continued in this authoritative mode. In practice, it depended upon the specialized application of technology (in the form of blood tests) and centered upon the nexus of the bodies of young men and women in urban locations with the epidemic. Not insignificantly, most testing facilities were located in urban areas, which meant that the objects of inquiry were near at hand. Three pieces of technology were the mechanisms through which the bodies (or, more specifically, the blood) of Tanzanians were used in the epidemiologic production of signs of AIDS: ELISA tests, so-called quick tests like HIV-Check and Testpack, and Western Blot blood tests (see Barin and Claire 1994). These tools of epidemiologic practice lay at the heart of medical authority over AIDS, and their importance to understanding HIV/AIDS in the context of a resource-poor health system such as existed in Tanzania cannot be overemphasized. Without the provision of these highly specific and sensitive diagnostic tools to local medical institutions by large donor organizations, the scope of the epidemic would have been nearly impossible to gauge.[11] In their absence, researchers would have had to rely nearly exclusively on much less specific and sensitive clinical case definitions of AIDS—a very inadequate basis for estimating the prevalence of a viral syndrome that only becomes symptomatic after years of infection. HIV-antibody test technologies literally illuminated the epidemic in the blood of thousands of Africans. Yet the pigment-seeking beams could be focused only on blood brought to or collected at the facilities where the technologies were installed. This fact, and the related logistical and ethical issues such as the conditions under which blood samples could be collected and tested, led to an important geographical fall-off effect in knowledge about the first several years of HIV/AIDS in East Africa; the further away one traveled from centers of intensive and technology-based research (i.e., capital cities and a few specific rural locations), the less could be said with certainty about HIV in African populations.

African cities, particularly capital cities like Kampala, Kigali, Kinshasa, Nairobi, and Dar es Salaam, were fundamental to an urban disease model of HIV and AIDS in the 1980s and 1990s (see, e.g., Kreiss et al. 1986; Mann et al. 1986; Merlin et al. 1987). In a chapter entitled

"The African Source" in a book about the history of AIDS, one observer engaged in remarkable hyperbole: "The main characteristic of the internal African population movements was a rush to the cities. . . . Small wonder, then, that today Kinshasa, Mombasa, Nairobi, Kigali, Kampala, Bangui, Lusaka—these megalopolises [sic] of the Third World where poverty and ghastly hygienic conditions reign over all—form the nurseries of the AIDS virus. . . . Liberated from the yoke of behavioral expectations imposed by the traditions of small village groups, the inhabitants of large cities abandoned themselves heartily to elaborate sexual play. . . . In such a new social situation the HIV virus found a propitious setting for its propagation" (Grmek 1990:176).

African cities were seen as shaping the course of the epidemic in advance of detectable patterns of infection in rural areas. According to the model, HIV first became established among urban populations and subsequently spread to peripheral areas via mobile sectors of the population, primarily along major transport routes (Chin 1991:15; de Zalduondo, Msamanga, and Chen 1989). The assumption that "the spread of HIV seems to be faster in urban areas, where sexual promiscuity is more common than in rural areas" (Merlin et al. 1987:507), typified some of the sociomedical assumptions inherent in this formulation of the East and Central African epidemic. "The character of sexual relations within major cities," it was argued, "will continue to determine the prevalence of infection throughout nations because a rural epidemic will not be able to sustain itself until a significant proportion of the rural population is infected" (Larson 1989:717).[12]

Through the first decade of AIDS in Africa, the quality of the social research upon which epidemiologists drew was hampered by the continued reliance upon "second-hand data" rather than upon original research, designed and conducted specifically to comprehend AIDS (Obbo 1995:12). The public health community, which stressed up-to-the-minute knowledge about the clinical pathology and molecular biology of the virus, seemed content to cite ethnographic and historical accounts of African sexuality conducted twenty to forty years before without considering the shortcomings of such material in the face of one or more generations of enormous social, political-economic, and cultural change across the continent.[13] The representations of epidemiologists of AIDS as a disorder of the African social body were directly descended from those of other diseases during the colonial era (see Packard 1989; Vaughan 1991).

On one hand, African culture was causative of disease; it was blamed for starting a global pandemic through dubiously argued theories of exotic cultural practices that effected a simian to human transmission of a human-compatible, mutating retrovirus (see Rushing 1995:45–50). To make matters worse, Africans were portrayed as being especially susceptible to disease through polygyny and a "loosened" sexual morality generated by their inability to cope adequately with modernity and change. African cities were written into the urban disease model of AIDS as spaces of sexual "promiscuity," devoid of "traditional" cultural restraint in sexual matters. Rural areas, on the other hand, with their supposedly tradition-bound peasant populations, were thought to have remained relatively untouched by the epidemic. Africans in towns, it appeared, "got sick essentially because they had forgotten who they were" (Vaughan 1991:202). "Those who [threw off] the moral and material shackles of the old rural milieu and tribal customs now fell into the trap of a relentless new social system. One of the results of this release was a wildfire of classic sexually transmitted diseases," opined Grmek (1990:179). Others offered a narrative of the bright lights of cities and their Western ways attracting women like moths to the flame: "Exotic sexual practices are unknown in traditional settings. Traditional society tolerates and indeed encourages multiple wives (sexual partners). In traditional society, prostitution is a perversion. . . . Western influence through acculturation in the 60s and 70s has brought on significant changes in sexual ethos in urban centers. . . . Girls migrated to urban centers or to neighboring countries where they were 'faceless' to engage in prostitution [in cities]. They were not considered deviants. They gained respectability when they visited their communities (villages)" (Pela and Platt 1989:4).

In village settings, where Africans supposedly retained self-knowledge, practices such as scarification, circumcision, the levirate, and healing modalities that entailed cutting or injection were vilified as "cultural risk factors" (Hrdy 1987) in the same way that Chagga lifeways were criticized by Bailey as unhygienic earlier in the century.[14] This quest for "the peculiarities of African behavior" structured much of the early medical research (Packard and Epstein 1991:771). The weaving together by medical scientists of a partial epidemiologic knowledge base and a simplistic concept of culture linked to "racial" otherness into a narrative of "cause" in Africa paralleled the early construction by Americans of AIDS as a Haitian disease (Sabatier 1988:45; Farmer 1992:208–28), as well as many previous Euro-American associations of "race" with pathology among slaves and immigrants of African or Afro-Caribbean descent (Gilman 1985).

The existence of several historical cases that have demonstrated the sustainability of rural epidemics of sexually transmitted diseases in Africa in tandem with those in urban locations (e.g., Jochelson 1991; Vaughan 1991:129ff.; Kaijage 1993) should call into question the ability of an urban model in its conventional form to account for the complexity of the interaction among mobile young people, a new disease entity, and the variety of sexual and reproductive networks in East and Central Africa. Even in countries where vastly more resources have been brought to bear on studying and monitoring the epidemic, the interpretation of prevalence and incidence rates "is an imprecise science at best" (Altman 1994). The unique population dynamics and economic histories throughout regions and subregions in East Africa make the fundamental variables for epidemiological inquiry in the urban disease model (*who* was in urban areas and for how long, *where* they were from and where they moved on to, and *when* exposure and infection occurred) very difficult to operationalize. These variables fluctuate widely given historical and cultural variability in patterns of productive and sexual relations from city to city, and variations in the relationship of cities to their hinterlands (Cooper 1983). The confidence with which a general model can be assembled for East and Central Africa is diminished still further by the inherent ambiguity about the onset of HIV infection (Benenson 1990:1–7; Volderbing and Cohen 1990:4.1.1–3; Ainsworth and Over 1994). In the absence of baseline blood tests and detailed sexual histories, it would be nearly impossible to determine where and when individuals became infected.

Although there was an awareness among epidemiologists that some rural locations, such as the border area of Tanzania and Uganda, represented a wholly different dynamic from that of cities (Mann 1987:114), for most of the 1980s, the evidence to assess HIV risk among urban versus nonurban dwellers within individual regions and to gauge the risks associated with duration of urban residence was scanty. In the early 1990s, in both Arusha and Mwanza regions, samples were drawn from among urban, semi-urban or "roadside," and rural communities (Barongo et al. 1992; Mnyika et al. 1994). In Arusha, only those in urban areas defined as of low socioeconomic status had significantly higher risk relative to rural dwellers after controlling for other risk variables. No information was provided about the duration of residence of these individuals, although it should be noted that the poorest urban dwellers are frequently the most mobile. Some epidemiologists, however, were aware of the fact that social conditions could be distorting their understandings of the spatial dynamics of the epidemic (Barongo et al. 1992).

Results from a survey of STDs among rural youth in Kilimanjaro suggested that residence in towns was not a factor in generating rates of infection comparable to many urban "risk groups" (Kessy 1995), and elsewhere in Africa parity in STD rates between towns and hinterlands has long been documented (Jochelson 1991). Furthermore, self-reported sexual behavior in the nationally representative samples of the Demographic and Health Survey flatly contradicted the widespread presumption that multipartner sexuality was more a feature of urban areas than of rural: "Except among urban formerly married women, the results suggest that those who reside in rural areas are more likely than urban residents to have multiple sexual partners or to be married to someone who does" (Rutenberg, Blanc, and Kapiga 1994:192–93). Although many writers subscribed to the protective / rural / traditional notion of sexual risk in Africa (e.g., Pela and Platt 1989), Tanzania was not unique in having little or no measured differences in self-reported sexual behavior in urban and rural areas. A cross-national review of WHO survey data resulted in the finding that "urban-rural disparities were less pronounced than expected and there was a strong correlation between behavior in rural and urban areas" (Caraël, Cleland, and Ingham 1994:170; also Orubuloye, Caldwell, and Caldwell 1992:287).

At this point it is worth emphasizing that having multiple partners is not a risk for HIV transmission per se. The risk is having unprotected sex with multiple partners. Given that behavior in the early years of the epidemic "must be seen in a condomless context" (Obbo 1995:81), however, these nearly amounted to the same thing. In Africa, where there has been historically low condom use, poor treatment of STDs, and a general preference for penetrative vaginal sex (as opposed to types of sexual or erotic contact that might be less risky), multipartner sexuality among some can be statistically related to increased risk of being infected with HIV. Such correlations led some in Kilimanjaro to the mistaken implication that having multiple partners is inherently risky. In the emerging consciousness of risk, as we have seen, it was thought that certain "types" of people represented a threat. Some people, in fact, began to define risky sex as "not necessarily sex with several partners, but sex with the 'wrong' partner which basically [meant] sex with a foreign man or woman or with prostitutes" (MUTAN 1993: 7–8).

The question of urban versus rural risk behavior aside, an even more basic question to be asked of the urban disease model has to do with the relative weight given to urban versus rural prevalence figures.[15] While urban prevalence and incidence rates may be critical for projecting the effect of the epidemic on more highly educated women and men, and upon econometric measures of productivity (Ainsworth and Over 1994), they do not necessarily illuminate the trajectory of the epidemic or inform the responses of local populations to it. They also may hide the scope of the rural epidemic. Despite rapid (though slowing) urban growth rates, roughly 80 percent of the Tanzanian population were categorized as rural residents in 1988 (United Republic of Tanzania 1992:5). Thus, HIV prevalence rates in rural areas that were a fraction of those in cities represented a far greater total number of incipient AIDS cases. For example, in Kilimanjaro region about 9 percent of the regional population were enumerated (and assumed to reside) in urban areas (approximately 104,700 persons), 14 percent were residing in areas designated as "mixed" (158,500) and 76.3 percent were living in rural areas (845,400). Applying sentinel incidence rates to the respective populations of men aged fifteen to sixty-four and women aged ten to fifty-four yields a rough estimate of 5,000 HIV infections in Moshi and other urban areas, and 28,000 in rural districts (Figure 6.2). Thus, there may have been up to six times more infected rural residents than urban residents in Kilimanjaro in the early 1990s. Furthermore, each increase in prevalence of 1 percent in rural areas would have represented vastly more HIV infections than equivalent increases in urban locations.

The urban disease model in its straightforward application in much of the epidemiology of AIDS in Africa has oversimplified urban-rural dynamics from early on in the epidemic, giving a false impression that

a. HIV seroprevalence rates for urban versus rural antenatal clinic attenders, 1992

b. Percentage of HIV cases living in urban versus rural areas, 1993

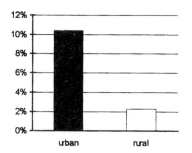
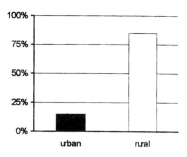

Figure 6.2. Two ways of representing the urban and rural AIDS epidemics in Kilimanjaro. (Sources: (a) Klepp et al. 1995; NACP 1992. (b) Author's calculations based on HIV seroprevalence rates for male and female blood donors in 1993 in Klepp et al. 1995 and Census 1988. Estimates are based on census figures for men aged 15–64 and women aged 10–59.)

rural areas had an early window of safety. Even if the studies conducted in large cities had represented a general set of urban dynamics in the East and Central African epidemic, one must still consider to what extent this research was applicable to smaller cities and towns, and to an understanding of the heterogeneity of risk that has emerged as a hallmark of the longitudinal picture of HIV and AIDS. In rural areas of Rakai, Uganda, for example, researchers reported an overall seroprevalence of 12.6 percent for all adults over thirteen years of age, yet the rates among sample clusters in the survey varied enormously, from 1.2 percent to 52.8 percent (Wawer et al. 1991:1303).[16] In order to account for such variations, an analytic epidemiologic history of AIDS must be viewed in the context of a spatiotemporal continuum built around social and cultural networks.

From this standpoint, the epidemic could be seen to as spreading through a series of overlapping "socio-geographic networks" (Wallace 1991; Obbo 1993) or interconnected "risk foci" (Barnett and Blaikie 1992:69ff.) in which cities represent especially concentrated points of intersection for sexually active people who are tied in with other networks in other locations. The explanatory assumptions built into the urban disease model invert a reasoning process that ought to center, as Barnett and Blakie argue, on "an understanding of the social, economic, and historical factors that have produced this particular spatial distribution of risk." This spatiality has nothing to with inherent effects of urbanity per se. Barongo et al. hinted at this point in their interpretation of higher HIV seroprevalence in urban Mwanza than in rural areas. "It is unclear whether seroprevalence is higher in towns because HIV-1 infection was introduced earlier, or because risk behaviour is different" (1992:1526). Thus, communities in which risk behavior takes place ought not to be conceptualized as traditional versus modern, promiscuous versus monogamous, or urban versus rural. Rather, sexual risk can be understood to vary for individuals according to context, and to require a model that accounts for the character of risky contact among infected and noninfected persons in the early stages of a lengthy epidemic, a political economy of itinerancy, interaction with cash economies, and social dislocation. Unfortunately, connections between a contextualized model of sexuality, different modes of mobility, and risk of HIV have remained largely uninvestigated. Instead, epidemiologists both popular and professional have tended to operate with loose and inaccurate dichotomous categories, variants of the urban disease model.

In the Kagera region of western Tanzania, however, the urban disease model never gained ascendancy. Stories of the experience of AIDS from this part of the country informed a great many epidemiologies of expectation around Tanzania. In Kagera, political economy, youth, and vulnerability to and blame for the epidemic all found expression in local discourse (de Zalduondo, Msamanga, and Chen 1989; Kaijage 1989; Lwihula 1988; Weiss 1993). In the early 1980s, a fatal wasting syndrome was "first noticed in young businessmen . . . trafficking illegal and scarce goods" (Lwihula 1988:3). One of the earliest colloquial names for this condition stemmed from its perceived association with the "quick-money" lifestyles of these young men: "Restrictions on foreign-currency exchange and imports and the scarcity of essential household commodities as well as luxury goods in the 1970s and early 1980s increased incentives for people to travel and trade with countries where goods were in greater supply. Before AIDS was called 'Slim,' it was referred to as 'Juliana' in Tanzania, named after a brand of illegally imported clothing that for awhile was a status symbol among young men who were successful in the illicit cross-border trade. Unlike the majority of the population, whose subsistence activities and cash-crop production were disrupted in the late 1970s and early 1980s, the Juliana traders had cash and access to valued goods that could not be obtained locally for any price" (de Zalduondo, Msamanga, and Chen 1989:183–84).

The Juliana nickname for AIDS could hardly tie its cultural meanings more closely to processes of commodification, importation, and heightened acquisitive desires. This epithet implied a folk epidemiology of AIDS in Kagera built upon qualitative notions of sociogeographic networks in which both the young Juliana traders and older elite businessmen moving between Kampala and Nairobi were seen to be at risk (Weiss 1993:24). As the epidemic progressed, the emphasis shifted to a different gendered axis, and local actors began to stress the role of female desire and itinerancy in the spread of the epidemic (Weiss 1993:24).

## HIV in Kilimanjaro: The Epidemiology of Expectation

In various forms, the urban model was shared by many informants and medical researchers in Kilimanjaro. This was in line with the established wisdom that "a major cause of the African AIDS epidemic has been social dislocation due to rapid urbanization" (Larson 1989:719). In Kilimanjaro, however, this formulation is more accurately put the other way round—as rapid urbanization due to social (and demographic) dislocation. Although there were few longitudinal studies in Africa that revealed an unambiguous pattern in the epidemic, from the perspective of epidemiologists, the urban disease model bridged available local data and expectations about the regional trajectory of AIDS. Residents of certain sections of Moshi appeared to be more prone to infection than others: "The pattern of HIV in this town varies considerably from one place to another with the highest prevalence near the market area" (Nkya et al. 1988a). This statement was not merely epidemiological observation, but it also confirmed the presumed symbiosis of social and medical disorder in specific locations culturally associated with subversive sexuality. Taken as a whole, however, the serological studies conducted in Kilimanjaro between 1987 and 1993 indicated a complex and diverse engagement with the AIDS epidemic, "a mosaic of disparate data" rather than "a monolithic blight" (de Zalduondo, Msamanga, and Chen 1989:166).

The first case of AIDS in Kilimanjaro region was diagnosed at the Kilimanjaro Christian Medical Center (KCMC) in March 1984. Tests of frozen sera, however, indicated that HIV was present in northern Tanzania since at least 1979 (Howlett and Nkya 1987:1). In 1984 Kagera, Tabora, and Kilimanjaro were the only three regions in Tanzania reporting cases of AIDS to the Ministry of Health. They were certainly not the only regions affected by HIV; after the establishment of the National AIDS Task Force in the Ministry of Health in 1985, all twenty mainland regions reported cases. By 1987, cases were being identified at KCMC at roughly the same rate as at Muhimbili Medical Center, the university's teaching hospital in Dar es Salaam (Howlett et al. 1988; Howlett, Nkya, and Mmuni 1987). In 1989, the NACP implemented a centralized, computerized case-reporting system that brought a degree of improvement to data collection. The forms, however, were not used at all health facilities where AIDS cases were being diagnosed (Klepp, Ngaliwa, and Ole-Kingori 1993:73; author's field notes).[17]

Because of uncertainties in the national picture of the epidemic in the early 1990s, it is difficult to know precisely how Kilimanjaro fit into the broader context of AIDS in Tanzania as a whole. In 1992 the NACP ranked Kilimanjaro as the seventh most severely AIDS-affected region on the mainland, with a cumulative case rate of 134.2 per 100,000 population (NACP 1992:15); by 1994 it had climbed to fifth, and by 1997 it was third (NACP 1994:22, 1997:6).[18] Yet over the period from 1987 to 1997, the region ranked sixteenth in seroprevalence among male blood donors, and twelfth among female blood donors (NACP 1997:19–20). Such a disparity in case reporting and seroprevalence among sentinel groups suggests that the detection of people with AIDS has been much better in Kilimanjaro than elsewhere in the country, or that many people with AIDS were coming home to die in Kilimanjaro, or both. The idea that large numbers of infected Chagga were returning from elsewhere in Tanzania after becoming ill with clinical AIDS fit with the cultural preferences of people to die and be buried on their land and their obvious needs for care during the terminal stages of illness. However, it also bolstered fears about how the epidemic might spread in Kilimanjaro.

During the 1980s, most of the epidemiological and clinical information about AIDS in Kilimanjaro was produced through the joint efforts of an expatriate physician, William Howlett, and a Tanzanian microbiologist, Watoki Nkya, at KCMC.[19] From 1989 to 1995, the joint Tanzanian-Norwegian AIDS Project, MUTAN, conducted many long-term research and intervention projects in Kilimanjaro and Arusha regions (see Klepp, Biswalo, and Talle 1995). After 1991, MUTAN was responsible for most AIDS- and STD-related research and for monitoring the epidemic in Kilimanjaro and Arusha on behalf of the Ministry of Health. Between 1987 and 1993, HIV/AIDS studies were performed among selected sample populations in Kilimanjaro, and sentinel surveillance of pregnant women and blood donors was established. Table 6.1 summarizes data for all serological studies and surveillance (excluding those among hospital inpatients) conducted from 1987 through 1993. Overall it seems clear that the epidemic was growing steadily from year to year. The best-defined trends in HIV increase appeared to be among women tested in Moshi. HIV seroprevalence among pregnant women seen at an antenatal clinic at the regional hospital rose from 1.0 percent in 1987 to 11.0 percent in 1992, more than doubling each year. Among female bar workers in Moshi, rates rose from 11.0 percent in 1987 to 32.6 percent in 1992, an addition of nearly 4 percentage points per year. There were no discernible trends among urban blood donors, and there were no time-series data collected on men other than male bar workers (which showed no trend). Among blood donors at rural hospitals, there was a clear trend of rising HIV prevalence, which increased by 0.46 percent per year between 1988 and 1992. No time-series data exist for other rural populations.

In 1988, Nkya and colleagues (Nkya et al. 1988a:1) presented a paper at the International Conference on AIDS in Stockholm in which they spoke of conditions in Kilimanjaro as giving an "impression of an urban disease model" for the spread of AIDS. They based their impressions on the prevalence of HIV among random samples of adults in

Table 6.1 Summary of HIV Prevalence Studies in Kilimanjaro, 1987–93 (in percentages, N in parentheses)

| | 1987 | 1988 | 1989 | 1990 | 1991 | 1992 | 1993 |
|---|---|---|---|---|---|---|---|
| **Urban** | | | | | | | |
| Self-identified prostitutes | 58.0 (51)[11] | 64.1 (65)[11] | 62.7 (51)[11] | 69.0[f] (45)[4] | 71.4[f] (35)[11] | — | — |
| Female bar workers | 11.0 (225)[1] | 21.0 (NA)[6] | — | — | — | 32.6 (426)[12] | — |
| Male bar workers | 5.0 (205)[1] | 5.0 (NA)[6] | — | — | — | 6.8 (340)[12] | — |
| Pregnant women | 1.0 (180)[1] | — | — | — | 7.5 (600)[10] | 11.0 (418)[10] | — |
| Men | — | — | 2.5 (200)[7] | — | — | — | — |
| Urban population | 7.3 (1,365)[2] | — | — | — | — | — | — |
| **Semi-rural or "roadside"** | | | | | | | |
| Men, 15–30 | — | — | — | — | 3.4 (NA)[6] | — | — |
| Women, 20–24 | — | — | — | — | 5.8 (NA)[6] | — | — |
| Women, 25–30 | — | — | — | — | 8.5 (NA)[6] | — | — |
| **Rural** | | | | | | | |
| Pregnant woman | — | — | — | — | 2.3 (128)[5] | 6.4 (251)[13] | 15.8 (101)[13] |
| Rural population | 0.2 (496)[1] | — | — | — | — | — | — |
| **Blood donors** | | | | | | | |
| Urban blood donors[a] | 7.0 (285)[1] | 4.9 (NA)[8] | 3.8 (NA)[8] | 2.8 (1,692)[9] | 4.2 (1,844)[9] | 3.2 (1,192)[9] | 5.0[b] (1,479)[12] |
| Urban blood donors[c] | 3.9 (NA)[6] | 4.4 (389)[9] | 1.7 (1,594)[9] | 1.9 (929)[9] | 3.1 (777)[9] | 3.0 (538)[9] | 3.3[e] (264)[13] |
| Urban blood donors[d] | — | 0.9 (440)[9] | 2.2 (782)[9] | 2.7 (1,977)[9] | 2.9 (2,066)[9] | 3.2 (1,607)[9] | 3.9 (2,085)[12] |

Source: [1]Nkya et al. 1987; [2]Nkya et al. 1988; [3]Howlett et al. nd; [4]Nkya et al. 1991; [5]NACP 1992; [6]MUTAN 1993; [7]Howlett et al. 1989; [8]Klepp et al. 1993; [9]Seha et al. 1992; [10]MUTAN unpublished data, 1993; [11]K. I. Klepp, unpublished data; [12]Klepp et al. 1994; [13]NACP 1994.
[a] Kilimanjaro Christian Medical Center.
[b] This figure is a composite of blood donors from KCMC and Mawenzi hospitals.
[c] Mawenzi Regional Hospital.
[d] Rural hospitals.
[e] Male blood donors only.
[f] Sample size less than 50.

Moshi and two rural locations, ten and fifteen kilometers from the center of town: 7.3 percent of the urban residents were found to be HIV-positive, while none of the rural residents were infected. To the researchers, these results suggested a mechanism for the spread of AIDS that involved "infected pools of people and mobile transmitters. The infected pools which are established in major towns or affected countries include the prostitutes and barmaids. . . . The mobile transmitters mainly include the truck drivers and young businessmen" (Nkya et al. 1988a:6).

The authors did not claim more than suggestive results from this exercise and made the critical observation that the study, "while not comprehensive shows that adjacent groups chosen on the basis of their geographical location may show enormous variation in seropositivity" (1988a:7). Nkya and colleagues' modified urban disease model for AIDS in northern Tanzania began to evoke the notion of sociogeographic networks. At the time, however, there was not a sufficient number of studies conducted elsewhere in the region to allow a more cogent interpretation of the spread of the epidemic. Versions of this impressionistic urban disease model were contained in subsequent publications by these authors (e.g., Nkya et al. 1988b). Furthermore, the interpretations must have informed early AIDS education and information in Kilimanjaro region. KCMC staff, primarily William Howlett, gave at least twenty-eight informational lectures to various audiences on AIDS and AIDS prevention in the Moshi area between 1986 and 1988 (William Howlett, personal papers).[20] The talks were given to health-care workers, at schools, to women's organizations, at local conferences and workshops, to Lutheran ministers and youth leaders, and to Catholic priests.

In this way, a modified urban disease model, with Moshi as a secondary node to larger and more distant cities, was a fundamental part of the emergent scientific epidemiology of AIDS in Kilimanjaro region. In this project of scientific interpretation, young, mobile men (typified by truck drivers and businessmen) and urban women operating outside marriage and families (typified by prostitutes and barmaids) were identified as the core transmitter groups, as the embodiments of disease and the history of regional social process. AIDS, having reached a certain prevalence in Moshi town, would, if not controlled, begin to move out into rural areas, the model predicted. Such "waves" of AIDS cases in rural areas were a feature of the epidemic in parts of Uganda (Obbo 1993:952). When MUTAN became responsible for monitoring the progress of the epidemic in Kilimanjaro and Arusha regions for the NACP

Epidemiology Unit, they conducted targeted seroprevalence and STD studies in Kilimanjaro region (notably among bar workers and in the roadside village of Kahe), in addition to maintaining sentinel data.[21] In 1993, they summarized the apparent course of the epidemic in the region and confirmed again that townships and communities along transport routes had higher rates of HIV seroprevalence than rural areas (MUTAN 1993:15). Yet because there are no adequate retrospective time-series data to prove the case one way or another, the scientific epidemiology of AIDS from its early days will never be known with certainty. Given that non-blood-donor data for various sample populations and locations were reported in only one year since 1987, there are obvious hazards in proposing a diachronic model on the basis of disparate cross-sectional studies. For example, in 1991 among semi-rural women aged twenty to thirty in Kahe village, HIV prevalence rates were as high as those in the sentinel population of pregnant women in Moshi town in the same year. In the absence of longitudinal prevalence studies, how can one interpret this finding as part of the urban disease model with any certainty?

Retrospectively, rates reported from existing studies may be more productively seen in the context of an understanding of the cultural processes and institutions that contributed to the unequal distribution of risk among young Tanzanians of both sexes in many locations. The sociogeographic and sexual networks that operated in Kilimanjaro may indeed have concentrated in and around Moshi town early in the epidemic. However, given Kilimanjaro's unique population dynamics, it seems equally likely that the epidemic had important rural manifestations at the same time. The city may have been bypassed since early on, and vulnerability to HIV influenced far more by one's proximity to certain networks that have borne the brunt of rigidifying gender hierarchies, economic disenfranchisement, and demographic dislocation than by urban locations, transport routes, or stereotyped notions about the links between moral character and sexual deportment. Nevertheless, among those who were engaged in speculating about the epidemic, there were very precise expectations about its trajectory and probable casualties.

The urban disease model was not just one of spatiality; it implied a great deal about the kinds of persons being infected in towns. In 1987, Howlett and colleagues (Howlett, Nkya, and Mmuni 1987) generated a risk profile of attributes more commonly associated with patients in KCMC who had AIDS than with a group of seronegative controls. Some of their results are presented in Table 6.2. The sociological vari-

Table 6.2 Characteristics of Patients with AIDS at KCMC, 1988

| | Males (N = 129) | Females (N = 71) | All (N = 200) |
|---|---|---|---|
| Mean age | 32 | 30.5 | 31 |
| Unmarried or divorced | 52.0% | 75.0% | 61.0% |
| Main occupation[a] | Business (25.5%) | Housewife (9.5%) | |
| Resident outside Kilimanjaro | — | — | 62.0% |
| Ten or more reported sexual partners over previous five years | — | — | 41.5% |
| Treated STD during previous five years | — | — | 44.5% |
| Extensive travel[b] | — | — | 52.5% |

Source: Adapted from Howlett et al. 1988:14.
[a] Only the modal responses were given; no other breakdown by occupation was specified.
[b] Defined as "regularly traveling and sleeping away from home" (Howlett et al. 1988:4).

ables, the embodied signs of risk, that the researchers chose to examine were marital status, occupation, and history of extensive travel. In terms of both the medical and social discourse about AIDS, the most salient findings were that persons with AIDS in Kilimanjaro were predominantly young, well-traveled men, only a slight majority of whom were unmarried. The average age of the persons was thirty-one years old, implying that they had become infected in their early to mid-twenties. Among men with AIDS, 25 percent reported being businessmen (versus 10 percent of HIV-negative controls), while among women with AIDS, 75 percent were single, separated, or divorced (as opposed to 48 percent of the controls). Overall, more than 40 percent of AIDS patients of both sexes reported having had ten or more sexual partners over the previous five years and having had a treated STD. Such a profile naturally fit many young adults in Kilimanjaro, many of whom were not primarily urban residents. It was also general enough to mesh with the cultural profile of the *mhuni* and thereby strengthened local concepts of risk and contagion.

## Knowledge and Expectation in Early Responses to AIDS

There were two central features of early expectations of the AIDS epidemic in Kilimanjaro: a reliance upon the urban disease model as configured in scientific narratives of AIDS in East and Central Africa, and images of mobile young adults and urban elites as harbingers of disease and contagion. Medical research and popular inquiry in the first years of the epidemic aided in the production of a particular cultural memory, an embodied social history of dislocation latent in the experience of young adults. This was accomplished through the metaphorical connections made between the bodies of adults and a new disorder of social and sexual reproductive capacity. A local historical consciousness of population dynamics was bolstered by epidemiologic inferences about AIDS as a disease of the city, mobility, and development. The scientific epidemiologic use of signs that "indexed" AIDS through techniques such as blood tests and case-control studies gave a growing and compelling (if occasionally shaky) physical and statistical substance to the epidemic, a substance that was taken up by a situated cultural inquiry into modern forms of sexuality that gave AIDS its symbolic and metaphorical meanings.

For those in Kilimanjaro concerned about AIDS in the mid-1980s, the situation in Kagera was particularly poignant. Some major themes in the emergence of conditions of risk for HIV among Haya in Kagera echoed conditions among Chagga in Kilimanjaro. The parallels included a local economy that had been enriched by coffee cash, and a small city, Bukoba, that grew as a center of regional commerce. In Kagera, a waning system of residence and farming with similarities to the *kihamba* system had given way to increasingly dislocated and highly mobile cohorts of youth, many of whom engaged in business activities and cross-border trade. Furthermore, as in Kilimanjaro, a cultural association between money, commodities, and local notions of desire had provided a preexisting conceptual framework for a disease such as AIDS (Kaijage 1989; Weiss 1993). This framework informed the sociomedical discourse about youth, gender, sexuality, risk, and disease.

A concatenation of historical forces, including fluctuating economic conditions, social stratification, and circumstances conducive to previous epidemics of sexually transmitted disease, were thought to have brought high rates of HIV to Haya areas. Given the emerging understanding in Kagera that AIDS was primarily sexually transmitted, the behavior of Haya with the disease was conceptually linked to that of sectors of the population who had suffered from high rates of syphilis from the 1930s through the 1950s (Kaijage 1989).[22] Indeed, much of the "blame" for AIDS attached to Haya women by Haya men was an elaboration of patriarchal critiques of transformations in gender authority and productive power in Kagera symbolized by female mobility and sex work (Weiss 1993).[23] In the context of AIDS, an acquisitive desire

among Haya women—what would have been called *tamaa* in Kilimanjaro—was akin to a death wish: "In rural Kagera women who return
from their urban labors are resented by men because they use their
funds to acquire land for themselves and their family. Land purchased
in this way, in most cases, eventually becomes the site of burial for the
woman who acquired it. In such an instance a woman is literally 'buying her grave,' purchasing a place of burial and the memorialization
it brings with it" (1993:30).[24]

The image of the "AIDS patient" in Kagera was easily associated
with "the traveled: the professional prostitute, the commercial travel-
ler, the itinerant trader, the participant in the illegal trans-border trade
. . . or indeed the town worker who is brought home in the terminal
stages of his illness" (Kaijage 1989:58). In this emerging "ecology of
risk" (Barnett and Blaikie 1992), the image of the AIDS patient ultimately began to change as more and more individuals who had not
traveled outside Kagera fell ill and died. Although conditions in Kagera seemed to fit neatly with the aspects of the urban disease model
that revolved around mobility, youth, and assumptions about their
"promiscuous" lifestyles, skepticism about AIDS education messages
based on this model began to grow around Tanzania: "It was said that
not everyone known to have died of AIDS was promiscuous, and that
many promiscuous people continue to enjoy good health. This engen-
ders the belief that there must be some other ways, hitherto undetermined, through which HIV is transmitted, and that there must be some
peculiar characteristics about people who get infected" (Muhondwa
1991:2).

In Kagera, there was a growing awareness that "individuals who
were not perceived to be at risk for STD were seen to fall ill with Juliana
or Slim, while others known to engage in multiple sexual encounters
remained symptom free" (de Zalduondo, Msamanga, and Chen 1989:
184). This nascent "counterepidemiology" succinctly expressed the dissonance that Tanzanians felt between the expectations engendered by
the urban disease model and their own experiences with the epidemic,
and the fallacious presumption that "promiscuity" was somehow inherently risky. From the standpoint of experience, this hypothesis was
true given low rates of condom use. The popular perceptions embedded in the presumption, however, did not admit the possibility of
meaningfully altering risk without altering numbers of partners.

Transformations in productive and reproductive relations that preceded the epidemic in Kagera were brought about in part by processes
that were also at work in Kilimanjaro: the lucrative sale of coffee and

the decline of the *kibanja* system (in many ways analogous to the *kihamba*). A similar formulation of the pathology of desire and young adult lifestyles was latent in local understandings of AIDS in Kilimanjaro that would emerge a few years later—though the signification of AIDS and gender in northeastern Tanzania was quite different from that of Kagera.

In the early 1990s, those entering into discussion about AIDS in Kilimanjaro plunged into a vast ocean of debate awash with medical fact and fiction, religious judgment, cultural assumptions, rumors, denials, and confusion. Epidemiological narratives of AIDS in Kilimanjaro were tacked on to preexisting conceptual frameworks about the moral character of mobile young people and urbanized elites. Confusion and rumor pervaded even the highest profile AIDS education efforts. The following exchange was characteristic of literally hundreds of question-and-answer sessions at public AIDS seminars and workshops:

> Questioner: Can goats spread the disease? [laughter]
> Regional AIDS Official: There is no evidence.
> Questioner: I heard that cats can get AIDS.
> Regional AIDS Official: We've heard this, but there is no proof.[25]

Despite the conceptual ferment and ambiguities surrounding the experience of the epidemic, by 1993 few people in Kilimanjaro were prepared to maintain that AIDS was only a matter of returning businessmen and the small cadre of Haya prostitutes in Moshi. Gradually, AIDS took on such an important place in the local social imagination that it was simply referred to as *ugonjwa huo,* "that disease." Yet the cases of people with HIV/AIDS presented at the end of the chapter illustrate how the disease remained an illusory presence, even when those afflicted with it were inexorably drawn into the end stages of disease.

People in Kilimanjaro began to make connections between episodes of morbidity and mortality in their immediate social environment and their knowledge about the emerging epidemic; the process was not the result of a concentrated media campaign or local AIDS education. Origin stories about AIDS in Moshi often revolved around the widely talked about deaths of two prominent members of the community. As Schoepf has pointed out, the death of high-status men has tended to make the epidemic particularly visible (Schoepf 1995:7). In Kilimanjaro, origin stories had many variations. The following version was told to me by a carpenter who had been acquainted with one of the two culturally acknowledged "index" cases of AIDS in Kilimanjaro.

[When did you first hear of AIDS?] We learned of AIDS long before it came to Tanzania. In 1982 and 1983 we heard of this strange disease from San Francisco and New York. [And when did it arrive in this country?] In 1985, the government mentioned cases in Bukoba.[26] The first victim in Kilimanjaro was in Moshi. [When was that?] January 1986. [Who was it?] The Secretary General of the Kilimanjaro Youth League. He was thirty-five years old. He had gone to Bukoba to attend a conference and gone to Dar es Salaam next. By the time he came to Moshi one year later, he was falling sick. He lost a lot of weight. He was living at the Police College then. The doctors diagnosed a problem with the whole intestinal tract, and so he was sent to Britain for treatment. Most people didn't know he had AIDS, but when he died, they said not to open the coffin. This caused a lot of problems as he was Muslim and they were supposed to wash the body.

[Was this the first case in Kilimanjaro?] This was the first case of a well-known person dying of AIDS here in Kilimanjaro. But in June of 1986 the Director General of the International Co-operative Alliance, a guy called Nasoro, went to Ethiopia, and while he was there he developed terrible diarrhea. I saw him when he came back, and I immediately said, "This guy has AIDS or cancer." I went to KCMC to see him. I'm very popular there because I've dated many of the nurses. I asked them if he had AIDS. They said he probably did, but that he was told that he only had some sores in his throat and that he should take some tablets. After he was discharged, many people came to visit him. He just deteriorated bit by bit until he died on June 26. He was forty-six when he died.

His wife had also lost a lot of weight. People knew that guy was very promiscuous—very, very promiscuous. Moshi was gripped by fear because his girlfriends were all around town. People said "Ooo! That guy is going to die because his girlfriend was Nasoro's girlfriend." Then people started talking. "Where did he get it from?" People speculated he got it from Europe; every few months he traveled to Britain, or Denmark, or Holland. People were expecting his girlfriends to die one by one. But they didn't. They are still in very good health. They say that AIDS is transmitted through small bruises. If this is so, he must not have been inside long enough to bruise them.

[How did AIDS affect things here in Moshi?] Prostitutes went underground and stopped going to places officially for them. [Did it change your actions?] I changed my behavior in 1985. I didn't trust condoms—to me it seemed like putting on a bullet-proof vest, but still going into a gun battle.

That's how it was when these great guys fell down.[27]

By the late 1980s, images of young men and women at risk for AIDS were swirling around the social landscape while the disease itself, with all its inherent ambiguities, slowly and almost invisibly began to create a different kind of awareness. Using medically tinged prose, the physicians at KCMC who were conscious that the spread of knowledge was preceding the presence of the virus regarded the late 1980s as "a window period from the onset of the awareness of the AIDS problem" to the implementation of a fully fledged prevention effort, and the inevitable arrival of AIDS in a more significant way into the disease ecology of the region (William Howlett, private papers).

The majority of people sampled in a nonrandom household survey in Moshi conducted between 1991 and 1992 (N = 152) got their first information about AIDS through the mass media (Setel and Kessy 1992). Yet the stories and informational pieces on radio and in newspapers left them with the impression that AIDS was not a significant threat to small regional capitals such as Moshi. In 1991 many informants denied that AIDS was present in Kilimanjaro other than among prostitutes or those who had resided in major urban centers and had returned to die. Chagga medical practitioners participated in this early discourse of AIDS as a "disease of elsewhere." In 1991, one Chagga physician asked and answered her own rhetorical question, "Where do most AIDS patients in Kilimanjaro get their infection? 90 percent is from outside the region."[28] Similarly, during a seminar about AIDS in Kilimanjaro held in Dar es Salaam in 1992, a Chagga microbiologist was adamant that those who had been diagnosed with AIDS in Moshi and environs had acquired their infections while away from the region. It was not until after the beginning of 1988 that more than half of the survey sample of Moshi residents said that AIDS had arrived in Kilimanjaro (Figure 6.3). Although awareness of the disease as present in Kilimanjaro had climbed to more than 90 percent by 1991, most be-

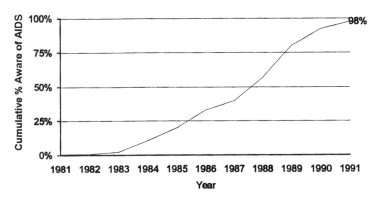

Figure 6.3. Cumulative awareness of AIDS in Moshi, 1981–92; N = 127. (Based on household survey conducted by Setel and Kessy, 1991–92)

lieved it was due to the return of the AIDS ill from large cities. In 1992, 94.2 percent of respondents stated that there had been an AIDS death in their neighborhood, while 59.2 percent said they had seen or visited someone they believed to be suffering from AIDS. Thus there was an important distinction in Kilimanjaro between knowing that AIDS existed and acknowledging it as a present force in the community or in social networks.[29]

The talk of AIDS in Moshi in the early 1990s was talk of a hovering, invisible malevolence, dangerous and immanent, everywhere and nowhere. As AIDS became more apparent to Chagga through both direct experience and education that emphasized its growing presence in the region, some engaged in a reassessment of their self-perceived risks. Women like Happiness, Martina, and Mariamu felt an acute sense of vulnerability, reasoning that their husbands' movements between Dar es Salaam, Mwanza, Nairobi, and home represented an immediate threat to their well-being that they were powerless to confront. One day in 1992 I paid a sympathy visit to the home of a friend, Luther, whose wife had been suffering from a heart ailment. The family had moved from high on the mountain to a fairly prosperous suburb west of Moshi because of Luther's business activities; he owned a petrol station near Arusha and a spare-parts store in Moshi and was also engaged in importing beer from Kenya. When I arrived at the house I found his wife, Esther, at home by herself; Luther had gone to Dar es Salaam. I asked Esther about her health, and she said she had improved quite a bit. Then her face became a tight mask of anxiety and, using the common euphemism for AIDS, she suddenly blurted out the question, "Do you think he's going to bring me 'that disease'?" I was taken aback and asked her what the source of her concern was. "Well, he travels so much, doesn't he?" I asked Esther whether she knew for certain that Luther had other partners. She waved her hand impatiently at the naïveté of my question. "He stays in guest houses," was her answer.[30]

Some in Kilimanjaro were so steeped in the cultural intuition represented by the urban disease model that they were unable to comprehend that there could be more total AIDS cases in rural locations than in towns. An officer of the local chapter of the ruling party's women's organization was incredulous at the regional AIDS coordinator's 1992 figures, which showed precisely such a condition to be the case:

> Woman: According to your statistics, there are more people with AIDS in the rural districts than in Moshi. But Moshi is the place where there is more opportunity and more promiscuity and adultery—how can this be?

> AIDS Coordinator: Because there are so many more people living
> outside the city, and because they are close to the city—a place
> where people can pick up their infection.[31]

Early on in the epidemic the cultural response to AIDS was about rhetoric, the inherently cloudy realities of AIDS, and the processes by which the two were mediated through lived experiences with and observations of those suspected of having the disease. Between 1992 and 1993 AIDS was interrogated, debated, denied, exaggerated, and mystified daily, the cultural engines of image production and ideology working full tilt as institutions and individuals strove for clarity and control. Regardless of whether the ambiguities and variations were clinical, cultural, social, or somatic, they were all part of the experience of AIDS in northern Kilimanjaro. Yet the plurality of perspectives was daunting, and they were repeated and reproduced in many contexts. Information was withheld from families of people with AIDS, leaving them unsure but suspicious about their son's or sister's illness; ministers said, on one hand, that AIDS was punishment for moral laxity and, on the other, that those who suffered from it must be shown compassion and Christian love; condoms were lauded as protective by some parties and derided by others as having been impregnated with HIV by manufacturers in the white world (*ulaya*).

The experiences of those for whom the disease had become a personal reality were an important part of the cultural signification of AIDS. While a plethora of voices joined in a chorus of concern and speculated about how AIDS might be entering into the Chagga social world, men and women suffered with this disease in uncertainty and silence. The uncertainty of AIDS was threefold. It was unclear to clinicians (Altman 1994; Benenson 1990:1; Chin 1991:203–4; Nkrumah et al. 1990), to those who had acquired it, and to those who encountered it in their social networks. In Kilimanjaro some of those with HIV disease described their own doubts about the accuracy of their diagnosis. Having been near death, they had regained such good health and were so symptomless and in such good spirits that surely they must be cured. Given the variation and complexity in the clinical presentation of the disease, the fact that few of the total number of actual cases were diagnosed or identified and that, once diagnosed, almost no one was willing to speak openly about his or her condition, how could people outside the clinic and the lab possibly recognize their illness and that of others as caused by an acquired immune deficiency? The answer, in general, was that they did not—but they often suspected (see Hooper 1990:30–31, 37–39). These suspicions were played out in the inner dialogues of persons who felt they might have been infected, and among lineage and *mitaa* members of ill individuals. At a broader level, the formal properties of the syndrome were determined by its pathology. The insidious, creeping character of HIV lent itself to the metaphorical associations discussed above and to the ideas that AIDS had "a long story." This story is one of AIDS having gradually and stealthily entered into the Chagga social body while Chagga were going about the business of development.

Ambiguity and uncertainty have been features of the cultural encounter with AIDS elsewhere in Africa, the rule rather than the exception. As Fleming noted, the expectation that AIDS would somehow stand out clearly against a background of prevailing misery and affliction is singularly ethnocentric: "Brought up without the Western assumption that disease is something alien to the pristine clarity of the ideal body, in a world where access to health care cannot be guaranteed . . . it seems to me that Rwandans do not conceive of life as the perpetual motion machine we imagine it to be in the West" (Fleming 1990: 449). The variations in the clinical manifestation of the disease have only contributed to the complexities of cultural recognition (Conant 1988a). Obbo (1988) hypothesized that AIDS might be incorporated into preexisting cultural categories of wasting syndromes in high prevalence areas—a phenomenon that might work against developing awareness of the disease. Indeed, AIDS has been classed with the long-standing wasting illnesses of *bagoumelé* among Bété in Ivory Coast (Caprara et al. 1993:1233) and *chira* among Luo in Kenya. Both of these conditions have been associated with sexual causation. In Zambia, AIDS has been enrolled in medical syncretism through the redefinition of local categories of disorder often, though not necessarily, caused by improper sexual relations that have been available in the past to encompass conditions such as tuberculosis (Mwale and Burnard 1992; Mogensen 1997).

Ambiguity and uncertainty have played a major role in the social handling of AIDS in Kilimanjaro and in coping strategies at the individual, household, and community levels there. In particular, the murkiness of the cause and course of AIDS often left it open to witchcraft accusations and curses. The exigencies of fieldwork, however, did not enable me to examine this facet of AIDS and ambiguity in depth. Between 1991 and 1993, most of my contact with people with HIV and AIDS was facilitated through contacts with AIDS counselors at the regional hospital and physicians at KCMC. The clinical and pastoral counseling available through the formal health sector discouraged the notion that HIV and AIDS were caused by witchcraft and cursing. Most of the HIV-infected people I spoke with had been counseled, and they generally adhered to what they had been told about AIDS being caused by "tiny bugs" (vijidudu) or a virus (virusi). As I have mentioned, I was often seen as part of the expatriate-led anti-AIDS effort in and around Moshi, and the fact that I contacted people through their counselors may have inhibited them from sharing their concerns about a more mystical etiology of their disease. Of the ten or so people with HIV/AIDS whom I came to know intimately, however, none indicated that they believed their suffering was caused by witchcraft. To the extent that the topic could be sensitively probed, all of them attributed their infection with HIV to past sexual behavior, either their own activities or those of an unfaithful partner. Nevertheless, witchcraft and, less often, cursing were invoked in connection with AIDS, on the part of both the ill and their families. One village study from Arusha found a similar pattern of causal theories in which notions of individual moral culpability predominated, tuberculosis was frequently invoked as an explanation for illness, and witchcraft beliefs played a minor role (Lie and Biswalo 1995:169).

## Ambiguity and Silence: Early Experiences of AIDS

From early on in the epidemic, the idea of AIDS generated a combination of fascination, horror, sorrow, despair, and curiosity. Before the physical manifestations of the epidemic were widely encountered, the brashness of young people seeming to live in denial of it was bewildering, irritating, or puzzling in light of the enormity of its expected effects. While verbal and textual representations of the illness proliferated, many people wanted to see it embodied before them. The confidentiality of those with HIV or AIDS in hospital was said to be routinely violated by health-care workers who might point out an affected individual to curious friends. AIDS educators and audiences often expressed the opinion that prevention messages would be innately more compelling if delivered by someone living with the disease. Part of this dynamic was set up by the fact that AIDS education posters and speeches, on one hand, repeatedly stressed that AIDS was a disease that could not be seen and, on the other, depicted people with AIDS as wasted, remorseful wraiths. Furthermore, the formal health-care sector claimed not to be able to visualise AIDS but had located it in the bodies of particular men and women with particular ways of life. In the early 1990s, a few persons with AIDS agreed to speak in public about the condition on behalf of the Kilimanjaro Women's Group against AIDS (KIWAKKUKI). On one occasion, when I arrived at the regional hospital to pick up a young man with AIDS and take him to an education speech, the medical assistant on duty attempted to refuse to let him go, saying, "He is not a movie." His comment was a frank statement of the potential for the symbolic life of AIDS to override the humanity of the ill in a stampede of signification, of a popular will to knowledge that could objectify the bodies and persons suffering with AIDS as a source of macabre voyeuristic entertainment.

Yet AIDS stubbornly retained its ambiguities for many years after its arrival in Kilimanjaro. Such ambiguities are an essential theme of the short story "*Kifo cha AIDS*" ("Death from AIDS" [Merinyo 1988]). In the story, young businessmen meet in bars and puzzle over their risks, their knowledge of the disease, their doubts about their own health, and contradictions in their own actions. Having slept with a woman who was rumored to have died from AIDS, the story's protagonist, a young civil servant-cum-businessman named Pinda, is admitted to hospital suffering from a severe case of malaria—or is it? Pinda suspects he might have AIDS, as do his friends, who gossip and joke about it in private but continue to visit him in hospital and care for him. Eventually, Pinda succumbs, consumed to the very end with doubt about the real cause of his illness: "It would come about that he himself would not be certain. Even if Pinda were to die from malaria aided along by an unusual weakness of the body, they [his friends and family] would all believe, without knowing for certain, that he had died from AIDS" (1988:51; my translation).

The circumspection required in confronting this entirely new illness in the context of research is well described by Farmer in his case studies of three Haitians who were among the first in their village to fall ill and die from AIDS (1992:59ff.). In both Haiti and Kilimanjaro, however, the confusion stemmed from more than the sensitivities required in interviewing those who suffered from a fatal and potentially stigmatizing disease and those who cared for them. It was part of the cultural process of recognizing the arrival of a much-heralded and unwelcome entity that confounded straightforward categorization. If anything, AIDS was more of a concern in Moshi and surrounding areas before its "noticed" arrival in the 1990s than it was before it emerged in rural Haiti in the early 1980s. Much more time had passed since the start of the epidemic, and media reports that covered the international climate of blame over the disease and the specter of an African pandemic were well known. As in Haiti, a fairly rapidly evolving set of associations between AIDS, more familiar disorders, and press reports of high levels of AIDS in cities and among homosexuals characterized the early understandings of the disease in Kilimanjaro. This merely added to the confusion in confronting AIDS as an experienced disease rather than as a perceived epidemic.

It is important to point out that despite the heavy morality surrounding AIDS in Kilimanjaro, as in Haiti (Farmer 1992:120) and Uganda (Barnett and Blaikie 1992:60; Seeley 1993:58–60), persons with AIDS were generally as well looked after by those near to them as circumstances would allow. Only in one of the cases discussed below, that of Ezra, was someone in good enough health during the entire course of my fieldwork to be able to live with HIV and conceal the gravity of his condition from his nearest kin. He did so both out of his sense of shame and from fear of being ostracized. His family knew that Ezra was unwell, but the nature of the opportunistic infections that were afflicting him at the time did not usually necessitate long periods of bed rest. In nearly eighteen months of fieldwork, I encountered only two cases in which individuals were shunned or abandoned by their families once their diagnosis with AIDS became known. Although violence against women who disclose their HIV status has been reported from elsewhere in Africa (e.g., van der Straten et al. 1995), I did not encounter this during the course of fieldwork in Kilimanjaro. In one case, the father of a twelve-year-old girl rejected her for having been promiscuous and bringing the humiliation of AIDS to the family. The girl, who was very ill at the time, was admitted for a lengthy stay at the regional hospital while AIDS counselors, the police, and workers from the social welfare office attempted to reconcile the family to caring for her at home. The counselor who was working on the case later suggested that despite the father's bluster, his main concern was that having his daughter at home might somehow lead to the infection of other family members, but other sources disputed this version of events. Eventually, however, the girl was returned to the care of her family. The second case involved a young man, Godlisten, in his early twenties from the central region of Iringa.[32] Godlisten had fallen ill and was sent by his family to an uncle in Kilimanjaro who lived near a hospital. That hospital referred Godlisten to the regional hospital in Moshi, where he was counseled and tested. When Godlisten returned to his uncle's in southern Kilimanjaro region, his uncle rejected him. He arrived back at the regional hospital destitute and far too ill to travel. Godlisten was cared for by the women of KIWAKKUKI and was allowed to remain as an inpatient at the regional hospital. KIWAKKUKI members provided him with food, clothing, soap, and, above all, with solace. While on the ward, Godlisten accepted the ministrations of one of the evangelists who visited the sick and was "saved." "Jesus is near me, and now I get his help," he explained. He also joined KIWAKKUKI's support group and agreed to speak publicly about having AIDS. He did so partly out of the desire to educate others and partly out of a sense of appreciation that he "might not be here without KIWAKKUKI."

The other people whose experiences are recounted below spent varying amounts of time away from Kilimanjaro during their youth. In this regard they fit the early perceptions of AIDS as a disease of returning migrants, a disorder of those who embodied dislocation. Yet their personal histories of displacement from the region were the only clear similarity among them. During the course of visits with Glory, Ezra, Anna, and others directly affected by the disease, it became evident that even in the end stages of the disease there was often a great deal of ambiguity among family members, neighbors, and not infrequently among the AIDS-ill themselves about the nature of their illness. In several cases there was uncertainty because individuals suffering from AIDS had not been given blood tests, were not told by physicians that there was a suspicion of HIV infection, or insisted on alternative explanations for their illness, such as witchcraft or cursing. These conditions have not abated and, partly owing to the departure of MUTAN and a reduction in the activity of counselors, the concealment of HIV serology from HIV-positive patients was still taking place in 1996.[33] Since early in the epidemic, people in Kilimanjaro were aware of the ambiguities of the disease, and some suggested that its uncertainties might offer protection from stigma and blame, should they fall ill.

> Interviewer: To whom would you turn if you are worried about being infected by the virus causing AIDS?
> Interviewee: I would not turn to anybody. I would keep the worries to myself and I would not be tested.
> Interviewer: Would you be willing to explain why?
> Interviewee: Yes, I would not like anyone to know that I am HIV+ because they will think bad about me. They will think I have been misbehaving. . . . I do not trust people in the hospital to keep the secret, that is why I will not be tested. I will keep the secret to myself even when I start developing AIDS; people may suspect, but the symptoms can be other diseases. I do not deserve the blame. (Thirty-six-year-old female health worker, quoted in Lie and Biswalo 1993:12).

The narratives of Glory, Ezra, and Anna (and those of others not recounted here) attest to some of the silences and ambiguities—both protective and harmful—that characterized the lived experience of AIDS on a case by case basis in Kilimanjaro in the early 1990s. The silences of AIDS were as manifold as its ambiguities; there was the internal silence of the disease itself as it depleted the immune system, the silence of unvoiced suspicion, and the silence of those who knew and did not wish to speak. Each case represents a different pathway by which the disease was (and in one case almost was not) identified. Most people diagnosed with AIDS in Tanzania have been identified very late in the course of their disease. In 1990, 70 percent of those diagnosed with AIDS at one hospital in Dar es Salaam reported having had generally good health until two to three months before their diagnosis, but only 7.5 percent remained alive three months after their diagnosis (Mbaga et al. 1990:95). Among patients at KCMC, the median survival time for people with AIDS from onset of major symptoms was 7.5 months (Howlett et al. 1988).[34] Glory fit this pattern. In 1991 she presented with end-stage disease at the regional hospital after having been sent home to Kilimanjaro from Mombassa. She died less than three months later. Ezra, however, was diagnosed as HIV-positive in 1991 and, as of March 1993, was continuing to work part-time despite being in constant pain from a skin ailment. Anna, meanwhile, probably would not have received a confirmed diagnosis had I not helped her contact MUTAN AIDS counselors. She and her family doubted that her only affliction was tuberculosis, as she had been told at KCMC. Together, they asked my assistance in finding out what Anna "really" was afflicted with; she died within a few weeks of her diagnosis.

*Glory*

Glory was buried on January 31, 1992.[35] They buried her in solid rock, stained with the sweat of the diggers who cursed the stone with every swing of the pick and the sledge. Glory did not know her age but was probably in her forties when she died. Her neighbors and family had either surmised or been told of the nature of her illness, but Glory never complained to me or her counselor of being ostracized or neglected when she was alive. Her funeral was similar to many I attended and was remarkable only for the side talk about AIDS among mourners and the whispered jokes about which of Glory's former lovers had been brave enough to attend. And how nervous they looked. At the funerals of those who had died of AIDS, presiding religious leaders occasionally delivered homilies that drew the thinnest of verbal veils over what most of the mourners knew to be the true reason for their gathering.

Standing over Glory's empty grave, the pastor warned that "the time for playing around is over for all of us. . . . We must recommit ourselves to leading clean lives. There are many kinds of filth. There is bodily filth, mental filth, and spiritual filth. We may have been able to go on with laxity in the past, but those days are gone, and anyone who says otherwise is fooling himself."[36] At this point, an older man leaning on a cane bent toward me and whispered a question.

> "You have this in your country, too?" Clearly he meant AIDS.
> "Yes," I said.
> "They burn in fire, don't they?" he asked.

More ambiguity; did he mean hell or cremation? The casket was lowered into the grave. In a matter of minutes and in a cloud of dust, the men filled it in. Then all the mourners helped decorate the margins of Glory's grave with stones and made a pattern of rocks in the shape of the cross atop it. Large branches from a woody succulent were planted at the four corners, and sprigs of purple-and-white bougainvillea were strewn on Glory's grave.

The gravedigging had gone on continuously since early that morning, just outside Glory's hut. It had to be dug the day of funeral, explained a mourner; if left empty overnight it calls death down upon another. While the men worked in shifts crushing stone and removing it from the deepening pit, the women sat on mats beneath an awning erected for them on the side of Glory's hut. Inside, her family lay weeping on mats spread on the dirt floor, accepting the condolences of those who entered to view Glory's *khanga*-wrapped body in the impossibly narrow open casket. Glory's hut was the feeblest I had ever seen, constructed of mud and sticks, with walls that readily admitted any wind that might blow. The tin roof, weighted down by stones, rattled in the breeze and radiated waves of heat during the day. There were no proper hearth stones, but a small fire was kept in the corner of the hut adjacent to the door. Glory lived amid withered stalks of maize on a dusty patch of *shamba* land. When I first met her in her tiny hut, she was sitting on her cardboard bed, laughing about the seemingly preposterous amount of food and exercise her hospital AIDS counselor was encouraging her to take.

On Christmas eve five weeks earlier, Glory's counselor, Pendo, and

I arrived at her house in the early afternoon. We called out "hello" and entered the room. Pendo had asked Glory in a previous visit if she wanted to receive me and explained that I was doing research on AIDS. Glory sat on the bed and clapped her hands together—a familiar gesture of welcome that punctuates a warm greeting in East Africa. A bag of used clothing lay on the dirt floor next to her, and behind the door sat a pail of water and an empty soda bottle that had been filled with milk. Glory shared the hut, no bigger than eight by ten feet, with her daughter and her daughter's three children. Glory's main concern when we arrived was that they had no food for a Christmas meal. Pendo avoided this topic and began to talk to Glory about her diet, exercise, and hygiene and presented her with a bar of soap and a sweater.

Glory removed the tattered brown sweater she was wearing when we arrived and put on the one just given her. She fingered the holes in the old one and puckered her dry lips. Glory looked up at me and began to explain that once she had been a fine tailor: "I could sew anything. I sewed caps for Muslims. I sewed socks. This was when I went to Mombassa when I was pregnant with my daughter. My daughter has three children by her husband, but she has left him now and lives here with me. I was the third born of seven. When I was a child we had a huge *kihamba,* so big that we had to hire neighbors to harvest, but my father sold it and we moved to this God-forsaken place."

Glory's narrative was jumpy and jumbled, interspersed with questions and comments for Pendo about her health. In one breath she explained that she liked living on the mountain as a child, and then switched to a series of questions about her persistent coughing. Abruptly, she returned to telling her about her personal history: "I wanted a church wedding to my husband, but we never had one and ended up splitting. By then I was pregnant, and I went to Mombassa to stay with my father's sisters. They could not afford to keep me, so I returned with my baby girl, left her with my mother, and went back to Mombassa. I was working as a tailor there, and I stayed with whoever could help me. First there was a bus conductor, then another man. I stayed with who would help me."

Glory had returned in poor health from Mombassa in November 1991 and was taken to the regional hospital by her family. She was referred by the clinician who examined her to Pendo, who gave her pre- and post-test HIV counseling, performed her serology, and later gave her the results. For her own part, Glory was quite clear about the source of her illness and about her feelings toward having AIDS: "I am the not first," she said simply, "and I will not be the last. Isn't it so, doctor?"

When Pendo and I visited Glory for the last time, she had become much worse. She was no longer able to sleep and had become too weak to walk. She complained of constantly feeling cold, and of the inadequacy of her bed. Pendo sat beside Glory, stroking and gently massaging her arms, then her feet. Glory winced at even Pendo's gentle touch. That day we had planned to talk more about Glory's time in Mombassa but spoke instead about how to keep Glory comfortable. Pendo promised to bring her a proper mattress from her own house. We ended the visit, as usual, with a lengthy prayer led by Pendo, a fervent Seventh Day Adventist. As the prayer ended, Glory looked up at Pendo and quietly asked, "Doctor, when will you come to stop my heart?"

As we left, Pendo was very upset. At her urging, we drove to a nearby dispensary, where I purchased a phial of an injectable tranquillizer, a pair of latex gloves, and a disposable syringe. We then returned to Glory's house so that Pendo could administer an injection that would let Glory sleep.

### Ezra

Ezra was forty-seven years old and the firstborn in his family.[37] Both his parents were from Kibosho, where his father was given a *kihamba* upon his marriage in 1945. In 1962, Ezra was given his own one-acre plot by his grandfather. The plot, he said, was big enough for a house, but Ezra had to purchase a larger plot on which he could farm.

> My father had many problems in providing for his eight children. Those days, in addition to his *kihamba* he had a three-acre *shamba* below the old Arusha road, where he grew maize and beans. In those days you could just take land, but it had to be farmed by hand, and we all helped. Each of the boys was eventually given a section of that *shamba* as well. The land way down there, there was no problem with asking the *Mangi* about it; it was all animals and it wasn't even safe to stay there. It was all animals until I was fifteen. They are gone now.
>
> I had only a few friends growing up; for the most part, your "friends" were your parents. Maybe there were one or two older boys whom I would help to herd the goats, but in general you didn't stray too much outside the *mtaa* [neigborhood]. You know, people didn't understand the benefits of friendship in those days. If you have lots of friends, you get lots of news and information.

In my family, we had little education, and social mixing was very limited, aside from immediate family. We never slept over at other people's houses, for example. When you came home from school, there was plenty of work to do, and my father was very strict. I started near home, and after that went to middle school up to standard eight, but I always lived at home. My grandfather was Muslim, but gave all his children the choice of being Muslim or Christian. My father is a Christian, and that's how I was raised.

I moved to Moshi after finishing school, and I worked with an ex-Nazi. He was very strict, but we understood each other. I stayed in Majengo in a rented room, and went home to the mountain every weekend. I was eighteen and already depending on myself for everything—I hadn't gotten my *shamba* or *kihamba* yet. Living was cheap, but my salary was also small. I earned 125 shillings per month. My room was 15 shillings, and I spent another 15 shillings on food. I sent 50 shillings home every month, and the money helped my father a lot.

The situation was very different those days compared to now. I didn't know anything about sex. When I was in the book shop, I read about love in books. My father warned us against bringing home a legal case about a woman.[38] "If you do," he said, "I'll make you marry her."

There was one woman in town who took an interest in me. She was half Goan and half Chagga, and we got used to each other and started a relationship [*urafiki*]. We had a son. The restrictions on making love were so severe that this relationship had to be kept a secret. But that woman had four children by two other men, a Greek and an Arab. But *she* was jealous! We bothered each other a lot.

She was a Muslim, and eventually people at work started whispering, "This guy is going with a Muslim woman. . . ." This brought me trouble. There was a guy at the shop who wanted my job, and he started to feed this private information around. I ended up leaving there. The situation wasn't good; people knew my private business.

So, I went to Arusha to look for work. I got work in a hotel, which I really liked. In Arusha, I started with another woman, and she was like a wife. In order to advance, I had to go to Dar, though. In Dar I didn't see any opportunities at first, but I landed a job that gave me chances to advance. I was in Dar at the end of the 1960s, and while I was there, I admit I had several girlfriends. Then I went to a hotel in a National Park for awhile, and eventually got transferred back to Dar. I quit that work eventually in 1975.

After 1975, Ezra concentrated on his own businesses. He traveled often between Dar es Salaam and Kilimanjaro and managed well enough to buy a plot and build a house that he rented to family members in Dar es Salaam. He and the woman from Arusha with whom he had an unsealed marriage had seven children. In 1991, the oldest was in his early twenties and lived in Moshi; the youngest was five and stayed with her mother.

In 1990, without any warning, Ezra's wife left him. She had gone to the regional hospital to have a tubal ligation performed and never returned. Instead, she left the hospital and went to her family in Arusha. In hindsight, Ezra suspected that during her stay at the hospital his wife must have discovered that she had been infected with HIV— although at this time Ezra did not know himself that he was infected. At roughly the same time that his wife left, Ezra experienced an excruciating inflammation of the skin on his side (herpes zoster, or shingles). He was seen at a hospital in Dar es Salaam and given medication. The problem persisted for weeks, and on a visit to Kilimanjaro he was seen at KCMC.

> I had been seeing Dr. W. about this problem for some time, and one day he said, "Let's sit and talk." It was November 1991. I said, "You've always been telling me you have something to say—what is it?" He told me. He told me that I could live for perhaps four or five years. I had to accept it.
>
> Nobody at my home knows. I don't want them to. I am the first-born. Everybody depends on me—my father, my mother, those I bore . . . ten people including myself, right now. I have strengthened myself not to tell them. I didn't want them to know because they would only worry and be bitter. I fear being ostracized, and the family would feel a terrible shame. Now I just pray for a remedy from God through the doctors. My promiscuity would be a shame upon the whole house.

From 1992 to 1993, Ezra's health prevented him from working full-time on his businesses. By mid-1993, he estimated that he was unable to work more than half-time. At the same time, other family members were in need. Nearly singlehandedly he supported thirteen children (his and those of four younger siblings), his parents, and four younger siblings. When he fell ill he had more than two million shillings in a savings account; by 1993 the money was gone. Most of it went into the construction of his house in Kibosho, a project that Ezra wanted to complete before he died. Even if his family became destitute, he felt, at least they would have a decent and secure place to sleep.

Medicines and treatment were another major expense for Ezra. He had spent more than TSh 50,000 on medicines from an herbalist in Dar es Salaam that initially had given him a great deal of hope. He had even passed samples of the medicines that he felt were most beneficial on to his physician at KCMC. In 1993, Ezra regarded the money as having been all but wasted. Nevertheless, he continued to take some kind of medication almost every day. Most of it was nonprescription patent medicine, but some of it was expensive prescription medication to control the unrelenting pain of his skin condition. Next to Ezra's bed stood a stool covered with bottles.[39] "*Dawa* is a part of my life," he said, "It's not easy to go a day without taking some. If I am feeling very good, maybe I can go three days. But no more than that."

After the physician who had been treating him left Kilimanjaro, Ezra rarely went to hospital. He had begun to find it humiliating and annoying to make the long trip from his *kihamba* to the regional hospital only to be shuffled around to different medical assistants, none of whom could really help him anyway. He rejected the idea of attending a nearby Lutheran hospital on the mountain because he knew several of the staff and was worried that his condition would be discovered and his confidentiality would not be protected. Ezra accepted a home visitor from KIWAKKUKI, who became one of his few confidantes. He began attending a confidential support group in Moshi run by the group, becoming quite active in it, raising the concerns of income support to people with AIDS and helping them obtain medical supplies. Meanwhile, Ezra continued to work on his house when he could and had started a small timber business. When we said our farewells in June 1993, Ezra asked me to wish him well on the completion of his house. Recalling his physician's prognosis that he would live for four or five years from 1991, he said quietly, "I am in a race, you see, with my health."

*Anna*

Anna was a neighbor of the family with whom I often stayed in Mbokomu.[40] She had been ill on and off for the previous five years, and by early 1993, rumors were beginning to circulate that she had tuberculosis and was probably dying of AIDS. I was urged by one of her family members to fulfill an important duty in East African social networks of making a sympathy call (*-mpa pole*). I agreed to go despite being aware that the invitation was a pretext for getting me to offer an opinion on Anna's condition that I was not qualified to make—and so confirm or refute the rumors. As we approached the house, I realized that I had visited this family on a previous occasion. I had been directed to this household more than a year before this sympathy call when I had asked the ward secretary for introductions to households in which

women had been left by their husbands. The *kihamba* belonged to Ngahenda, a successful butcher, with three shops in Kiboriloni. At that
time, in December 1991, there had been several children and grandchildren of the *kihamba* owner living in the three buildings that made up
the homestead. Anna was one of Ngahenda's daughters and had been
staying at the house, though I did not meet her at the time. Ngahenda
usually stayed with his other wife on a farm nearer to the market. During my visit the previous year, members of his household told me that
they had heard of AIDS and that three people so far had died of it in
the village. They also said that they had never knowingly seen anyone
with the disease.

In 1992, Anna was thirty-two years old and before she fell ill was
doing small business in Kiboriloni. She had been married in a church
wedding but hadn't seen her husband for a long time. She was staying
at her mother's home with her five children, aged four to fourteen.
Her husband, David, was forty years old and was selling locally made
alcohol called *ulanzi* in Mbeya in southern Tanzania. She had met and
married him at home in Mbokomu, and, Anna said, "he kept the first
two children well. Then he fled." Initially they had stayed in Kilimanjaro and worked in Kiboriloni market. In the mid-1980s Anna accompanied David to Mbeya but stayed for only five months: "We parted because I couldn't help him sell beer with a small child around." For a
while in the later 1980s David sent home about TSh 3,000 per month
for his children but had only been back to visit twice in the previous six
years. Anna, meanwhile, had returned to her occasional small business.

> While he was away I sold erasers and foam rubber thongs in Kibor-
> iloni. It was just enough to clothe the children. By this time I was
> living at home.
>   I started to fall ill in 1988. It started with my stomach, and I was
> in very bad shape. I was admitted to Mawenzi hospital almost ev-
> ery other week. It was on and off for a very long time. Then, at
> the end of 1992 I went to see my brother in Dar es Salaam, and I
> started to feel dizzy. I fell down and lost the use of my arm. Now
> I have TB.
>   It has been such a long time [since falling ill]. My father hired
> an *mganga* to come from Tanga to try and cure me. He spent TSh
> 15,000 on the *mganga,* but it did no good. His *dawa* didn't help at
> all. He said I had been bewitched by people at home, but I don't
> believe him any longer. I took his *dawa* for witchcraft for two years
> and there has been no effect.

"When her illness started, they kept telling her it was amoebas," explained Anna's mother. Anna was still able to work sporadically until

three months before our meeting but then became too ill to leave her bed. First her father took her to be prayed over, and then she was admitted in KCMC for two weeks. From there she was returned home with a course of injections to be administered by the nurse from the local clinic. Anna's father also spent a great deal of money on an *mganga,* who had divined that Anna was suffering as a result of a curse. When I asked Anna whether she believed she had been cursed, she replied that she had doubted from the first that the *mganga'*s ministrations would have an effect on her illness. But what about a curse or witchcraft? I inquired. Anna equivocated. At first, she explained, she was willing to accept that there might have been cursing or witchcraft involved. Over time, and with the failure of a renowned *mganga,* however, she came to discount the possibility. She reasoned that she had more than made amends with anyone who could have been holding a grudge against her serious enough to warrant such an assault. Her grave state, she believed, was caused by tuberculosis. Not witchcraft or cursing.

I visited the house a number of times over the next few weeks and, as I feared, was prompted a number a times to offer my opinion about the nature of Anna's illness. At one point Anna's mother drew me aside. We stepped out into the *kihamba* behind the house. The brief, whispered conversation that ensued beneath the banana leaves was one that I was to have many times, in many different versions.

"What is it really, doctor?" she asked. (I was often called "doctor" by people in Kilimanjaro despite frequent explanations that I was a student and that my research was not medical or clinical.)

"What do you think it is?" I replied.

"If I knew what it was, I would tell you. . . ."

I shrugged my shoulders. "Isn't it TB?" I asked, not believing a bit of it.

"It's, um, it's that, it's uh, it's AIDS, isn't it?" she stammered.

"It seems possible," I said reluctantly, adding quickly, "But I'm not a doctor, you know. If you, and more importantly, if Anna wants to know if this is the case, I will bring someone from Mawenzi tomorrow whom you can speak with." Anna's mother didn't respond immediately. She seemed very far away, although our heads were bent close.

"How are you?" I asked her.

"Me?" she snapped her head back and stared at me wide-eyed— as though I were making an accusation about her health rather than inquiring about her state of mind. "Oh! I'm fine," she said defensively, "I told the man of this house—the butcher—that I'd seen enough of his *mhuni* ways. He'd better stay far away from me." She laughed nervously and began to back away as her voice drifted off.

A few minutes later, Anna's mother asked me the name of the person I had offered to bring from the hospital. That afternoon Anna's father was summoned. They bundled Anna into the back of a pickup and had her admitted to Mawenzi hospital. A few days later she was released and returned home with a supply of gentian violet paint for bedsores and an intravenous drip that no one in the household had the skill to install. Anna was unable to eat and was vomiting constantly. She died two weeks later. During these two weeks many people went to pay sympathy calls, including home visitors from the KIWAKKUKI group and a MUTAN counselor. Although she was married, Anna refused to be buried in her husband's *kihamba,* and instead was interred in the banana grove of her father's *kihamba* in Mbokomu. Her five children were taken in by their maternal grandmother, all attempts at contacting David having failed.

## Clarity, Confusion, and AIDS in Kilimanjaro

The experiences of Ezra and Glory are a corrective to the unreliable clarity of expectation that characterized most local discourse about the HIV epidemic in Kilimanjaro, while that of Anna fits more closely with cultural predictions about the epidemic. The personal struggles of these people with a confusing, recalcitrant, and fatal disease epitomize several facets of the cultural and demographic context of the AIDS epidemic developed throughout the book and sum up many of the gendered paradoxes of signification and praxis that the AIDS epidemic posed for people in Kilimanjaro. For Chagga, a deceptively confident discernment about AIDS was fashioned from the scientific epidemiology of the disease and from domains of experience that were closely linked to sexuality, to social reproduction, and to concepts of personhood, moral character, and desire. Beyond the irony of nostalgia for a constructed image of the past, these domains of experience have proved to be complex in their historical character. Yet despite the clarity of the vision of vulnerability, causation, and risk evoked by moral demographies and epidemiologies, the majority of those affected by AIDS have remained unsure of the cause of their suffering.

Like so many other Chagga men his age, Ezra left his small plot on the mountain for the opportunities presented by entering the world of business. Although he came to feel ashamed of the "promiscuity" he associated with his own disease, his life's labors had enabled him to provide for his extended family, even through his protracted illness. Above all, Ezra's concerns were for accomplishing this duty of the firstborn son toward his parents, children, and siblings. If anything ameliorated his physical pain and emotional anguish during the months of our acquaintance, it was the thought that he was able to struggle on long enough to ensure some lasting security for his family. Glory, meanwhile, was promised a proper wedding but was eventually jilted and sent to stay with her paternal aunts. She too left the mountain, but her departure was connected to her precocious fertility. Her vulnerability stemmed from another dynamic of dislocation, and her relative dependence upon men in Mombassa to supplement what she could provide herself from her tailoring work. Some aspects of Anna's story evoked the popular epidemiologies of AIDS. Certainly it evoked the association of AIDS with the dislocation of young people, and with the itinerancy of a life in petty trade. Indeed, as her family spoke of him, the simple fact of Anna's untraceable businessman husband (who exists in her life story like an echo of the vanished youth in "Hey, Listen!") portended doom for other young women. The open-endedness of Anna's contact with him up until her death also reminds us that into the future, the course of epidemic will remain indistinct, filled with challenges for understanding and action.

In many ways, Anna's experience encapsulates the conundrums of AIDS when seen as a crisis of social reproduction and representation. At first, much of the dangerous "Otherness" of AIDS (Gilman 1985) was kept at bay with the notion that AIDS was a disease of elsewhere, of Kagera and Dar es Salaam. Quickly, however, this notion was supplanted by the fears of rural women that their migrant husbands might infect them and by the growing expectations of a local epidemic that would sweep away "people of a certain lifestyle," leaving others unscathed. Local moral demographies, in which a self-conscious push toward development and modernity accelerated the pace of cultural change and moderated the effects of population pressures, were reformulated in light of eroding domestic gender relations and decreasing security of productive lifeways. Desire was no longer merely a personal quality to be held in check or harnessed to a push for development. It had become mortally dangerous. All of its representations suddenly betokened deadly excesses of personhood, a perception strengthened by popular and professional epidemiologies of AIDS.

Yet as the three cases above illustrate, the signification of AIDS in Kilimanjaro has never been a homogenous process of reaching cultural consensus about the disease and its meanings. Among researchers and clinicians, ambiguities persisted as the overall severity of the epidemic in Kilimanjaro, the total number of AIDS cases and infections, and the trajectory of the epidemic in the region could only be guessed at in the early 1990s. Meanwhile, the management of someone's series of increasingly debilitating illnesses might easily elude the part of the health-care system designed to identify cases of HIV infection, accusations of witchcraft arose while remedies failed, and rumors flew at funerals or circulated in the street behind someone's back. AIDS was shrugged off as a World Bank phantasm designed to make Tanzanians accept structural adjustment or was said to be curable by local *waganga*. At AIDS education talks, presenters were asked whether AIDS could be transmitted by fish caught in Lake Victoria into which the bodies of the AIDS dead were supposedly thrown, or whether the communion chalice could transmit it to those attending mass.

Throughout the debate and ferment of the encounter with AIDS, however, formal and institutionalized responses have built upon the themes of development and dislocation in various ways, drawing discussions of AIDS into preexisting frameworks. In the form of cultural texts such as reports, journal articles, speeches, plays, songs, sermons, and poems they have been highly articulated and focused and so have been amenable to analysis as discourse (see, e.g., Seidel 1993). On the other hand, an important range of informal responses existed outside any disciplinary or discursive practice. These more inchoate cultural rhetorics of AIDS cannot simply be totted up as misinformation or misconception to be rectified by better AIDS education, for they reflect a much more profound process of the application of cultural logics to an unprecedented type of social disorder. Amid these explanations, origin stories, expectations, and recriminations, the voices and experiences of those who were contending with AIDS within their own bodies or their own families were by and large silent. Had they been given a forum, they might have further muddied the waters by pointing to the gaps between lived experience and cultural and epidemiological expectation.

As a final comment, I resist giving any sense of closure to this account of a process that is not complete—indeed grows more severe—for those in Kilimanjaro. My thoughts return often to the heartbreaking solemnity of a Lutheran pastor who stood in the December sunshine at a World AIDS Day event in 1991 and begged the young people gathered there not to let their parents die of broken hearts. Even though many of the parents of those young men and women had risks of their own, his words conveyed the depth of concern and anguish that the first seven years of the epidemic had wrought. I also recall the young adults and older married women who confronted AIDS and ambiguity in their families and networks of friends. These people, and many others I lived with, continued to seek for ways to make sense of and respond to AIDS in conditions of hardship, to respond in ways that would allow them to lead full, secure lives, and to fulfill their personal ambitions and their unique human promise.

# CHAPTER 7

## Conclusions without Closure

> The urgency or immensity of a practical social problem does not entail the assurance of its solution.
>
> Merton (1949:8)
>
> Anthropology is uniquely equipped to investigate a new disorder, but the anthropological study of AIDS should be more than a search for "cultural meaning," that perennial object of cognitive and symbolic inquiry.
>
> Farmer (1992:253)

### A Plague of Paradoxes and Concentric Catastrophes

In this book I have attempted to show that AIDS in Kilimanjaro has been an outgrowth of culture, history, demography, and political economy. That it has been a disorder of social reproduction that emerged through the intersection of HIV with people engaged in a conscious struggle with forces both impinging upon and internal to their cultural worlds. Sexuality, of such proximate importance to the study of AIDS, has itself been framed as an outcome of sociocultural change in productive and reproductive regimes. I have argued that AIDS has been a plague of paradoxes, of concentric catastrophes, of disordered relations of power from the interpersonal to the international, the productive to the reproductive, the societal to the sexual.

In the years before I met Anna, Glory, and Ezra, they strove for survival without knowing that they carried the time bomb of HIV within them. At about this time an American anthropologist-physician on the other side of world was interviewing Haitian villagers about the arrival of a new disease, *sida* (AIDS), in their village (Farmer 1992, 1995). Many Haitians in the village of Do Kay, where Farmer worked, experienced AIDS as "the last thing," the final, "numberless misfortune" in a losing struggle with life (Farmer 1992:47). This Haitian village was, itself, literally a by-product of disordered development. The peasantry framed their collective encounter with AIDS in terms of the macro and the micro, of history and political economy, within Haiti and between Haiti and the United States (e.g., 1992:254–62). Following their lead, Farmer was able to assemble an interpretive cultural account of a syndrome involving a sexually transmitted pathogen with practically no reference to sexuality at all.

To some extent this may have been a reaction to the exclusive emphasis on sexuality on the part of the international health community during the 1980s. Although useful in countering the "gay plague" typification of AIDS, the concept of geographic patterns of spread based upon generalized links between sexuality and epidemiology (Piot et al. 1987: 576) and later notions of "geographic areas of affinity" (Mann, Tarantola, and Netter 1992:22; see Farmer 1992:123, 260) failed to highlight the connections between AIDS and global poverty.[1]

Schoepf has demonstrated that in the Democratic Republic of Congo, a narrow, decontextualized focus on sexuality as the central problematic in a social science of AIDS runs the risk of obscuring the historical synergies among political economic disenfranchisement, gender, and risk (1991a, 1991b, 1992, 1993a, 1993b; Schoepf et al. 1988). In Central Africa, Schoepf demonstrates, sexual diversity was a feature of social systems throughout the region. The slave trade and colonialism shattered this diversity and reordered the kinship systems in which it was embedded. Through the colonial era and into independence and the age of structural adjustment, men and women have adapted sexual comportment to conditions in which they have often been unable to establish stable, long-term relations (Schoepf 1992). The feminization of poverty, women's exclusion from economically secure lives, and their dislocation from cultural institutions that provided them with greater power in controlling their sexuality lie at the heart of this inequality of risk (Ahlberg 1991, 1993; Bassett and Mhloyi 1991; Anarfi 1992; Mann, Tarantola, and Netter 1992; Awusabo-Asare, Anarfi, and Agyeman 1993). Under such circumstances, "Failure to recognize the economic causes of prostitution and multiple sex partners, to address the structural causes of underdevelopment, poverty and joblessness, builds resentment among African[s] . . . and resistance to advice such as the need for condoms" (Schoepf 1992:363–64; see also Konoky-Ahulu 1989; Preston-Whyte 1995).

AIDS in Kilimanjaro has been suffused with a selective consciousness of local circumstance and a critique of the moral agency of certain categories of local actors. At the same time it has also been cast as a disorder of development in a way that has encoded a critique of postcolonial relations in the developing world. Tanzania, like Haiti and like most other countries severely affected by HIV, has labored with its own history of colonialism, postcolonialism, and neocolonialism. Chagga in Kilimanjaro, like Tonga villagers in Zambia, among whom Mogensen worked, cannot be portrayed in a simplistic "world systems theory" paradigm as members of a reactionary and traditionalist periphery; rather they must be seen as belonging to a "dynamic periphery in the midst of managing culture and meaning by responding critically to the charms of the metropolis, and in doing this they are revealing values essential to them" (Mogensen 1997:436–37). For many Tanzanians, the "charms" associated with modernity were very much a product of local cultural processes under way since early in the century. As a reviewer of Merinyo's *Kifo cha AIDS* commented in the Tanzanian press, "AIDS is only one among many tragedies that reminds man of his continual suffering due to a 'sick' society that he himself creates" (*Daily News* 1988b). While in much of Tanzania, AIDS was used to carry strong moral messages, Mogensen has argued that in parts of Zambia it was not: "Nobody is accused, nobody is blamed, nobody did this on purpose. AIDS is but one of those things that happen, because the world has changed. . . . The disorder is not caused by certain individuals— but by society as a whole" (1997:437).

It is worth noting different ways in which Chagga, Tonga, Haitians, and others have positioned the meanings of AIDS in relation to their structural positions in the local and global order. In Kilimanjaro, as elsewhere in East and Central Africa, various etiological rumors and slogans indicated that AIDS was explicitly related to a disorder of international relations. AIDS was said to have come from Uganda as a result of war. I was often asked if I thought it was possible that the CIA had manufactured AIDS and released it in order to rid the world of Africans. Some in Kilimanjaro doubted the existence of AIDS on the basis that it was yet another aspect of African suffering over which white people sought to claim absolute authority, and which they tried to foist upon a struggling and captive continent. One day, when discussing regional HIV rates at the home of a neighbor, who managed a tannery in Moshi, he became enraged.

> This is not true. I don't believe it. People have changed their behavior. I'm telling you. Ten years ago they said that all of Bukoba had AIDS and that we were all done for. If you believed them the whole country should be finished by now. It's these stupid World Bank people running around spreading false statistics. They don't have any reason for explaining how their whole development plan for Africa has failed, so they are blaming it on AIDS now. You can't

run in and tell Africa how to develop. These fucking little boys coming here from college, they have no experience with management here. You have no idea what it takes to manage a company here. No idea. It takes a hell of a lot I'm telling you. AIDS. No way. Twenty percent in Mwanza, you are telling me? That's the same as saying that everyone has it. If you work it out mathematically that means that after two years the whole population is infected. Impossible. Africa was here doing fine long before the Europeans came, and if you ask me it's Western Europe that's on the verge of collapse. Look at these stupid Swedes. They are telling me how to run my company and their country is a total financial disaster; they're bankrupt! No. It's the World Bank that's making all this up about AIDS to frighten us and to intimidate us. They have been totally wrong about everything and now they are lying about AIDS to somehow cover their tracks.[2]

Although this outburst was unique in my experience in Kilimanjaro, it echoed the cynicism of other friends and acquaintances there and corresponds with cultural conspiracy theories reported from elsewhere in the developing world. Often, as in Haiti and the Republic of Congo, AIDS was associated with something "sent" as part of the machinations of political regimes seen to be more aligned with the Western interests than with African citizenries. Rural Haitians theorized that AIDS was produced by Americans who purchased Haitian blood for their diabolical project from the dictator Duvalier. They reckoned that it was "collateral damage" of CIA germ warfare aimed initially at Cuban pig herds and speculated that AIDS was loaded into tear-gas grenades purchased from the Unites States and used by the Haitian constabulary in their repression of citizen protest. Others thought that it was the product of bacteriologically trained henchmen of Duvalier who had learned how to "disappear" dissidents through the manufacture of microbes and, most straightforwardly, that it was a genocidal plot of Americans to rid the world of Haitians (Farmer 1992:230–31).

In 1988 a Kenyan friend in Boston, for example, quipped that people at home "were beginning to wonder what kind of AIDS/aids people were getting from the government these days." A Zairian actor claimed that "taxi drivers in Kinshasa say that it [AIDS] comes from [Zairian President] Mobutu's mind. He has thought it up so that all the men will not spend their money on prostitutes." In the mid-1980s, "For a while the joke in Kinshasa was that SIDA—the French acronym for AIDS—stood for *Sydrome Imaginaire pour Décourager les Amoureaux,* or Imaginary Syndrome to Discourage Lovers. It was also about this time, so the story goes, that hundreds of T-shirts were distributed as publicity for the Swedish International Development Agency that boasted *SIDA, c'est moi!"* (Fleming 1990:449). A Ugandan anthropologist offered an alternative explanation for the nickname "Juliana" that was given to AIDS: "People see that this disease makes you very thin. The only people they know who are obsessed with being thin are the Europeans. This is why they call the disease by a European name, 'Juliana.'"[3] Condoms were another vehicle for linking AIDS to disordered international relations. No condoms are manufactured in Africa, and, as mentioned previously, American condoms were rumored by Tanzanians to be impregnated with HIV. In the former Zaire "nationalist sentiment . . . link[ed] contraception and condom use to Western population control strategies, which [were] viewed as a form of imperialism" (Schoepf et al. 1988:219). All of these conspiracy theories-cum-"rhetorical defenses" of some of the world's poorest people have been dismissed as scurrilous rumor in the West. Yet they have an eerie ring of truth about them when viewed in the specific contexts of histories of the effects of Western power relations upon Africans and their bodies.

The analysis of what AIDS means and how it is constructed in each of these concentric zones of catastrophe is not reducible to "crude formulations [like] 'imperialism causes AIDS'" (Farmer 1992:261). As Farmer has so fervently argued, anthropologies of AIDS demand more than investigations of meaning; they must be accountable both to history and to political economy. Above all, they must strive for an "interpretive anthropology of affliction, attuned to the ways in which history and its calculus of economic and symbolic power impinge on the local and the personal" (Farmer 1988:80). Such an insistence on a historical perspective of context and meaning has guided this analysis of the group experience of AIDS in Kilimanjaro.

## The Contested Place of Medicine in an Anthropology of AIDS in Africa

Medicine continues to occupy a dubious role in the cultural experience of health and illness in Africa, and in the AIDS epidemic in particular. Haraway (1987) has pointed out that Western cultural agendas have been implicit in the field of primatology. Primate studies in Africa, she notes, reached new and penetrating depths at precisely the historical moment that industrial, extractive capitalism was losing its grip on much of the continent through the demise of formal structures of colonialism. Similarly, AIDS opened up new frontiers for science in the developing world at a time when Cold War geopolitics had a diminishing influence in the continent, when structural adjustment programs had begun taking their toll on the health of Africans (Bierman and Campbell 1989; Lugala 1994; Sanders and Sambo 1991), and when the political pressure to transform single-party African nation-states into multiparty democracies was being ratcheted up by the West.

In the early 1900s Africa was a proving ground for advances in scientific techniques and technologies: "Africa was a laboratory in which the possibilities of the new bacteriology could be explored in a challenging way. Africa was a place in which scientific reputations could be made" (Vaughan 1991:37). As the millennium draws to a close in the shadow of AIDS, this adage pertains just as well to Africa and the new immunology and retrovirology. The biomedical narratives of AIDS in Africa in the 1980s and 1990s were an object lesson in the veracity of Haraway's dictum that "science remains an important genre of Western exploration and travel literature" (1991:205).[4] Some argued that the scientific inquiry and pursuit of AIDS across the African continent represented a new form of hegemony extended over Africans under the rubric of international health. As a recapitulation of industrial imperialism, which developed Tanzania in order to exploit it (Koponen 1994), this new "scientific colonialism" had a new twist; it has depended upon the active involvement (or, some would say, cooptation) of African scientific communities, ostensibly through "capacity building": "The systematic involvement of LDC [less-developed country] scientists as implementors of research designs or purveyors of unique datasets can be called 'scientific colonialism,' for it is typified by extraction and export of knowledge rather than fertilization and indigenous growth. Scientific colonialism involves . . . the gathering of data in LDCs, exportation of data from LDC in raw form, and processing (analysis and publication) outside the LDC. Unlike earlier stages of colonialism, however, the finished products (published papers) are often never marketed back to the countries that produced the raw data" (Trostle 1992:1322–23).

Furthermore, the ethics of vaccine trials conducted in Africa, and epidemiologic research on STD transmission carried out by Europeans and American researchers, have been questioned (Patton 1990:87–97; Schoepf 1991a:758–59). Researchers have been accused of using lowered standards for informed consent in research among Africans, of employing study designs that would not pass ethics reviews in Europe and America, and of using poor, vulnerable people to test drugs and vaccines that they could never afford. At one international conference, the authors of a Tanzanian study that proved the importance of STD treatment in lowering rates of HIV transmission (Grosskurth et al. 1995; also Laga 1995) were likened to those who conducted the notorious Tuskegee syphilis experiments in the United States.[5]

When viewed from a local perspective, however, the "biopower" dynamics of north and south were not so black and white. For at least fifty years, residents of Kilimanjaro have been invested in the use of biomedicine as an integral therapeutic practice. Despite the insidious side to what has been labeled "safari research" (Palca 1990), HIV/AIDS research and prevention programs in Tanzania offered African scholars important new skills and technologies for understanding health and disease in their own countries. It must be borne in mind that the practice of medicine and epidemiology in the context of Kilimanjaro's AIDS epidemic was generative of more than discourses of Otherness constructed solely for "First World" consumption (see, e.g., Treichler 1989; Watney 1989). Through the MUTAN project, several Tanzanian scholars were authors (and co-authors) of scientific papers, traveled to international conferences, and had opportunities to pursue professional studies and training in a number of fields. It is certainly valid to note that African medical schools and universities are often unable to afford subscriptions to the very journals in which their faculty members publish. However, to suggest that their participation was nothing more than the hegemonic appropriation of African intellectual capacity by the white West greatly oversimplifies the conditions of African scholars and overdetermines the outcomes and as-yet unrealized benefits of their participation in scientific research and training.

The fact that in the 1940s the Chagga leadership could articulate the idea that "progress cannot be expected of a people with unhealthy bodies," and that this idea was explicitly linked to Western medical services, speaks to the fact that in the "twentieth century, biomedicine is an African healing practice" (Vaughan 1991:206). It also serves to emphasize that medicine, as part of the cultural legacy of colonialism, has accomplished more than the reproduction of colonial power relations through the aggregation of embodied signs of cultural Others (thereby constructing them as "different" and "diseased" in a group, as opposed to an individual, sense [Setel 1991a; Vaughan 1991:11; Comaroff 1993]). One cannot overlook the effects of nonclinical forms of practice upon embodied African subjectivities. Christianization, education, maternal and child health education, urban planning, land alienation, and agricultural and industrial wage labor are the among the major forms of practice that refracted through populations and individual experience (see Beidelman 1982; Curtin 1985; Hunt 1992; Packard

1989; Turshen 1984). Anything that acted upon the persons of Africans also acted upon their sexualities (see, e.g., Ahlberg 1994) and senses of embodiment. Such "productive" consequences of colonial practices can be seen in Kilimanjaro's tuberculosis hospital. In 1949 occupational therapy, medical confinement, the faculty and students of a Lutheran girl's school, and colonial social clubs all converged in the treatment of diseased Africans. This convergence is an example of how "mutually constitutive relations of political economy, symbols and science" (Haraway 1991:208) can act in a highly orchestrated, institutionalized fashion.

In the age of AIDS international biomedicine has come into its own as a social force mediating bodily discourses, disciplinary practices, and subjectivities of persons in many locations in sub-Saharan Africa. The procedures of power operating through biomedicine there have relatively recently (albeit incompletely) made a jump from an emphasis on "regulative" to "productive" exercises of power. In other words, there has been a shift from a social use of medicine as a means of control within and among populations (but external to individual bodies) to one in which medicine has become an African technique of knowing and defining persons from the social spaces within (hence acting upon their subjectivities). However syncretically conceived, viruses, bacteria, parasites, hormones, hypertension, stroke, and diabetes have become as integral to the subjective experience of health, aging, and somatic disorder in the cultural context of Kilimanjaro in the early 1990s as any concepts that derived from more "local" forms of knowledge. In part, this accounts for the syncretisms of medical and local knowledges found not only in the AIDS epidemic in Kilimanjaro but also in many settings in Africa.

Despite its status, Western medical authority has been thoroughly challenged in the AIDS epidemic. Some in Kilimanjaro quoted a Swahili proverb in an ironic manner to emphasize that now that AIDS has proven too much for even the greatest medical minds, it will surely overwhelm African capacities. "The bone has bested the hyena," they marveled, "how will the dog possibly handle it?" (*Mfupa umemshinda fisi; mbwa atauweza?*) For Tanzanians, AIDS sometimes represented a challenge to African ingenuity in the healing arts. During the 1980s, a great deal of attention was focused on anti-AIDS drugs such as KEMRON and MM-1, both of which were developed in Africa and both of which have been proven to be either ineffectual or of limited long-term benefit in treating those with HIV. The discrediting of MM-1 by the international medical community occasioned a series of letters in the

Tanzanian press extolling the genius of Africans and the suspicious readiness of the north to discount their achievements: "These two from the African soil, one Zairian and another Egyptian have done it! . . . Africans should be conscious of their own strength. The myth that anything substantial must come from Europe must be eliminated. This is a result of the psychic destruction . . . during the colonial period. . . . It is no wonder that the WHO with its headquarters in a Developed Country refused to affirm the effectiveness of MM-1 because it was developed by African Doctors" (*Daily News* 1988a).

Thus, the symbolic life of AIDS in Kilimanjaro was not limited to its manifestation as the result of strictly local processes or to the incursions of the wider world into the Chagga community. It threatened moral, physical, political, and personal disorder, connecting mundane individual characteristics such as *tabia* and *tamaa* with ligatures of signification that extended to the United States and Geneva. Yet the bonds from Europe and America to Africa were not encoded in the symbolism of the AIDS epidemic alone. One merely needed to tour laboratories in Tanzania where AIDS research was being conducted to see their material manifestation. In Kilimanjaro, Norwegian funds enabled Tanzanian medical researchers to fill HIV test kits manufactured by British or multinational companies with African blood using Finnish-made pipettes beneath vacuum hoods of West German manufacture. The tests were read by means of Japanese spectrophotometers while researchers sat on chairs rumored to have been brought from Scandinavia, and rested their feet on boxes of American condoms and rubber gloves. For some, the importation of the equipment and the expertise through which AIDS was signified for science was virtually the same thing as importing the syndrome itself.

As we have seen, the unleashing of powerful epidemiologic technologies and comparatively large financial resources upon the epidemic in Africa has done little to uncover the true demographic and sociocultural dimensions of the disease. The misapprehensions of the urban disease model and the ramifications of conceiving the global pandemic in terms of patterns of sexual transmission revealed the relative impoverishment of epidemiologic interpretations of what have constituted conditions of risk for the majority of Africans. This dimension of the social production of scientific knowledge about AIDS continues to point simultaneously out and away from Africa and inward toward the bodies of individual African men and women. It demands more critical and reflexive accounts of international health that uncover the implicit cultural agendas and the explicit manner in which the practice of medicine, not merely medical epistemology, continues to create particular visions of health problems on the ground. Fieldwork will be essential to these accounts since medicine, with its strengthening status as an African healing system, must be examined as it operates in the dialogic encounter between its practitioners and the engaged subjects of its practice. The propensity of actors in Kilimanjaro to incorporate bits of medical knowledge into their own interpretive endeavors in grappling with a response to the epidemic speaks to the need for an anthropology of international health that situates medicine in a model of concentric or overlapping spheres of power and influence from the global to the local.

By necessity, this concluding chapter leaves many open questions about the cultural meanings of AIDS in northeastern Tanzania. No researcher writing about the epidemic in America in 1984 could have put a seal on what AIDS meant in American society and culture, or what it would come to mean ten years later. Likewise, it is impossible to extend an argument about AIDS and social process in Kilimanjaro beyond the historical moment with which this account of the epidemic has dealt. Thus, this chapter is a conclusion without closure. Nevertheless some things can be said conclusively, for as people in Kilimanjaro confronted AIDS, there was a definite cultural logic to their response.

The negotiation of experience and expectation, realities and rhetorics, and disease and development operated through existing networks of practice and power and shared conceptual frameworks to give AIDS meaning and to shape cultural and epidemiological expectations about the epidemic. People and institutions were not free to invent entirely spontaneous meanings or responses to AIDS, nor was the content of their responses and representations completely foreordained. In order to address the underlying conditions of AIDS—its meanings and its manifestations—one must begin to address the issue squarely as one of productive and reproductive power, economic security, and the nature of cultural programs for adulthood. Such an agenda is complicated by the momentum of forces in train that extend far beyond the short-term influence of policies and programs. Even under optimum conditions, the impact of targeted interventions such as those promoting condom use may be very limited (see, e.g., Higgins et al. 1991). Behavior change in this regard is subject to situational constraints (Allen et al. 1993a, 1993b; Setel 1995b), if it can be accurately measured at all (Cohen and Trussell 1996:141–49). The fact is that "individual, psychological intervention approaches will not promote optimum changes in behavior when structural and environmental constraints are not addressed" (Sweat and Denison 1995:S255).

In the absence of successful strategies that address the contextual issues of AIDS, the ultimate toll that the epidemic will take in northern Kilimanjaro is not likely to depend upon which intervention strategies are used; relatively few people ever come in contact with targeted interventions for a sustained period of time. A follow-on effect of consciousness raising and motivated behavior change for those who do seems improbable and would be difficult even to discern. The most substantial contribution the public health community can make may be service oriented rather than educational. Emphasis can be placed on STDs and AIDS as matters of reproductive health rather than as lifestyle issues of young adulthood. Reproductive health services and technologies and family-planning services can be addressed more effectively to men as well as women, echoing the AIDS-prevention theory of the man at an AIDS seminar who said that young people must be helped to realize the life that *they* see is good. The least that any AIDS-prevention program can do is to ensure that young people have the knowledge necessary to save their lives and the material means and the social support to put the knowledge into practice.

## AIDS: Demography, Bodies, and Culture in an Anthropology of Paradox

It is now a commonplace among social and cultural anthropologists that human bodies cannot "be adequately understood as ahistorical, natural, or precultural objects in any simple way" (Grosz 1994:x) and that forms of medical practice connected to reproduction and sexuality give an artificially "natural" quality to the production of historically and politically situated knowledges of bodies, to the experience of corporeality at its most root level (Turner 1984; Gallagher and Laqueur 1987; Laquer 1990). Thus knowledge in the form of medical truths "always remains *probable,* because it is always open to the criticisms of any future investigators" (Rochberg-Halton 1986:7; emphasis added). Nevertheless, it is necessary to distinguish between the concreteness of truths established through medical inquiry and the way biomedicine uses that knowledge. To conflate cultural knowledge and biological realities is to reassert a theory of sympathetic magic in which texts and language are the fetishes and personal bodies are the objects of the analytical spell. However "textualized" and "imag(in)ed" European bodies may have become through medical inscription and techniques of visualization (see, e.g., Vasseleu 1991), one need only consider the enormous demographic and epidemiological ramifications of "culture contact" (Kunitz 1994) to appreciate that the reduction of the somatic to the semantic is unsatisfying. As Foucault (1980a:151–52) stated: "Does the analysis of sexuality necessarily imply the elision of the body, anatomy, the biological, the functional? To this question, I think we can reply in the negative. In any case, the purpose of the present study is in fact to show how deployments of power are directly connected to the body—to bodies, functions, physiological processes, sensations and pleasures; far from the body having to be effaced, what is needed is to make it visible through an analysis in which the biological and the historical are not consecutive to one another . . . but are bound together in an increasingly complex fashion in accordance with the development of modern technologies . . . that take life as their objective."

In order to represent this nonlinguistic yet immanently cultural dimension of existence, I have suggested the concept of empersonation to complement that of embodiment. Rather than treating the body as the cultural repository of preconscious or habitual ways of knowing (see, e.g., Bourdieu 1977), the concept of empersonation configures personhood in such as way as to problematize the biologically immutable facts of aging, sexuality and sex, pregnancy and birth, morbidity and mortality. This concept has been used to understand the cultural history of personal development and sexuality in Kilimanjaro. The momentum of generations of regional population dynamics, demographic processes, and structural vulnerabilities became embodied in youth. At the same time, their bodies—habits of dress, diets, physiques, unstable physical locations, mortality, and, more recently, the diseases for which they have become at risk—became empersonated by a changing economy, disease ecology, and population structure. Indeed, none of these processes was or is consecutive to the others; they are mutually constitutive.

The response to the AIDS epidemic in Kilimanjaro was an openended inquiry into culturally shaped demographic and epidemiologic processes. This inquiry was made up of different kinds of signs, many of which derived from the bodies and actions of young adults. Given that there is never a "closed loop" between the corporeal and the cultural, or embodiment and empersonation, one may appreciate how individuals retained a degree of freedom in influencing the production of meaning, devising new interpretations of experience and generating new patterns of meaningful action. As Jackson insists, "Inasmuch as bodily praxis cannot be reduced to semantics, bodily practices are always open to interpretation; they are not in themselves interpretations of anything" (1989:134).

Hence, competing and indeterminate meanings of the AIDS epidemic emerged out of ideological contests over sexuality and disease, and out of pragmatic responses to self-perceptions of risk and to the agents of AIDS education. The meaning of what was being disordered and what was at stake in the AIDS epidemic in northeastern Tanzania was not the same to all parties. Nevertheless the bodies of youth came to personify risk, AIDS, dislocation, and diseased development. They did so through actions such as wearing certain types of shoes or sunglasses, through hairstyle and diet, through men's beer bellies and the pregnant bellies of young women, through selling bales of imported second-hand clothing in marketplaces, and through the demographic states of presence and absence of young men reflected in the age and sex structures of urban and rural wards. All of these bodily states served as changeable and unstable signposts in an ongoing process of giving meaning to basic elements of being a social person in Kilimanjaro in the late twentieth century.

The arrival of HIV in Kilimanjaro was a discrete event, yet the conditions revealed by the AIDS epidemic were not. In this way, AIDS has been a connected, unfolding process in the life of the Kilimanjaro community. As this study has shown, hierarchies of generation and gender, and demographic and political economic processes, have operated in an era of hardship in such a way as to place women and young adults at particular risk. This analysis of disease as social process has entailed a consideration of the conditions under which the epidemic of signification that inevitably accompanies AIDS unfolded in Kilimanjaro in the way that it did. AIDS threw a spotlight on processes that have been in motion for generations, giving an illusion of suddenness and entrenchment. While successful persons were loved and admired, they were signified not as repositories of cultural integrity but as agents of cultural loss. Previously the concept of dislocated men returning to Kilimanjaro was associated with a thin thread of tradition that still bound men in some mystical way to the mountain. In the late 1980s, men who went away were among the first wave of AIDS ill to return to the mountain to die. Both the present and past arrangements of productive and reproductive life stood out in stark relief against the backdrop of the looming expectations, moments of clarity, and the tenacious ambiguities of the epidemic.

Many of us have heard people with HIV, cancer, or even depression express an almost unbelievable gratitude, not for the infection, malignancy, or affliction, but for the insights and awareness illness has brought to them as individuals. AIDS forces such introspection on many levels. Even if an effective, inexpensive cure or vaccine were to emerge and the epidemic were to end, a process of social and cultural inquiry has been set in motion that challenges American anthropologists no less than young Africans to look forward, not only to understand the cause of disease and suffering in broader terms than that of individual behavioral choices and dangerous pathogens but also to frame prevention as an issue of social justice and human development (e.g., Preston-Whyte 1995). The emergent subfield of demographic anthropology has a great deal to contribute to this undertaking. A call for sets of middle-range theories, of situations, grounded in culture and political economy of reproduction and fertility, is a good beginning. Such a focus on the meeting of large-scale forces and the persons and bodies that inhabit these situations will allow, I believe, the contradictions of daily life, the paradoxes of culture and experience, to come to the fore and to be examined in a new light. For in such contested meetings are to be found truths about the universally shared and culturally divergent experience of sex and reproduction, of ill health and well-being, of death and life.

# Notes

## Chapter One

1. Chagga are the largest ethnic group on the slopes of Mount Kilimanjaro and in the regional capital of Moshi.

2. A person who has antibodies to HIV in his or her blood is said to be "HIV-positive" and is assumed to have been exposed to the virus. These antibodies are detected through any of several blood test technologies which are often (and somewhat misleadingly) called "AIDS tests." The term "HIV disease" is used to describe both the condition of an immunocompromised person and the various HIV-related opportunistic infections in people who harbor the virus but do not meet any of the numerous clinical criteria for having AIDS (see, e.g., Phillips et al. 1994). Although there have been reports of individuals developing AIDS-like conditions without the demonstrated presence of HIV in their bodies, such exceptional cases are not relevant to the AIDS situation in sub-Saharan Africa.

3. Intravenous drug use and infected blood transfusions account for a small proportion of HIV infections, and the rate of perinatal transmission in Tanzania has been assumed to be roughly 30 percent (NACP 1992).

4. These have included variables such as circumcised/uncircumcised, prostitute/nonprostitute, married/unmarried, history of STD/no history of STD, among others.

5. The shortcomings of the first generation of studies in which demographers sought to address cultural issues have been well inventoried by others (Hammel 1990; Le Blanc, Meintel, and Piche 1991; Lockwood 1995). More recently, a "culture and political economy" approach to demographic anthropology has been proposed by Greenhalgh. This approach "directs attention to the embeddedness of community institutions shaping fertility in structures and processes operating at regional, national, and global levels, and to the historical roots of these macro-micro linkages" (1995:13). Despite this progress in demographic anthropology, the subfield is only now attempting a synthesis of theories of patterned action, cultural reasoning, interpretation, and embodied experience (Kertzer and Fricke 1997a).

6. The Swahili acronym for AIDS, UKIMWI, stands for *ukosefu wa kinga mwilini*, literally "a lack of protection in the body."

7. "Discourse" refers to a cultural dialogue, whether across or within cultural frameworks, about bounded domains of knowledge or experience—from the mundane to the extraordinary. This dialogue inevitably involves diverse groups of actors with varying degrees of social and cultural power. Discourse, in the sense that I wish to use it, consists of the manipulation and communication of signs and symbols, including those of language, by these groups in order to work out contested aspects of experience, and to set the boundaries within which discourse itself takes place.

8. "Hey, Listen!" copyright © 1992 by Eziron Macha and Ben Lyimo. Lyrics used by permission; translation by author.

9. The local banana and millet brew of Kilimanjaro.

10. KCMC is the Kilimanjaro Christian Medical Centre, the zonal referral hospital in Kilimanjaro region. In 1984, the first case of AIDS in the region was diagnosed there.

11. In the late 1980s, there was considerable public and scientific interest in an alpha interferon–based drug called Kemron for the treatment of symptomatic HIV infection. The drug was invented in Kenya, and was hailed by many in East Africa who saw it as a triumph of African ingenuity and scientific skill. The drug was researched in clinical trials and was found to alleviate some symptoms of AIDS temporarily, but it did not affect the progress of the disease. Questions about Kemron were frequently asked at public AIDS education seminars from 1991 to 1993.

12. In epidemiologic terms, "prevalence" refers to the number of given cases of disease in a population at risk at a particular moment in time. "Incidence" refers to the number of new cases of a disease occurring to a population at risk over a specified period of time.

13. Pollock capitalizes "the Body" to distinguish it from "a body." As he notes: "The capitalized entity has emerged in the literatures of anthropology, sociology, history, and literary theory, among others, as a single abstract thing, usually (if implicitly) with universal applicability to all cultures at all times. The lowercased body is of variable composition, extension, and social significance both cross-culturally and across history" (1996: 338).

14. Again, this part of the discussion is aimed principally at anthropological readers.

15. I realize that the use of the singular term "sexuality" can be construed as implying that this aspect of human life is somehow unitary. Although I occasionally use the term in its singular form in this account, the reader is enjoined to bear in mind that "sexuality" as a concept must inherently embrace a plurality of forms, of sexualities as people live and experience them, if the term is to be of analytic use.

16. See, e.g., Bourdieu (1977) and Caplan (1987).

17. For examples of this debate, see Pellow (1990); Ahlberg (1991); Caldwell, Caldwell, and Quiggen (1991); Le Blanc, Meintel, and Piche (1991).

18. The population denominator for this figure was from the 1988 Tanzania census.

19. Research in western and northern Tanzania indicated that sentinel groups were likely to be reliable for only a few years and may have resulted in the actual prevalence of the epidemic being underestimated. Comparing sentinel rates to those from a community-based serosurvey in Mwanza, Borgdorff et al. (1993) demonstrated that by 1992, the sentinel rates among pregnant women already produced a severe underestimation of actual HIV prevalence among women of reproductive age.

20. By the late 1990s, UNAIDS recommended that only pregnant women be used as a sentinel population, since blood donors who engaged in high-risk behavior were meant to be screened out before their donations were accepted.

21. "Wewe, habari za kuchapa?" he asked, meaning, "Hey, you, how's the 'banging' going?" The verb he used as slang for having sex, -chapa, literally means "to hit" or "to strike."

22. It has sometimes surprised colleagues that I conducted interviews about sex and AIDS with women at all, given the potential for the overtones of sex and power, which did, in fact, occasionally emerge. On balance, however, there were few difficulties in conducting research in this manner (see Hammar [1996] for an example of successful sex research by a white man working with women of color in a developing country setting). In order to check how my conducting interviews might have affected the outcome, I compared transcripts of interviews that I conducted with those gathered by female research assistants (Gertrude Kessy and Sarah Kwayu), using identical questions, among women of comparable ages and social status. These comparisons revealed little

or no difference in the quality or character of the responses to most of the questions. I should also note that certain topics, including young women's personal narratives of specific sexual experiences, were almost always left to my research assistants.

## Chapter Two

1. It could, perhaps, be argued that the "true" local history of sexuality is of less immediate importance than how "traditional" sexual morality (whether merely nostalgic or wholly imagined) is used in local discourse about the disease. This not a defensible position if we wish to account truly for the cultural meaning of AIDS.

2. During the nineteenth century, the residents of Kilimanjaro resided in up to thirty separate chiefdoms. There are many indications that these people did not consider themselves to be part of a single cultural or ethnic entity; certainly they were never united linguistically (see Wilhelm, Möhlig, and Winter 1982) or politically (more than very fleetingly) before the colonial era. Although the use of the term "Chagga" to describe all the people on Kilimanjaro's slopes was very much a German colonial innovation (Kimambo 1996:75), it has been taken on board—along with its imprecision—by most writers this century, and to a large extent by Kilimanjaro-ites themselves both during and after the colonial period. I will follow this convention but also wish to emphasize that fairly wide variation in custom and cultural practice has always been evident among the populace. Thus, I speak of "Chagga men and women" and of "Chagga culture" in cases where the preponderance of evidence suggests the existence of widely shared institutions, practices, or beliefs. I treat the situation as pointing to local variation within the mountain system where evidence is patchy (particularly for the precolonial and early colonial eras), where sources contradict, or where my own findings indicate this to have been the case.

3. This ideology supported a system based on the valorization of heterosexual reproductive relations; there is no evidence that the pursuit of sexual pleasure among members of the same sex has ever been culturally validated in Kilimanjaro. For men, there may have been some form of institutionalized recognition of transgendered behavior, but only a single source contains this suggestion (Lemenye 1955:46). Furthermore, I was unable to locate any cultural memory of a general category of such "male-bodied" females during fieldwork.

4. Occasionally unions between certain clans were proscribed, and between others it was preferred. Marriage was patrivirilocal (near the husband's father's homestead) for first and last sons, and patrivirilocal or neolocal for middle sons. Allegiances to clan were crosscut by an age-grade system which incorporated men of many lineages within a chiefdom and by duties to the chief.

5. Aside from several varieties of bananas, the cultivands of the *kihamba* in the nineteenth century included beans, sweet potatoes, cassava, yams, pumpkins, squash, sugar cane, tobacco, cattle fodder, and vine potatoes (Moore 1977:21; New 1873:370).

6. Chagga descent is based on the patrilineage, and Chagga custom with regard to descent, inheritance, and marriage is renowned for its complexity. Two major works that deal substantially with the formal and social complexities of these issues are referred to throughout this book: Gutmann (1926) and Moore (1986).

7. Technically, all *kihamba* land was the property of the clan. Male members of the clan had permanent rights of use that approached outright ownership, including the right to rent out *vihamba* and to pass *vihamba* land to their sons. Within families, however, men did not have equal access to productive resources. In polygynous marriages, each wife was meant to have her own *kihamba* to farm and to reside on with her children. While there were many intricacies to laws and customs of inheritance, the essential principle was that control over a father's land was given to two sons: the first- and last born. Firstborn sons usually received their *vihamba* after initiation and before completion of marriage arrangements with a first wife. At the same point in their life courses, last-

born sons were given the *kihamba* that included their mother's homestead. They were also given primary responsibility for caring for their parents as they aged. When the firstborn son inherited full control of a *kihamba* following his father's death, he acquired exclusive rights to all his father's fields, fallow land, and deserted groves. Thus, under this polygynous system, the first son of the senior wife was the most structurally favored, while the first sons of other wives were entitled to inherit only their mothers' private property. Middle sons were provided for in a number of different ways (by favored siblings, grandfathers, or by being given a portion of their fathers' *kihamba* before it was turned over to the firstborn), and often managed to obtain *vihamba*.

8. Participating in the *kihamba* regime through establishing residence and engaging in agriculture on the mountain was an obligation surrounded by heavy morality. The exploitation of lands off the mountain could have easily challenged the cultural structures and authority rooted in intergenerational control of the productive mountainside; these spaces were stigmatized as "bush" (*-pori*) and hence unsuitable for human habitation.

9. The poetics are worth quoting: "Northwards the vast mass of the mountain stretched upwards into the heavens, its twin peaks shrouded in heavy cumulus clouds, and below the clouds, the billowy swell of hill upon hill and ridge succeeding ridge was a deep sullen blue under the shadow of lowering cumuli. Then came a few lines of dark purple-green forest, still in shade, and, in the middle distance, where the sunlight broke upon the scene, the gentle, rounded hills gleamed out against the sombre background with their groves of emerald-green bananas marking the commencement of the cultivated zone. Nearer to us succeeded deep ravines with thread-like cascades, clumps of tidy forest . . . just a few clumps left growing out of religious veneration . . . smooth, sunny downs, whereon flocks of goats were grazing, patches of freshly-tilled soil, cultivated fields, hedge-lined lanes, and lastly, the red denuded hill . . . on which we were standing to gaze on this Promised Land" (Johnston 1886:88).

10. The recognition of the interdependence between dominant and subordinate elements within Chagga hierarchies was often explicit. The advantage of those who were culturally empowered was tempered by clear-cut obligations toward the less empowered. In the nineteenth century, men learned that adopting an attitude of humility and responsibility toward social inferiors was one key to building a good reputation and a life free from curses. The abuse and neglect of children, wives, or siblings meant public humiliation and the temporary or permanent withdrawal of sanctioned reproductive potential; a wife could return to her birth clan, claiming to have been driven out by the brutality of her husband. Men with reputations for brutality, youths were taught, could find remarriage difficult. The abuse of sisters or elders carried the threat of powerful curses on a man's health and fertility or portended the death of his children (see Moore 1986). These punishments could bar one's entry into the revered ranks of the ancestors. The bodies of those who died without contributing their fertility to the clan were not buried on the *kihamba* with their forebears, but thrown into the bush, thereby breaking the chain of ordered succession and leading to the ultimate of social deaths. Kindness to inferiors was prompted by more than the threat of sanctions, however. The tactical and practical benefits of magnanimity were also stressed to men. Older sons were encouraged to set an example by displaying their generosity to younger brothers through gifts of land and cattle. Doing so would prevent quarrels and discord, and simultaneously place the younger in debt to their elder siblings.

11. The only comprehensive collection of initiation lessons was made by Gutmann in the three volumes of *Die Stammeslehren der Dschagga* (1932, 1935, 1938), of which only part of the first volume has been translated into English.

12. For the first several years of their lives boys and girls were referred to by a single term (*mwana*, in the Kichagga of Old Moshi) and performed similar household tasks. This combinatory state was stressed to boys, who were taught in grandparental songs

that "half of you should be a girl" (Gutmann 1932:203). Eventually, children began to diverge in the pursuit of culturally defined gender-appropriate conduct. Boys were meant to follow the sacred edict to imitate their fathers, who in turn intoned the following prayer: "Oh heavenly man, oh [chief], may this child again imitate something tomorrow so that I may again eat my fill from it" (231). Boys were also encouraged not to feel humiliated if they were mocked for copying the actions of elder siblings. For this was the way to grow in intelligence and to learn house building and cattle keeping. Girls went to market and imitated many of the actions of their mothers and grandmothers, including the weaving of toy market baskets.

13. The lack of a very strong tradition of local therapeutics (uganga) attests to this; the "traditional" healers with the greatest power came from elsewhere in the region. Specialist therapeutic knowledge among Chagga was more focused on the spiritual and divinatory than the "blood and guts" aspects of human existence.

14. Elemental forces like water, fire, blood, milk, and food might connote maleness in one ritual context, femaleness in another, and life or death in yet a third (Moore 1976: 365). Fundamental substances and processes derived their particular symbolic valences from the contexts in which they were evoked in song, or the use to which they were put in daily life; a single entity, such as the banana plant, took on different meanings in different ritual settings. In certain rituals, banana blossoms were symbolic brides for male ancestors who had died unmarried (Gutmann 1926:83), at other times they were symbolic penises for male children who were occasionally sacrificed to insure the integrity of chiefdom boundaries (1926:356). The growth of banana leaves was also used as a metaphor for the succession of male age grades (Gutmann 1932).

15. Although the *kihamba* itself appears not to have frequently been mentioned in ritual, its presence floated like an afterimage above every reference to mundane symbols of bananas, milk, beer, livestock, and houses. When it was referred to directly, the *kihamba* served as a metaphor for the entire clan or chiefdom, spotlighting its centrality to social reproduction. Children were taught that society, like the *kihamba*, had its winners and losers, and that those on top were the most essential to the proper order of things: "There are those who are taller and stronger, and those who fail to flourish. Do not remove these 'masters' of the grove, for it would be ruined" (Gutmann 1932:158). For boys, the extraction of their incisors at about age twelve coincided with their own removal from their mother's or grandparent's house. At this point in the life course, young men resided exclusively with members of the same sex and had a great deal of freedom. Most of their social activities revolved around the peers who were to form the next initiation age grade.

For young men and women alike, this was a time when a great deal of emphasis was placed on inculcating in them a suitably domestic disposition and a respect for marriage and generational authority. The majority of the songs in the translated sections of Gutmann's first volume of *Die Stammeslehren* dealt with these topics. Girls learned to have a sense of power and responsibility in certain domains of *kihamba* life and submissiveness in others. Work was stressed above all. A number of other lessons dealt specifically with controlling and directing young women's sexual desires. "As long as a little bird doesn't flutter about, no boy will catch and roast it" (Gutmann 1932:119), they were taught. Still, there was room to flirt: "Don't be shy and dumb in the company of boys. Laugh, be happy, make yourself pleasant! If you withdraw into yourself you will not get a husband!" (Raum 1940:182).

16. There appears to have always been a strong emphasis among Chagga on individualism and on seeing social power as pertaining to bounded sets of social relations. The power of others to issue sanctions against errant individuals was seen in quite situational terms: "In a 'constitutional' sense organizations of which Chagga individuals were not members had no directly effective authority over them" (Moore 1986:53).

17. There is some indication that these states may have much broader relevance. In Swahili, "to give birth" (-*zaa*) is commonly referred to as "opening oneself" (-*jifungua*).

18. Among young men, initiation also built the community of the *rika*, which remained a powerful organizing institution through the first part of the twentieth century. Since the initiation of a new *rika* implied a replenishment of the age grade that went to war at the behest of the chief, one might have expected the flourishing of the initiation ceremony to coincide with the period of greatest interchiefdom conflict. Yet this appears not have been the case. The height of the grove initiation ceremonies may have been during an era of relative peace, since boys from one chiefdom could be sent to participate in the grove proceedings of another (Gutmann 1932:4). For reasons that are not entirely clear, the grove ceremonies became shorter and shorter with each successive age grade and were eventually reduced to the minimum in the late 1890s by Chief Rindi in Old Moshi, who forbade overnight stays in the grove. At about this time, the military nature of the *rika* was suppressed by the German regime.

19. Female informants indicated that in the past, circumcision incorporated the wide excision of the clitoris and labia minora. In the 1990s, female circumcision was usually limited to clitoridectomy.

20. Even though initiation was pivotal to Chagga culture and the induction of young people into adult sexual life, it appears to have undergone a substantial decline toward the end of the last century. This is puzzling given that the apparent centrality of the *ngoso* might imply that this tradition would be an enduring one. Why abandon it if it did, indeed, mark the transition to adulthood in such a powerfully symbolic manner? The significance I have given to the symbolic anal closure is, in part, a product of the emphasis it has received in early ethnographic accounts. Previous accounts and analyses of the grove ceremonies indicate that the ritual was not merely an object of exotic fascination on the part of outsiders. It was, indeed, a critical step in becoming an adult man, in legitimizing men's general supremacy over women, and in acquiring virility and fertility.

21. As of 1998, in a few areas, *rika*s were still being inaugurated and *mregho* (see below) was still taught. In Old Moshi, the last full-fledged grove initiation took place around 1850 (Gutmann 1926:292), with truncated versions surviving until 1927 (Gutmann 1932). In Machame, the last camps were held in the 1890s (Raum 1940:320).

22. The earliest mission in Kilimanjaro was established in 1885 in Old Moshi. In 1892, the Church Missionary Society (CMS) missionaries there were evicted by the Germans, who sponsored the entry of the Leipzig Lutheran Mission. Meanwhile, Catholic missionaries had established a station in Kilema, Marangu (one of the large Chagga chiefdoms), in 1890 (Gogarty 1927:37–40; Moshi Diocese 1990).

23. The grove was both a liminal and superior location. Here, the initiates literally stood above even the *mangi*, the chief, at whose behest the initiations were called and to whose bidding the newly anointed *rika* would soon be committed.

24. It is useful to note that the homologies between *vihamba* and human bodies were emphasized through a symbolic system that was also inherently processual, situational, and multilayered. This symbolism made explicit the qualities of unequal interdependence within generational and gender hierarchies. As with many groups in Africa, Chagga houses were symbolically connected to female bodies. The conical beehive huts in which most Chagga lived and where reproductive sex was meant to take place were located in the sphere of inherited patriarchal authority (the *kihamba*), and primarily constructed by men. The careless execution of the important task of house building could affect women's bodies and female reproductive capacity; a house improperly built by a man for his wife was said to be "closed," a state which could easily transfer to her body and render her infertile (Raum 1940:326). This symbolic association persists to some extent; into the 1990s, people not uncommonly referred to the "door" (*mlango*) of the womb being "open" (*wazi*) during menstruation.

25. Before the passing of this "secret" fiction from the initiators to the incipient *rika*, two pits were dug, one for feces, one for urine. The feces pit was the deeper of the

two and received the masculine appellation "the steer," thus connecting male digestion, masculinity, and the major element of bridewealth (i.e., cattle) (Gutmann 1926:290).

26. Significantly, the *ngoso* could only be possessed by a limited number of *rika*s. The setting of the *ngoso* in one age set implied its removal from another. The relinquishing *rika* thereby removed itself from the reproductive regime and entered (or returned) to a state of combination with female actors whose fertility had also ceased through menopause. As the initiates were told, "Today I am handing the *ngoso* to you, for I have grown old. You preserve it, you and your older brother. The country is a succession. We leave it to you to seize the *ngoso* as we have kept it. Today I step aside and unite with the women. I withdraw the *ngoso* and hand it over to you. . . . I am now on a par with the parturient woman" (Gutmann 1926:303).

27. Men were not to perform these acts in the sight or presence of women and children, for they were now supposed to be possessed of the ability to completely digest their food. If afflicted by diarrhea, they were to be cared for by other men or women past the age of childbearing.

28. The act of closure bears more scrutiny, as its significance has been the source of some debate (Moore 1976; Stambach 1996b). The setting of the *ngoso* was only partly a sanction against homosexual intercourse, as Moore asserted (1976). Rather, the fiction of male self-sufficiency and total digestion appears to have been more significant than symbolic threat of anal intercourse. This threat is based on the presumption that anal sex represented a culturally "improper" combination of forces. It is unclear to what extent homoeroticism played a part in ritual, and to what degree same-sex sexual activity was part of erotic life for nineteenth-century Chagga men. If it was, however, the sanctions against anal intercourse in initiation ceremonies were some of the only recorded allusions to its existence.

More than an edict against anal intercourse, I see the fictionless fiction (i.e., that what was supposed to be a physical closing of the anus was actually a symbolic one) of *ngoso* as part of the system of interdependencies built into hierarchical gender relations. Obviously the maintenance of this empowering pretense required female complicity—it did not matter so much what women *thought*, as long as they *acted* as if adult men were literally closed at the anus. The erasure of men's defecation must have had precisely the opposite effect in day-to-day consciousness. It marked one of the most mundane and universal of bodily functions as requiring the participation of all household members in an elaborate, and unconvincing, ruse. From this standpoint, anal closure was more a charter for masculine reproductive capacity and social power than it was a sanction against male-to-male sexual activity.

29. There were at least two types of men's *mregho*, and the songs and lessons associated with them were meant to be learned by rote; initiates could be tested on them at any time after their instruction. The *mregho* collected by Raum describe in detail the development of the child in the mother's womb. The Uru type, a stylized version of which I collected, encapsulated clan history, focused on homologies between men's bodies and social order and how to maintain a balance between them. (According to Raum [1940], the women's *mregho* was carved with symbols of the female body.) In form, the Uru *mregho* represented the geography and topography of the chiefdom and the anatomy of the male body. The *mregho* also aesthetically reinforced the conjunction between anal closure and male fertility; the bottom of the *mregho* was called "the anus" but was carved in a way that clearly represented a circumcised penis.

30. In the 1990s men were still the active agents in the formation of the fetus: to impregnate a woman was "to give her your foetus/pregnancy" (*-mpa mimba yako*).

31. Raum, who offers the most complete account of *shiga* (1939, 1940), stated that the rites differed from the male initiation in two main regards: there were no female age grades, and the entire initiation process was accomplished in a much shorter span of time.

32. An older woman performed the *shiga* teaching for a group of newly circumcised girls. The leader began the lessons by "stealing back" the symbol of male procreative power: a grasshopper covered in a man's feces. Feces were also mixed with ocher and rubbed on each initiate's forehead before the lessons began. Thus, the initiates in their turn "hunted" the tokens of male fertility—the grasshoppers that their brothers had licked and released and that were now forbidden. The hunting of these six-legged "leopards" (as they were referred to) was accompanied by the telling of the story of men's treachery in having stolen the *ngoso*. In capturing the insects, women symbolically reappropriated the power to reproduce.

This act also materially subverted the fiction upon which the *ngoso* was based. Not only had women stolen back the symbol of the anal plug, but it was covered with the substance that men were no longer meant to produce (a myth which they pungently, if temporarily, exploded by smearing the evidence upon their foreheads). As Stambach put it, for women, the closure of men was nothing but an "open secret" for women (Stambach 1996b). Yet women were also meant to conceal the tokens of their own reproductive capacities. As the men were meant to hide the pretended secrecy of their symbolic closure, women were meant to obscure the evidence of their actual physical openness. The "unction of fertility, the blood which comes once every month," could be shown to no one; women were told explicitly to hide it from parents, siblings, and age mates (Raum 1939:559).

33. The French missionary Le Roy cites a figure of between 40,000 and 60,000 inhabitants of Kilimanjaro (Le Roy 1889:345), but this must be regarded as pure speculation. Similarly, Rebmann's note on *kihamba* size (an eighth of a mile on a side) is probably the only one recorded before the turn of the century, but similarly appears to be based on impression.

34. Like other aspects of reproductive life, birth spacing also reflected wider processes of social change. The three-year postpartum taboo was frequently violated (Raum 1939:88), and after the arrival of Christian missions, nominally monogamous Christian Chagga decreased birth spacing (presumably in order to maintain high total fertility or because men found it difficult to abstain with only one wife) and were told that having a baby a year was acceptable (Moore 1986:110).

35. Techniques for preventing conception included inserting rags into the vagina to stop conception. Abortion was induced by the ingestion of widely known abortifacients. Other techniques of abortion, such as the use of massage or the insertion of a sharp midrib of a leaf into the uterus, required expert assistance (Raum 1939, 1940:67–68).

36. Some chiefs were said to have carried out slaving among their own subjects (Stahl 1964:214), although the extent of slaving among Chagga is not accurately known. Without any acquired immunity, Chagga must also have been particularly vulnerable to severe attacks of malaria when off the mountain.

37. One lesson stated: "Do not lie with your boy friend. You will give him a disease, and he will not want to marry you at all!" (Raum 1940:182).

38. In 1893, Brehme, the German medical officer stationed in Marangu, wrote that malaria and respiratory infections were very common among visitors to the plains, and that transmission of malaria at high altitudes was beginning to occur as a result of increased traffic to off-mountain locations (Clyde 1962:12). My own calculations, based on data recorded by Brehme, indicate an incidence of 50–65 percent and case fatality rates of 15–20 percent among Chagga men conscripted for short military campaigns in the plains.

39. Gutmann states that there was an overall perception of a shortening life span, and linked this to a demand on the part of elders for young people to marry at an earlier age so that grandparents could participate in the rearing of their grandchildren.

40. I have been unable to ascertain any linguistic relationship between the words *ngosa* (bridewealth) and *ngoso* (the anal closure of men). As Päivi Hasu (personal communica-

tion) has suggested, however, the phonological closeness of the terms suggests intriguing interpretive possibilities about the connection between initiation and bridewealth, should a linguistic link be demonstrated.

41. In commenting on African marriage, it is a truism to say that it is far more a matter of relations and interests among lineages and clans than a private issue between two individuals. Chagga were no exception to this, and the numerous steps and stages of bridewealth marriages emphasized the group nature of *ngosa* through the carefully scripted involvement of specific kin of both the bride and groom.

42. The transfer of a woman to the home of her husband in an *ngosa* marriage was expensive, elaborate, and time-consuming (Gutmann 1926:39ff.). Betrothals were often made on behalf of young people of both sexes by their fathers, although young women supposedly had the right to veto the arrangements. The sublimation of self-interest by participating in *ngosa* marriage served as "an indication that the marriage does not take place for selfish reasons, but rather as an act that is of the utmost importance for society and its population" (1926:96). The importance of fertility within *ngosa* marriages was underscored by the custom of paying the final installment of the bride-price only after the fifth month of the bride's first pregnancy.

43. There was definitely a shortage of cattle due in large measure to the rinderpest epizootic.

44. It has been demonstrated in other parts of Africa, however, that sexual and reproductive relations can respond quickly to shifts in the political and social environment, while others remain remarkably resilient (Schoepf 1992:358). At the time when colonialists were making their first permanent presence felt in Kilimanjaro, the negotiation between Africans and Europeans over the domain of personal sexuality was already under way in other parts of the continent. Cultural interactions over sexuality in southern Africa are also illustrative of the way in which different power interests were asserted in the debate. Certain local stakeholders, notably the local patriarchs, sought to preserve culturally conservative forms of marriage and domestic arrangements. At the same time, men and women made tactical moves (both geographic and symbolic) in their efforts to exploit the accelerating pace of change in rural areas to personal advantage. Leaving rural areas and moving to towns or rural areas of labor concentration were made possible by changes in the material conditions of productive life. This, in turn, led to shifts in the short-term value of different kinds of nuptial transactions and marital arrangements (Jeater 1993).

45. In punishment, uncircumcised girls who became pregnant could be forced into marriage with older men. Most Chagga recount a more grisly fate for both the girl and her partner if both were uninitiated. Custom has it that the offenders were led to a special location in the forest, placed one on top of the other as if engaged in sex and impaled with sharpened stakes or spears. The bodies were left to wild animals. By the 1900s, however, this practice was abandoned by the *mangis* for fear of having to execute too many uninitiated boys and girls (Gutmann 1932:385). Unmarried lovers who were initiated and who were caught out through a pregnancy or birth were often forced to marry in a "wedding of shame." In this Chagga-style shotgun wedding, the infant, who was born "out of sequence," was meant to be put to death immediately after birth (Gutmann 1926:15).

46. Men were increasingly selecting their own partners. At one point early in the century many young women either felt the ability to opt out of marriage altogether or felt that a viable range of alternatives existed. In Old Moshi and other chiefdoms, an "entire generation" of young women was seized by a "spirit of revolt against marital ties" so widespread that the chief was eventually prompted to request the assistance of colonial officials to bring matters in hand (Gutmann 1926:58).

47. In one initiation lesson "tobacco" is an obvious euphemism for sex: "You see a beautiful woman newly married. She is used to taking snuff, and she asks for some. You

say you have none. She says 'why are you so stingy?' You say 'if I am so stingy, have I had any of yours?' She says 'did you ask me for any and did I refuse?' You say 'and if I ask you for some will you be willing?' She answers 'why should I not be willing?' This is how an affair develops. You will be ill from it" (Gutmann 1932:403–4).

48. A woman who married into a clan suspected of having either a curse or an inherited illness was tacitly permitted to become pregnant by someone outside her husband's clan. Although fully incorporated into the woman's husband's clan, the child, it was reasoned, would not be prone to inherit the disease or the curse. Also, in cases of suspected male infertility, a man might arrange for a *rika*-mate euphemistically to "visit his homestead." In both cases of sanctioned adultery, however, it was necessary to ensure secrecy, thereby preserving an impression of fertility within the context of proper reproductive unions.

49. "Outwitting the girl" *(ilemba mana)* and "the lifting up of the girl on the way" *(iiramana ndizien)* were the terms for bride capture. Such abductions were often concurred in by members of both clans, if not the woman herself (although unwilling women often had some recourse to nullify the union). This form of capture was used to truncate the payment of *ngosa*.

50. "The custom of bride-capture has become rather prevalent in Chagga territory, and in certain chieftancies one could get the impression that bride-capture was the only form of bride transfer," Gutmann noted (1926:131).

## Chapter Three

1. Changes in the epidemiology of smallpox in Kenya point to the responsiveness of disease to population dynamics. In the early 1900s the pattern of smallpox altered dramatically owing to population movement. Smallpox endemicity was low in the precolonial era owing to limited migration and trade. In the twentieth century, however, labor migration (including army service), longer distance travel for trade, increasingly crowded markets, circular migration, and commuting to urban centers all fostered the increased spread of the disease (Dawson 1992:97–102).

2. What they did, actually, was to blame one another. Some physicians blamed the Christian missions for removing severe penalties for extramarital sex, while missionaries blamed the suppression of the feudal political system (Vaughan 1991:133–34). What was not in dispute was the supposed way in which African women were incapable of encountering change without having their innate passions released. In Uganda and elsewhere, such explanations appealed to rural elders, for they provided ammunition in struggles to reassert patterns of authority threatened by social change.

3. Many of the Ghanaians were single mothers and had been displaced from nonmarital, cohabiting *mpena* relationships in their home areas. In Ivory Coast, as many as 75 percent of them engaged in one of several forms of commercial sex work. These women returned periodically to Ghana during the course of sojourns in the city. This movement was tied to the emergence of AIDS in home communities in Ghana, making it a disease of "elsewhere."

4. Indeed, early in the epidemic it was relevant to ask whether AIDS would even be recognized as a new illness at all (see, e.g., Obbo 1988). The concern was that preexisting cultural illness categories that described wasting conditions among adults and children in cases of sexual transgression within marriage (found in several East and Central African cultures) would simply be extended to cases of AIDS.

5. ELCT Northern Diocese AIDS education seminar, Machame, Nov. 1, 1991.

6. In Kilimanjaro, for example, informal or moral demographies acquired discursive ontologies because language and stories were the media in which people represented the meaning of population processes to one another, and were the media in which I elicited narratives for the purposes of fieldwork.

7. I do not view cultural phenomena associated with bodies as variants of "discursive practice," but rather of "signifying practice." A concept of discursive practice too seamlessly bridges a gap between concepts of corporeality, action, and discourse, a point at which great cultural and disciplinary battles of meaning are fought. Although actions mean nothing by themselves, neither is their meaning foreordained by a discursive set of concepts through which they *must* be comprehended. Before actions enter into discourse, they undergo a process of interpretation and evaluation which welds them (sometimes tentatively, or with very weak bonds) to particular meanings in particular times and places.

8. This was said without any hint of irony. The lack of a sense of contradiction in the idea of "traditional Christian Chagga culture" stems in part from the rationalization or understanding held by many Chagga that the era before missionization and conversion to Islam predated religion altogether. Thus there was no traditional religion to supplant, merely elements of local culture and custom (*utamaduni,* or *mila na desturi*) to be augmented, blended, improved upon, or discouraged.

9. It is also important to note that *tamaa* was not spoken of as inherently gendered; both women and men experienced it. The qualities of *tamaa,* and ways in which it placed them at risk and eroded their moral character, however, were thought to differ for men and women.

10. By "modernity" I refer to the host of forces and institutions imported during colonial occupation: from the church, the school, and the clinic to money, commodities, technology, capitalist modes of production, and the state apparatus itself.

11. The way in which desire operated as an aspect of moral character and sexual relations in the 1990s is also an important aspect of the concept of *tamaa* and will be discussed in chapter 4.

12. Esther Lema to nurses and medical assistants at Kilema hospital, Nov.12, 1991.

13. Interview, April 2, 1993. Unless otherwise indicated, the interviewer's speech is contained in square brackets.

14. Interview, Sept. 26, 1996, twenty-four-year-old man.

15. In the nineteenth century, many of the most desired and valuable objects (e.g., iron rings and implements, cloth, clay pots, salt and soda) were only obtainable through trade and an engagement with a wider world of things and people external to Kilimanjaro. The raw materials for pots, weapons, rings, and the like, and soda and salt, did not occur naturally on the mountain. Yet it was the commodified, money-linked, and mass-produced objects made available through colonialism and the introduction of agrarian capitalism and coffee cash cropping which many people spoke of as having instilled in Chagga a sense of *tamaa* for things.

In his examination of the meaning of objects, wealth, and power in Madagascar, Graeber (1996:20) points out that the desire for a particular kind of coveted object is an implicit acknowledgment "of the various acts of creation, consecration, use, appropriation . . . that make up its history." The cultural recognition of value in things, then, implies that those things have been generated by a unique historical crossing of personal desire and intention. Seeing something as desirable and valuable locates the beholder at the juncture of the past production of the value of that object and the future intention or hope to acquire it. In Kilimanjaro *tamaa* for objects can simply be seen as an urge to acquire new kinds of objects. Yet it also suggests the emergence of a shared cultural disposition, an aesthetic that arose out of the intersection of local demographic histories and a widening world of opportunity for new arrangements in domesticity and work.

16. Medicine, discussed later in the book, played a parallel and similarly important role, though in a somewhat subtler fashion.

17. For men, it appears that an education became a very desirable quality in a future wife. One can also imagine that a number of pressures must have been acting upon young women in mission schools, whose familiar timetables for marriage and mother-

hood were being altered. Commenting on the early years of schooling in Kilimanjaro, Shann (1956:26) observed that "before the girls had learnt much of their duties as mothers and housewives, they tended to run away in order to get married. Then as now a Girls' School was a popular matrimonial agency."

18. Interview, Jan. 30, 1992.

19. As one Chagga noted, "The growing opportunities for paid workers in mission and government stations to earn a regular wage and for . . . cash crop[s] created new consumer demand. In place of traditional weapons, tools, utensils and clothes—all made within the Chagga household—people began to purchase European manufactured steel axes, knives and cooking pots; china plates, cups and dishes; cotton shirts, trousers and dresses. A whole range of imported goods such as umbrellas, boxes, chairs, and leather goods, etc., also appeared in shops" (Lema, quoted in Howard 1980:55).

20. Writing in 1940, Raum noted that "the wholesale adoption of European standards by youthful members of the tribe is only apparent. . . . 'To turn European' is not an end in itself, but a means to realize the native national aspirations more firmly" (1940:290).

21. At a societal level, there were the concerns as lineages maneuvered for advantage in acquiring land. Within core lineages, there were both "vertical" and "horizontal" concerns. Men had to balance the need to display proper conduct toward parents and elders against the forces pushing them away from the *kihamba*. At the same time they had to contend with the stresses of defending their interests against the machinations of brothers or other agnatic kin (see cases in Moore [1975] and [1981] for examples). The material consequences of bad rapport with one's kin could be severe indeed. Given that so much depended on good agnatic relations, it is not surprising that moral character of migrants and desires associated with the off-mountain world should acquire such a powerfully negative set of overtones.

22. Interview, April 3, 1992.

23. There is not much consensus about the rate at which land pressures developed on Kilimanjaro. Although they are admittedly impressionistic, Johnston's observations in the 1880s suggest that even in the absence of any land alienation, little *kihamba*-zone land remained uncultivated. Despite an ambivalent policy of the German administration toward European settlement (Koponen 1994:153–56), by the early 1900s there was considerable alienation of arable land on the margins of the kihamba zone. After interchiefdom warfare had subsided, the German government limited land acquisition for Europeans to areas below the *kihamba* belt. Tracts that were put under crop by settlers were primarily used for rubber, sisal, cotton, and coffee (Green 1986:15), although much of the land is said to have remained uncultivated.

24. Coffee was introduced by missionaries in the chiefdom of Marangu about 1914 (at about the time of the British takeover of Tanganyika as a protectorate), although its cultivation as a cash crop was not emphasized until Sir Charles Dundas's tenure as district officer from 1919 to 1924. While land shortage became much more acute after the commercial viability of coffee had been demonstrated, the effects of land scarcity were not felt simultaneously in all areas. Gutmann stated that in the early 1900s every person in Old Moshi resided on a *kihamba* and estimated the size of a "decent" *kihamba* to be half a hectare (Gutmann 1926:367, 371). Yet the oral history I collected from a nearby area indicates that an acute land shortage emerged in the vicinity at roughly the same time. Still, other sources concur that land was generally available on many parts of Kilimanjaro through the first quarter of the century (Howard 1980:43) and that *vihamba* could be purchased for as little as a cow and a goat (Moore 1986:110). Kimambo has stated that through the 1950s land near the forest verge high on mountain could be easily converted to *kihamba* without even obtaining chiefly approval, although land lower on the slopes was subject to discretionary allocation (1996:79).

British policy, and Dundas's in particular, was to push coffee cultivation in every way possible—even to the extent of floating loans to *mangis* to purchase seedlings for resale to *kihamba* owners (Moore 1986:119). Even at this early point, the aggregate productivity of Chagga coffee farmers rivaled that of settler-owned estates (Howard 1980:52). Coffee was successful and popular among Chagga in part because it fit the social organization of land and labor under the *kihamba* regime; it intercropped perfectly with bananas and could usually be harvested without drawing upon labor of nonclans-folk.

In 1923 it was estimated that there were 3,300 Chagga coffee growers. By 1968, there were more than twenty times that number. Even the fleeting impressions of visitors to the *kihamba* belt indicate the scope, rapidity, and variability of change. By 1930 in Old Moshi, where intensive coffee farming had gone on for roughly fifteen years, the average plot size was only 500 square meters, yet in Kibosho where heavy farming began after 1920, plots were nearly ten times that size (Iliffe 1979:275). The homesteads that Rebmann estimated to lie an eighth of a mile apart in 1848 were said to be separated by only 100 yards in 1931 (Bailey 1931:1). By the middle of the century, plots allocated to newly married couples were often as small as 100 square meters. Moore's detailed maps of *vihamba* holdings in Marangu (1986:113, 230) give a graphic sense of the process of *kihamba* fragmentation.

There were strategies for increasing overall Chagga land holdings, but these benefited very few. One option was simply to buy land back from missions or planters, which was done in Marangu. Another option was to sue for the return of land. The Kilimanjaro Native Planters Association (KNPA) and, later, the Kilimanjaro Native Co-operative Union (KNCU) launched land-claims cases for the return of mission and plantation land alienated by the churches and by German planters. They met with some success, and several thousand acres of land were returned to Chagga ownership (Maruma 1969:14).

25. In some areas women and younger children, rather than men, took up labor on plantations (Meghji 1977:34).

26. Population growth and changing land-use patterns led to a greater reliance on food crops such as maize grown at lower altitudes—a demand for the kind of agriculture that some of the expanding population were in a position to take up. This bit of ecological and economic serendipity was one way in which growing populations were initially absorbed. Indeed after World War II, grain production rivaled coffee production in scale. Many others sought new horizons through education and employment in the civil service, through churches, or in education or health.

27. A caveat about the use of census data in this chapter: the reliability of censuses and published analyses of them is uncertain. Operating on the assumption that early censuses are minimally useful (especially for rural areas) and that enumeration has improved over the course of years, I place more weight upon demographic studies and census material since the 1960s. Nevertheless, a certain lack of precision (even if it exists in more recent demographic studies) is tolerable. Whether, for example, the "true" rate of male out-migration for educated young men from Kilimanjaro in the 1960s and 1970s was closer to 70 percent or 90 percent than to the 80 percent figure given in the text is not nearly as important to this account as the fact that male out-migration was a demonstrably significant aspect of population dynamics in the mid-to-late twentieth century.

28. Reproductive sexuality has changed a great deal in Kilimanjaro over the past forty years. Between the 1950s and the late 1980s, Kilimanjaro maintained among the highest total fertility rates in the country, though significant decreases in the crude birth rate suggest that fertility may have been falling. The crude birth rate (defined as the number of births in a given year divided by the midyear population) went from the nation's second highest in 1967 (51) to the third lowest (38) in 1988. Married women in Kilimanjaro have had the country's lowest desired fertility (as measured in surveys) and by far the highest rates of modern contraceptive use (Bureau of Statistics 1993). The total fertility rate (the total number of children born to a woman over her lifetime) was estimated at 7.1 in 1988, even though by 1992, the mean desired fertility of women of all ages in

Kilimanjaro was 4.3 (United Republic of Tanzania 1994: Tables 8.3, 8.4; Bureau of Statistics 1993:49, 66).

Between 1967 and 1988 the region also had by far the nation's highest mean age at marriage. It was twenty years of age in 1967 and twenty-seven in 1988 (United Republic of Tanzania 1994: Table 8.7). The usual cautions about the dangers of measuring the age at marriage in Africa must be borne in mind here. The processual and protracted nature of marriage arrangements in most of the continent make the category a dubious one. If we assume that the inaccuracies in measuring age at marriage are spread more or less evenly throughout the Tanzanian census data, however, Kilimanjaro stands out as consistently having the highest mean age at marriage in each of the three censuses since 1967.

29. Calculated from data in Table 4.1 (United Republic of Tanzania 1994:50).

30. Wages on coffee and sisal plantations dropped through the first part of the century from 18 shillings per month to a low of 8 shillings during the Depression (Green 1986: 47). Urban wages, meanwhile, had outstripped rural wages by 1928 and may have encouraged young Chagga men to move directly to town, bypassing agricultural wage labor altogether. Casual labor at the Moshi railhead, for example, paid 4 shillings per day for loading and unloading rail cars, enabling men to earn in a week of work in town what they would have had to labor months for on a plantation. Such work was very insecure and required men to maximize every opportunity. One strategy for doing so in the rail yard was to delay loading the cars until shortly before a train was due to depart; the loaders were then able to force forwarding agents to pay higher wages in order that their shipments not miss the train and the ship.

31. A rail link connecting Moshi to the coast was completed in 1911, and by the 1920s Moshi became a hub for the extraction of raw materials such as sisal, coffee, ballast and stone, timber and cotton (Green 1986:19).

32. Urban overcrowding was a complaint of health and sanitation officials into the late 1950s as the African sections of town grew and expanded (Tanganyika Territory Medical Department 1950–57). Effluent from a tannery and soda and cheese factories polluted the urban water supplies and fouled the air around the market (TNA J.1.11841). This particular part of town, the vicinity of the African market, gained a bad reputation early on among Europeans and Chagga alike. In 1930 the president of the Moshi Chamber of Commerce complained that "the practice of natives taking liquor and frequently being in a state of intoxication in the Bazaar is a danger to the morals of the community" and successfully lobbied for the removal of the beer shops to a location "not frequented by Europeans" (TNA J.1.11841). Chagga religious leaders also sought limitations on hours of operation for *mbege* bars, although urbanites defended their prerogatives to drink and defied the new ordinances by refusing to leave the bars (Samoff 1974:68). Although the district officer claimed Moshi was comparatively free from commercial sex work, the two general forms of prostitution in East African cities, *watembezi*, or streetwalkers, and *malaya*, women who received customers in their homes (White 1990:13–15), have been present in Moshi since the 1950s, and probably before; in the 1930s, the area around the market was also alleged to be the location of "a native brothel" that Europeans were seen to frequent (TNA J.1.11841).

33. Interview, Dec. 6, 1996.

34. In several small convenience samples taken during fieldwork (the mean sample size was seven), an average of two women in each group had children and claimed they had been left by their husbands or by the men they identified as the fathers of their children.

35. The numerical predominance of women in rural areas and the social significance attached to their plight masked an important dynamic of migration in Kilimanjaro: the movement of women to town. Since the 1970s, there have been relative deficits of *both* men and women of reproductive age in many rural locations. Compared with rural areas,

women between fifteen and thirty-five years of age made up a larger proportion of the total population in all urban areas. Similarly, men between the ages of fifteen and fifty were a proportionally larger part of the urban population compared with their rural counterparts. Nevertheless, there was a distinctly gendered character to rural and urban populations in the reproductive age groups. In 1988 women had become numerically predominant in rural Kilimanjaro, while in urban areas men dominated the adult population. See below, table 5.1.

36. The perspectives of long-term migrant men were not obtained during fieldwork.

37. Interview, May 28, 1993.

38. Responses from group discussion with Kirua M., Mwanahawa M., Gloria O., Eli G., Esta N., Lily M., Rosy K., Jan. 30, 1992.

39. Interview, Dec. 17, 1991. The slaughter of a goat in the *kihamba* has long been common propitiatory rite in Kilimanjaro.

40. Interview, April 17, 1993.

41. Interview, April, 17, 1993.

42. The figures were 60 percent male, 45 percent married; 40 percent female, 30 percent married.

43. In Arusha, the adjusted odds ratio was 5.16 (significant within 95 percent confidence limits) after controlling for age, sex, and area of residence. In Mwanza, the adjusted odds ratio was 3.4 (significant within 95 percent confidence limits) after controlling for age group, area of residence, travel to Mwanza town, marital status, number of partners, STD history, and history of injections.

44. The adjusted odds ratio was 1.71 (significant within 95 percent confidence limits) after controlling for more than twenty-one variables. In this study, the authors did not describe how they distinguished between women who were currently "married" and those who were "cohabiting," or what the relationship was between the categories of "cohabiting" and "polygynous." They did point out, however, that roughly half of the HIV-positive women were in monogamous marriages at the time of the survey (Kapiga et al. 1994:302).

45. Relative to single men, the adjusted odds ratios were 18.7 (currently married, monogamous or polygynous), 24.7 (widowed / divorced / separated), and 18.0 (nonmarital relationships, casual and steady). Relative to single women, the odds ratios were 2.4 (currently married, monogamous or polygynous), 2.7 (widowed / divorced / separated), and 6.9 (nonmarital relationships, casual and steady).

## Chapter Four

1. In the moral anatomy of the *kihamba* regime the liver was the organ associated with "spirit"—especially in the context of personal trials such as warfare and initiation. In the twentieth century, heart, or *roho,* became associated with spirit. *Moyo* refers literally to the heart muscle, while *roho* pertains to sentiment and spirituality, as in the Swahili translation of "holy spirit": *roho mtakatifu.*

2. Christians pointed out that the Bible's commentary on *tabia* is contained in the story of Cain and Abel, implying that good and bad are the only two true kinds of *tabia.*

3. None of these rituals were looked upon with much favor by the Christian establishment, and so were often performed furtively in the *kihamba.*

4. Dr. Doris N., at an AIDS seminar, Kilema hospital, Dec. 12, 1991.

5. Interview with Freddy S., May 24, 1992.

6. Interview with Gabriel M., Mar. 26, 1993.

7. Interview with Issa L., April 15, 1993.

8. The very old aged *(wakongwe),* however, returned to childhood. When speaking of them, women used the verb *-lea,* which literally means "to nurture or raise a child." "An *mkongwe* is exactly like a child of four or six years old. They eat, speak, and want attention

for themselves exactly like a child of that age. They do everything like a child," I was told by a woman who cares for her centenarian mother-in-law in Mbokomu.

9. Although the word *"kijana"* (plural: *vijana*) can refer to a young person of either sex, in practice it usually refers to a young man.

10. Interview with Freddy S., May 24, 1992.

11. Interview with Mariamu K., June 2, 1991.

12. Interview with Ishindi I., conducted by Sarah Kwayu, May 12, 1993.

13. Interview with Lilly K., June 2, 1991.

14. Interview with Freddy S., May 24, 1992.

15. Interview with Michael N., Oct. 13, 1991.

16. Interview with Japhet M., Sept. 26, 1996.

17. Ibid.

18. Much of the case material on the lives of young women reported in this chapter was collected by two research assistants, Gertrude Kessy and Sarah Kwayu.

19. Meghji's interviews with female workers who moved to work in various industries in Moshi during the 1940s and 1950s (1977:111–21) show that many of the patterns said by informants in the 1990s to be recent and male-inspired were well established more than forty years ago, and that they appealed to women as well as men. Several women were cohabiting with male partners, and only a few reported being "legally" married. Some women with children sent them to live on the mountain, while they themselves stayed in town either alone or with their partners. Others were happily unmarried or divorced single parents raising children by one or more men.

20. Undated, unsigned letter written in Kiswahili to Eliza M.; author's translation.

21. The word *starehe* retained the meaning of entertainment or recreation and did not necessarily imply sex. Going to a movie or video bar could also be *starehe*.

22. A note about language: many young people used the English noun "sex" as a Kiswahili verb. The cognate, *-sexi*, was conjugated like any regular Kiswahili verb, although there was no passive form. The person who is doing the "sexing" is the one who assumes the superior position in the act.

23. Interview with Masanja R., May 15, 1993.

24. Interview with Vero W., conducted by Sarah Kwayu, May 6, 1993.

25. Among twenty to twenty-four year olds, 65 percent of women were ever married, and 25.3 percent had experienced at least one live birth. (Unfortunately, it is not possible to determine the overlap of these groups, and nuptiality has been a notoriously poor indicator of entry into sexual and reproductive life in Africa.) These figures contrast sharply with the 57.9 percent of ever-married women aged forty to fifty-five who reported having experienced a pregnancy by the age of twenty, and the 81.2 percent who had been pregnant by the age of twenty-four. These figures may be affected, however, by respondents' misdating events long past.

26. In African countries such as Tanzania that were rocked by recession from the late 1970s through the mid-1980s, estimating the effect of recession on ages at marriage and the timing of first and second births has proved extremely difficult (Working Group on Demographic Effects of Economic and Social Reversals 1993:166–70). A major cross-national comparison, however, tentatively concluded that age at first marriage, which was rising across the continent independently of the 1980s recessions, may well have been further postponed for many owing to economic hardship. Furthermore, the odds of having a first or second birth appeared to have fallen as economic indicators declined (1993:166). The relationship between these factors and the rates of voluntary abortion in Tanzania at the time requires further study.

27. Many people interviewed estimated that young people were becoming sexually active at about fifteen years of age.

28. Some adults partially absolved young women of this misdeed by arguing that their pregnancies were a strategic response to the limited marriage market. They reasoned that

the cultural value of children to men was strong enough to cause them to acknowledge paternity of their children and so prompt them to provide in some way for their children's mothers, regardless of whether there was any kind of sanctioned union between the two.

29. For example, among men with any children, 68 percent (N = 168) had their first children before entering into marriage, and among those who had their first children after marrying, twenty-one of fifty-eight men stated that their spouses were pregnant at the time the marriage was "sealed."

30. Interview with Ishindi I., conducted by Sarah Kwayu, May 12, 1993.

31. Technically, abortions for other than grave medical reasons have been illegal in Tanzania. However, they have commonly been performed at hospitals and private clinics (Mpangile, Leshabari, and Kihwele 1993). The cost of the procedure was between TSh 10,000 and TSh 12,000 in the late 1980s.

32. Letter from Upendo M to Laura K., May 14, 1993; author's translation.

33. Interview with Saba C., April 28, 1993.

34. Interview with Abdul Ali F., June 6, 1993.

35. A common form of elopement was for a woman to stay "publicly" with a man for an entire night. After they spent the night together, the parents of each partner were meant to come to an understanding about a "fine" and a brideprice.

36. Interview with Alice U., Dec. 27, 1991.

37. About $7.00 in 1991.

38. Christine Trupin, personal communication.

39. See Moore's discussion of the secularization of ritual foods (1996:131–33).

40. *Urafiki* (friendship) and *rafiki* (friend) are words that denote entirely nonsexual relationships when applied to members of the same sex. When the speaker refers to a member of the opposite sex, however, they readily take on more ambiguous connotations.

41. Interview with Sharifa S., Feb. 22, 1993.

42. Interview with Marita M., June 11, 1993.

43. Interview with Sharifa S., Feb. 22, 1993.

44. Interview with Gloria F., Feb. 19, 1993.

45. Interview with Tina J., June 8, 1993.

46. Interview with Fortunata G., May 12, 1993.

47. Janet Lefroy, personal communication.

48. Interview with Devota S., by Gertrude Kessy, May 30, 1993.

49. Interview with Ufoo L., by Sarah Kwayu, May 9, 1993.

50. Interview with Abdullah, Sina, and Garo, Mar. 29, 1993.

51. Interviews with Helen T., May 31, June 1, June 4, and June 20, 1993.

52. Interviews with Rahman K., May 29, 1992, and Mar. 1, May 18, and June 24, 1993.

53. This idea counters somewhat the notion that circumcised women had decreased desires.

## Chapter Five

1. The World Bank, meanwhile, suggested that the prevailing outlook for the AIDS epidemic would improve mainly by pursuing the policies entailed in structural adjustment programs (World Bank 1993:107).

2. The term "informal sector" refers to small, unregistered, and generally nonagricultural private-sector income-generating activities. In Tanzania the main informal activities have included: food vending, operating small kiosks, small retail trading, providing small-scale fabrication and repair services, woodworking, working in domestic service, and operating small hotels and restaurants (Luvanga 1996:4–6). Activities not usually enumerated, but important in the local narratives of AIDS in Kilimanjaro, were tacit and

open commercial sex work for women and a highly male-dominated smuggling trade across the Kenyan border.

3. Lilly M., speaking to Community Development Committee, Mbokomu, Jan. 30, 1992.

4. Interview with Samuel H., Oct. 13, 1991.

5. That is, relative to women, men accounted for roughly a third of those who nominated themselves as working in agriculture, two-thirds of those engaged in commercial and business activities, and just over half the skilled labor regardless of whether they were living in Moshi Urban or Moshi Rural District. The exception to this pattern was among the unemployed, where women accounted for 63.1 percent of rural jobless and 51.0 percent of those without work in town. The significance of the category of "other" occupations can be discounted since it represents 5 percent or less of the labor force. The complete breakdown of occupational categories by sex is shown above in Table 5.2.

6. According to a household survey conducted in two urban and one peri-urban ward (Setel and Kessy 1992), "business" was by far the most common occupation from which Moshi respondents derived most of their income (39.5 percent, N = 157). Skilled and manual labor accounted for 25.5 percent of the sample, and farming accounted for 17.8 percent. Yet more than 70 percent of respondents indicated a secondary source of income, primarily additional small businesses (such as selling used clothing or running a kiosk) or casual labor (kibarua).

7. The category "unemployed" in the 1988 census is particularly suspect. During the 1980s, petty traders were harassed and vilified by the government as part of the Nguvu Kazi (Hard Work) program, largely because they had become the lowest level of distribution for smuggled consumer goods (Kerner 1988:45). According to one man responsible for regional census enumeration, this encouraged many people to conceal their petty trading activities during the census for fear of discovery.

8. Mirungi, or miraa, is a popular recreational drug among Muslims. The stimulant effect is achieved by chewing the leaves and barklike skin of the miraa plant, which is sold in bunches.

9. Interview with Jackson Jacob M., June 1, 1993.

10. Interview with Jonas U., May 24, 1993.

11. Interview with Lewis K, May 27, 1993.

12. As Raum noted, "In the market the female sex has evolved a social institution, with its own laws and secrets, to which men are not admitted. There judgement is pronounced on the conduct of husbands. . . . Those men who do not pass this examination experience the humiliation of being publicly mocked" (1940:183).

13. The material basis for markets has been discussed mainly in connection with outside trade and with periodic shortages of common foodstuffs in microecological pockets around the mountain. During the precolonial era, the most significant trade with outsiders entailed the provisioning of slave and ivory caravans of up to a thousand men from Mombassa and Zanzibar (Moore 1977:12). The volume of goods required was "a big business that must have required a marked increase in Chagga food production" (Moore 1986:31). If the presence of markets was a straightforward issue of supply and demand in relation to the provisioning trade, it was more puzzling when viewed in the context of the mountain system. First of all, if Chagga culture was straightforwardly configured in terms of male domination, why would women be ceded control over such a lucrative sphere of activity? Furthermore, aside from the provisioning trade, the very existence of the markets for local consumption was something of a conundrum since there was such uniformity of produce sold there. If each family was growing and selling more or less identical crops, what was the need for a market? Previous explanations for the local relevance of women's markets have stressed that they provided variety in an otherwise monotonous diet, and the observation that the microecologies of the mountain create delays in ripening times for certain produce. Hence pockets of demand were created for

various commodities throughout the year (Moore 1986:23). Agricultural surpluses from *vihamba* and seasonally cultivated *shamba* fields supplied markets attended every three days by women of many chiefdoms. By the mid-nineteenth century there are accounts of more than 500 women attending a single market (Moore 1986:23). Throughout this period women appear to have solidified their control of an arena of economic activity that increased in significance over time. Women were predominant in the agricultural work of the *kihamba* before the acute land shortages of the twentieth century, while men were more often engaged in the production of wealth through cattle and goat herding, raiding, hunting for ivory, and longer-distance trade for soda, iron, and clay (Iliffe 1979: 18–19; Moore 1986:28–29).

The extent to which women controlled produce and the profit from its sale is unclear, although they did seem to control the milk trade. In addition to milk, women appear to have had control over field produce and yams. They also decided when bananas were ready for cutting. The ability of women to direct profits to their own uses depended partly upon age; before initiation, anything a young woman generated belonged to her father (Gutmann 1926). Between initiation and marriage, a woman's earnings were hers to keep. This right continued, at least nominally, into marriage, although women rarely seem to have been able to acquire much personal wealth beyond some jewelry and clothing. After a woman's circumcision and before marriage, all produce grown by her was her property to dispose of as she desired. The market provided a means for her to profit from this period of economic autonomy. Young women were encouraged to invest their proceeds from food sales in leaden rings, a form of currency and adornment with high exchange value. The rings, which were hedges against times of trouble, occasionally helped a young woman amass a small herd of livestock. These animals were concealed with friends or maternal relatives to protect them from claims by brothers for assistance in raising a bride-price (Raum 1940:311).

Part of the relevance of markets to Chagga women themselves may have rested on some important noneconomic functions that they performed. Were it not for the market and a few other forms of corporate female labor, the margins of the *kihamba* may have marked the edge of the known universe for many married women. After all, in Old Moshi, the word for wife, *mka*, was said to denote "the one who is chained to a place" (Gutmann 1926:153). The vast majority of women's routine activity could be conducted with a minimum of movement off the *kihamba*; cattle were kept in stalls, much fodder was readily to hand, water ran nearby in rivers or irrigation channels, and wood and food staples were obtainable from the *kihamba* and immediate environs. Private communication may have been very limited on the *kihamba*, where married women were physically separated from women of neighboring clans by groves and hedgerows. Because of the virilocal residence pattern of the *kihamba* regime, women were likely to be even more distant from their birth-clan relations. Lessons of grandparents to uninitiated children acknowledged the potential for grown women to withdraw and become isolated on their *vihamba*. They frequently stressed the theme of neighborliness and foretold dire consequences (including hunger and starvation) for those who kept to themselves too much. In the market, however, women could presumably re-engage with family and friends from their home districts, and women of other chiefdoms.

14. As Moore notes, "Women flocked to the grounds where many dozens of caravan porters camped and there conducted their own exchange directly with the coastal visitors" (1986:37).

15. Gutmann does not indicate the clan affiliation of such children, nor how such "children of the market" were incorporated into social groupings later in life. Who performed the rituals on the father's clan's behalf? If the child was male, who would stand him the bride-price? If female, who was entitled to negotiate for and receive the bride-price? These questions are unanswered.

16. *Dawa* is usually inadequately glossed in English as "medicine." A more accurate

rendering might be "remedy" or "substances used in preventive or remedial action." In the 1990s, *dawa* encompassed everything from pesticides, toothpaste, shoe polish, and narcotics to traditional *materia medica* and modern pharmaceuticals.

17. Interviews with Gertrude K., April 23, 1992 ; Mariamu K. and Lilly L., May 31, 1992.

18. One man cut his wife's face with glass; the other knocked out some of his wife's teeth (author's field notes).

19. Interview with Tina N., May 31, 1993.

20. Interview with Stephen L., Feb. 20, 1993.

21. Interview with Mariamu M., May 31, 1992.

22. The verb *-sexi* behaves like a regular Kiswahili verb. "*-Sexi*" is the active form and refers to the person in the superior position. Thus a woman can "sex" a man if she is on top.

23. Like the use of "boyfriend" and "girlfriend," the latter term (pronounced "*piz*" in local slang) has a Kiswahili antecedent; *-kojoa*, "to urinate," is also slang for having an orgasm.

24. "*Kishingo fani* [fan], *macho balbu* [bulb]."

25. Interview with Amadi T., May 28, 1992.

26. Ibid.

27. Interview with Jonas U., May 24, 1993.

28. Interview with Amini K., April 17, 1993.

29. Speech by MUTAN AIDS educator to secondary school girls, May 28, 1992.

30. The full list of occupations is as follows: accountant, bank manager, bar worker, builder, bus driver, business/factory owner, car mechanic, cook, doctor, driver, factory worker, farmer, gemstone miner, guest-house worker, herdsman, nurse, police/traffic officer, politician, post office/bank employee, priest/minister/sheikh, school teacher, shop owner, small businessman/market woman, soldier, student, tailor.

31. Interview with Adela M., May 8, 1993.

32. Lilly M., speaking to community development committee, Jan. 30, 1992.

33. KIWAKKUKI AIDS seminar, Uraa, Machame, Mar. 13, 1992. The grammatical construction is particularly interesting. The speaker could have said "*wahuni wagonjwa*," which would have meant, literally, "the sick *mhunis*." Instead, he constructed the epithet in such a way that *wahuni* modified the noun *wagonjwa* (sick people), thereby giving the connotation that there is something essentially "*mhuni*-ish" about the sickness as well as the sick people.

34. Interview with Rose M., April 8, 1992.

35. KIWAKKUKI drama competition, Feb. 25–26, 1993, YMCA, Moshi.

36. Untitled *ngonjera*, performed by a group from the Police College, Moshi, Feb. 25, 1993, YMCA, Moshi.

37. The first working group on AIDS was formed in the late 1980s and consisted of personnel from KCMC. In 1988, they received more than $160,000 for their activities. These included protecting health workers at KCMC and acquiring a videocassette player to begin public AIDS education (William Howlett, personal papers).

38. Here she was reminding the girls that should they become pregnant, they would be expelled.

39. Speech by Nancy M. to secondary school girls at Mawenzi Secondary, Moshi, May 28, 1992.

40. Rev. Daniel L., Nov. 29, 1991, KCMC.

41. Pastor Romanos R., Moshi, June 10, 1992.

42. In the 1990s bride-price, while still in existence, was never cited to me by any young man as an obstacle to marriage. Landlessness posed far more complications.

43. Man at AIDS Seminar, Kalali Machame, Nov. 1, 1991.

44. Author's field notes.

45. Voluntary abortions are illegal in Tanzania, yet they are not difficult to procure from health-care workers, especially in urban areas. The first study on this topic in Tanzania reported that among a sample of women who had undergone induced abortions in Dar es Salaam, 87 percent of those performing the abortion were identified as doctors or health workers (Mpangile, Leshabari, and Kihwele 1993).

46. During 1992 there was a growing resentment among the other hospital staff about the preferential shift assignments given to MUTAN AIDS counselors. The counselors were aware of this resentment and asked my assistance to prepare a letter arguing their case to the hospital administration. They showed me a memo from the MUTAN director thanking the hospital's medical officer in charge of assigning the counselors only to daytime shifts so that they could perform their counseling duties after work hours. Non-MUTAN hospital workers often complained to me that the counselors had the additional privilege of signing in and out of work during their day shifts in order to conduct home visits. In addition, the counselors were given one day per week to conduct home visits in rural areas and met twice a week for several hours in the middle of the day to review cases. Many of the hospital staff simply viewed the meetings as marathon gossip sessions and felt that the privilege of signing out for home visits was being thoroughly abused.

47. MUTAN/NACP seminar for bar and guest-house workers and owners, Mawenzi hospital, Dec. 4, 1991.

48. Interview with Gabriel M., May 17, 1993, Moshi.

49. Because many people understand UKIMWI as a disease that weakens the body's ability to resist and recover from sickness, they reason that if the wound heals quickly and without infection then they are seronegative.

50. Interview with Gabriel L., April 20, 1991.

## Chapter Six

1. Pastor Romanos R., June 10, 1992.

2. Dr. Wilfred N., Mar. 24, 1992.

3. One's progeny and reproductive capabilities were especially susceptible to mystical attack, for these were the very essence of one's ability to make a complete circuit through the life course. A childless death was a total death, condemning the deceased to an eternity of spiritual limbo (Moore 1986). Of all physical trials, infertility and the threat of dying childless were existentially the greatest, even if they were not necessarily the most physically debilitating. Thus, cursing the offspring, fertility, or reproductive well-being of malefactors or errant kin has remained one of the most powerful of coercive tactics in times of intra- or interfamilial strife. In the nineteenth century, a variety of materials, including cursing stones, cursing pots, and shards of cooking pots, were used to curse antagonists. Unfired clay pots styled in human form and embossed with exaggerated male and female genitalia channeled "the slumbering forces of perdition" (Gutmann 1926:559) that could render the target of a curse sterile or infertile.

4. *Waganga* were sometimes Chagga but more often from among the neighboring Pare or Sambaa. Sambaa and Pare *waganga* are still thought to possess the strongest "traditional" *(kienyeji)* powers either to harm or to heal. Among Chagga themselves, categories of healing practice were (and, to some extent, have remained) discrete but overlapping, and much medical knowledge circulates among folk independent of the agency of *waganga*. This has been particularly the case with *dawa za miti shamba*, remedies made from parts of plants and trees. Women have often traded the ingredients for medicaments, and in Kibosho a man with no particular specialization in healing was said to have discovered a "vaccine" for smallpox early in this century (interview with Xavier M., Dec. 21, 1991). Another way in which Chagga responded to disease was to reject as marriage partners women (and sometimes men) of clans thought to carry

"blood diseases," including leprosy, chronic leg ulcers, smallpox, and ringworm (Gutmann 1932:62).

5. Various techniques of divination remained in use into the early 1990s. Some diviners read markings on the torn edge of a dracaena leaf plucked from a hedgerow, while others diagnosed and prescribed using small wooden pegs floated in a bowl of water and stirred with a porcupine quill. Remedies frequently involved the performance of a ritual to remove curses or to propitiate ancestors.

6. As with the crowded wards of the Kibong'oto tuberculosis hospital before it, the maternity clinic in the rural area of Machame quickly gained in popularity after it opened in 1924. Demand steadily increased into the 1950s; more than 15,000 women visited prenatal clinics, and more than 6,000 women gave birth in mission and government facilities each year between 1950 and 1953 (Tanganyika Territory Medical Department 1950–53).

7. Most of the African wards were ramshackle mud and wattle huts and were infested with "body vermin" (TNA J.3.26178). The heat on the other wards was "frightful," and the medical officer ordered all the patients to be put on the dirt floors, as far away as possible from "the almost red hot tin roof" (TNA J.3.26178).

8. As the 1956 Medical Department report stated, "This institution is now virtually the largest in the territory . . . the outpatient department which, being the busiest in the territory, is completely incapable of coping efficiently with the very large attendances. Overcrowding is extreme and discomfort to patients considerable. . . . Provision of a new, much larger and efficiently designed department on the lines of the dispensaries in Dar es Salaam is an urgent necessity" (Tanganyika Territory Medical Department 1956:25).

9. Elsewhere, the rhetorical deployment of concerns over health and hygiene led to more coercive measures such as the alienation of land and the displacement of urban food sellers in Moshi through public measures to promote a "sanitary human environment." Early in the century, nearly a third of all African houses in the vicinity of Moshi train station were destroyed, ostensibly as a malaria control measure (Green 1986:41). Later, annual reports from Moshi District fairly boasted of demolishing pole-and-thatch eating places in the 1950s in favor of ones built according to plans laid down by the Health Department (Tanganyika Territory Medical Department 1953). Elsewhere, a confidential letter from the provincial commissioner written in 1945 indicated that sanitary surveys were used throughout the Northern Province to facilitate "expropriation of land from natives under tribal tenure" (TNA J.1.11841). It is unclear from these documents how the use of surveys for land seizures relates to the documented history of land alienation in Kilimanjaro, which had supposedly been curtailed. Given this use of sanitation surveys, it is ironic that the eradication of tsetse fly habitats and control of sleeping sickness were officially tied to "the problem of providing a safe and attractive outlet for the Wachagga as they overcrowd their present cultivation zone," a problem anticipated to confront all the communities on the mountain (TNA 5.449). Indeed the rationale for clearing tsetse habitat for human occupation may have been somewhat disingenuous to begin with, considering that it was the Moshi Maize Growers Association that requested the tsetse research be carried out.

10. The initial communiqué requesting administration support for the committee claimed it would "express the wishes of the Chagga people on health matters . . . in order to let the Wachagga feel that the Committee is truly the voice of the people and their representatives in all health matters" (TNA 5.12.12, letter of 20 September 1950). The specific objectives were enumerated in the letter as follows: "1) to set up new dispensaries. 2) to give advice on infectious diseases. 3) to give advice on venereal diseases. 4) to undertake preventive health measures and propaganda. 5) to manage staff and orderlies. 6) to manage sanitation, and 7) to advise the Native Council about their requirements to accomplish the above" (TNA 5.12.12, letter of 2 June 1950).

11. I am indebted to William Howlett for several discussions on this and related topics.

12. The logic of this argument is based on the assumption that in order for the epidemic to continue in a given locale, the mean number of new infections from each index infection must be greater than 1.

13. In an effort to assist epidemiologists and other researchers, one anthropologist (Conant 1988b) developed a set of rating scales to help scholars evaluate the reliability of historical and ethnographic data that might be used in the study of AIDS.

14. This outlook reached a pernicious extreme in the scholarly literature with the publication of racist sociobiological theories of evolutionary susceptibility that placed Africans at the bottom of the ladder of human development and so prone to infection (Rushton and Bogaert 1989).

15. This general topic arose out of conversations with Ulrich Laukamm-Jostin, to whom I am grateful.

16. Wawer and colleagues stratified their sample clusters according to a three-tiered ranking: main road trading centers, rural agricultural villages, and rural trading villages. They emphasized that the typology was based on a priori community characteristics and not on population seroprevalences (1991:1304). Their results showing the relative risk for men and women in the different types of rural communities give some idea about the potential for variation in such settings—possibly along the lines of sociogeographic networks, as suggested in the text.

17. The Ministry of Health has estimated that only one in every four to six cases of AIDS in Tanzania was being reported to the formal health care sector (NACP 1992, 1997). Based on these statistics, Figure N.1 shows the cumulative number of AIDS cases in Kilimanjaro from 1983 through 1997, along with high and low estimates of unreported cases. By the end of 1991, 33,699 cases of HIV from across the country had been reported to the Ministry of Health (NACP 1992). In sub-Saharan Africa, only Uganda had more reported cases of AIDS (Mann, Tarantola, and Netter 1992). By the end of 1997, Tanzania had one million estimated AIDS cases; only Uganda and Ethiopia were thought to have more (UNAIDS 1998). Kilimanjaro accounted for approximately 6 percent of nation's the total. The highest case rates among both sexes were in the thirty to thirty-four year age group; between forty-four and sixty-six of every thousand men and thirty-six and fifty-four of every thousand women in this age range had clinical AIDS (NACP 1997:14). Among reported cases, the sex and rate ratios were approximately 1, suggesting roughly equal numbers of men and women were being infected overall.

18. This ranking, based on cumulative case reports, was subject to biases of unknown magnitude on the basis of factors such as time delays in case reports, unreliability in regional totals due to logistical problems in compiling accurate figures using the NACP

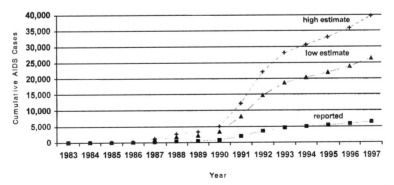

Figure N.1. Cumulative AIDS cases in Kilimanjaro, 1983–97. (Source: NACP 1997)

case-report forms (see Klepp, Ngaliwa, and Ole-Kingori 1993), which year case-reporting procedures were implemented from region to region, and how efficiently these procedures were carried out (assuming high levels of underreporting of cases).

19. Nkya and Howlett developed numerous research projects and articles on clinical manifestations of AIDS and community and hospital-based HIV-1 epidemiology, and contributed to early discussions about AIDS prevention and education (Howlett and Nkya, n.d.; Nkya et al. 1991; Nkya et al. 1988a, 1988b; Nkya et al. 1987; William Howlett, personal papers).

20. In addition to public lectures, medical staff at KCMC "produced 30,000 pamphlets, *AIDS Na Wewe* [AIDS and You], 15,000 posters on AIDS (4 different designs), 650 pamphlets 'Some suggestions for teaching about AIDS in schools,' . . . [and ] 200 handouts on condom use" ("AIDS related activities KCMC, Moshi," William P. Howlett, personal papers).

21. In the early 1990s, two population subgroups were selected by the NACP for surveillance as so-called sentinel groups: pregnant women and blood donors. These populations, it was felt, could provide some indication about the state of the epidemic in the population as a whole without having to launch difficult and expensive population-based serosurveys. This strategy, however, has been called into question. By 1992, the NACP noted that seroprevalence in blood donors must be assumed to have been decreasing even though the prevalence in the population was increasing (NACP 1992:7). Furthermore, a population-based serosurvey conducted in Mwanza Region in 1992 indicated that the figures for pregnant women may have seriously underestimated HIV rates among women of reproductive age in that population (Barongo et al. 1992).

22. These earlier epidemics of sexually transmitted disease had been associated with coffee businessmen and disempowered, acquisitive women seeking material gain in urban areas: "Moreover, there had in Haya society developed 'a standard of values in which money reigns supreme,' and money tempted those who did not have it. Women became accustomed to black figures draped in perfumed silk and supported proudly, if painfully, on a pair of high heels. The poor woman was dazzled by the finery of the rich man's wife and hankered after the latest fashions" (Kaijage 1989:54).

23. While some wrote about the cultural precedents for commercial sex work (de Zalduondo, Msamanga, and Chen 1989:182), the suggestion that Haya had more "permissive" traditions than other groups was criticized as a by-product of the focused AIDS-related research conducted in this high prevalence area and the overdetermined reputation of the far-flung Haya prostitute: "There were East African societies where women were equally or even worse oppressed but they did not produce prostitutes in the same period. Prostitution everywhere has always been a socio-economic phenomenon. Resentment of sexual oppression was an important dimension but the quest for economic opportunity in a society deeply penetrated by the cash nexus was an even more crucial factor in Haya Prostitution" (Kaijage 1989:57; also see Ahlberg 1994:222; and White 1990).

24. In this context "buying her grave" was a euphemism for being at risk for dying of AIDS.

25. MUTAN/NACP seminar for bar and guest-house workers and owners, Mawenzi hospital, Dec. 4, 1991 , Moshi; speech in Kiswahili, my translation. This confusion about whether cats can get AIDS may have been about feline leukemia, one of the first diseases to have been shown to be caused by a retrovirus like HIV.

26. In fact, it was 1983.

27. Gabriel L., Apr. 20, 1991.

28. Dr. Nila L., Oct. 12, 1991.

29. This latter issue has not typically been part of Knowledge, Attitudes, and Practices (or KAP)-style questionnaires in East and Central Africa (e.g.. Wilson, Msimanga, and Greenspan 1988; Adamchak, Mbizvo, and Tawanda 1990; Kapiga, Nachtigal, and Hunter 1991). One study conducted in Arusha and Bukoba (Ndeki et al. 1994) approached this

issue by asking schoolchildren if they had ever seen an AIDS patient. In Arusha, 36.2 percent of girls and 39.2 percent of boys responded yes (cf. Figure 6.2).

30. Esther L., Mar. 27, 1992.

31. MUTAN/NACP AIDS seminar for *Umoja wa Wanawake wa Tanzania,* Moshi branch, held at Mawenzi hospital, Nov. 25, 1991.

32. Godlisten H., Mar. 28, 1993.

33. Author's field notes.

34. There is no indication at what point during this period diagnosis occurred.

35. Interviews with Glory N., Dec. 24 and 27, 1991, Jan. 10 and 26, 1992.

36. Pastor M., at the funeral of Glory N., Jan. 31, 1992.

37. Ezra's narrative is a synthesis of formal interviews on April 3, 1992, April 30, 1993, May 7 and 17, 1993, and many informal meetings.

38. That is, getting a woman pregnant.

39. Each day Ezra used one or more of the following medications: Tegretol, Panadol, Valium, APO Chlordiazepoxide, petroleum jelly and tineafax powder, Scott's Emulsion (a vitamin syrup that Ezra said gave him a good appetite), and Ribena (a cordial made from black currants and fortified with vitamin C that promotes itself with the claim "gives energy").

40. Interviews with Anna S. and family, Dec. 10, 1991, May 10, 20, and 21, 1993, and June 18, 1993.

## Chapter Seven

1. In their volume *AIDS in the World: A Global Report,* Mann et al. (1992:19) divided "the new global geography of HIV/AIDS" into ten geographic areas of affinity. These were identified "by considering four factors: the evolving epidemiology of HIV/AIDS in each country; the type and level of response to the pandemic; societal vulnerability to further spread of HIV; and the relevant geographical realities." "Societal vulnerability" was the only criterion in which some economic factors were taken into account (1992: 21). Table N.1 places the average per-capita GNP for countries covered in each of the

Table N.1  Epidemiologic Characteristics and Average Per-Capita GNP for Three Patterns of HIV Transmission, 1989

|  | Pattern I | Pattern II | Pattern III |
|---|---|---|---|
| Distribution[a] | Western Europe, North America, some areas of South America, Australia, New Zealand | Africa, Carribbean, some areas in South America | Asia, the Pacific region (excluding Australia and New Zealand), Middle East, Eastern Europe, some rural areas of South America |
| Main affected groups[a] | Homosexual/ bisexual men, intravenous drug users | Heterosexuals | Both homosexuals and heterosexuals |
| Sexual transmission[a] | Predominantly homosexual | Predominantly heterosexual | Both homosexual and heterosexual |
| Average GNP (US$)[b] | 12,531 | 608 | 3,200 |

[a] *Source:* Piot et al. 1988, Table 2.
[b] *Source: World Development Report 1989.*

three "patterns" of Piot et al. (1988) alongside the variables the international health community chose to highlight instead: the predominant mode of sexual transmission in each country

2. Interview with Vincent B., April 12, 1993.

3. Christine Obbo, at American Association for the Advancement of Science meeting, Boston, 1988.

4. Chirimuuta and Chirimuuta (1989) and Treichler (1989) have thoroughly explored the ethnocentrism embedded in this genre.

5. From 1932 to 1970 in Macon County, Alabama, the United States Public Health Service and the Tuskegee Institute denied treatment to a group of African-American men infected with syphilis by lying to them about their condition (they were told they had "bad blood") and gaining the complicity of the local medical establishment. The Tanzanian study design called for recruiting a series of matched pairs of villages and then randomly assigning one village of each pair to receive improved STD treatment services (Grosskurth et al. 1995:530–31).

# References

## Tanzania National Archives and Other Unpublished Sources

TNA 5.449. Kilimanjaro Regional Files.

TNA J.1.11841. Medical and Sanitary Arrangements: Northern Province, 1935–1938, vol. 2.

TNA J.3.26178. Native Hospital Moshi 1939–1942, vol. 2: Secretariat Files.

TNA 5.312. Medical—Native Sanitary Inspectors, 1927–1947.

TNA 5.12.5. Medical Infectious Diseases, 1951–1957.

TNA 5.12.12. Chagga Medical Executive Committee, 1950–1951.

William P. Howlett, personal papers.

## Books and Articles

Adamchak, D., M. T. Mbizvo, and M. Tawanda. 1990. "Male Knowledge of and Attitudes and Practices towards AIDS in Zimbabwe." *AIDS* 4:245–50.

Ahlberg, Beth Maina. 1991. *Women, Sexuality, and the Changing Social Order: Impact of Government Policies on Reproductive Behavior in Kenya*. Philadelphia: Gordon & Breach.

———. 1993. "AIDS Prevention with Women and Youth in Nairobi and Njeri." Paper presented at African Studies Association Annual Meeting, Boston, 1993.

———. 1994. "Is There a Distinct African Sexuality? A Critical Response to Caldwell." *Africa* 64 (2): 220–42.

Ahmed, Samira Amin, and Al Haj Hamad M. Kheir. 1992. "Sudanese Sexual Behavior: Sociocultural Norms and Transmission of HIV." In *Sexual Behavior and Networking: Anthropological and Socio-Cultural Studies on the Transmission of HIV*, T. Dyson, ed., pp. 303–14. Liège: Editions Derouaux Ordina.

Ainsworth, Martha, and Mead Over. 1994. "AIDS and African Development." *World Bank Research Observer* 9 (2): 203–40.

Allen, Susan, Antoine Serufilira, Valerie Gruber, Susan Kegeles, Philippe Van de Perre, Michel Caraël, and Thomas Coates. 1993. "Pregnancy and Contraception Use among Urban Rwandan Women after HIV Testing and Counseling." *American Journal of Public Health* 83 (5): 705–10.

Allman, J. 1980. "Sexual Unions in Rural Haiti." *International Journal of Sociology of the Family* 10:15–39.

Altman, Lawrence K. 1994. "Obstacle-Strewn Road to Rethinking the Numbers on AIDS." *New York Times*, March 1.

Anarfi, John. 1992. "Sexual Networking in Selected Communities in Ghana and the Sexual Behavior of Ghanaian Female Migrants in Abidjan, Cote D'Ivoire." In *Sexual Behav-*

*ior and Networking. Anthropological and Socio-Cultural Studies on the Transmission of HIV,* T. Dyson, ed., pp. 233–47. Liège: Editions Derouaux Ordina.

Anderson, Benedict. 1983. *Imagined Communities.* London: Verso.

Ankrah, E. Maxine. 1989. "AIDS: Methodological Problems in Studying its Prevention and Spread." *Social Science and Medicine* 29 (3): 265–76.

Awusabo-Asare, Kofi, John K. Anarfi, and D. K. Agyeman. 1993. "Women's Control over Their Sexuality and the Spread of STDs and HIV/AIDS in Ghana." *Health Transition Review* 3 (supp.): S69–S84.

Bagachwa, M. S. D., and A. Naho. 1995. "Estimating the Informal Economy in Tanzania." *World Development* 23 (8): 1387–99.

Bailey, B. T. 1931. "Report on the Work of the African District Sanitary Inspectors in the Northern Province (Kilimanjaro Area) and General Sanitary Report." Tanzania National Archives, Kilimanjaro Regional Files, Accession Number 5.312.

Barin, Francis R., and Mulanga Kabeya Claire. 1994. "Diagnostic Tools for HIVs." In *AIDS in Africa,* M. Essex, S. Mboup, P. J. Kanki, and M. R. Kalengayi, eds., pp. 109–31. New York: Raven Press.

Barnett, Tony, and Piers Blaikie. 1992. *AIDS in Africa. Its Present and Future Impact.* New York: Guilford Press.

Barnum, H. N., and R. H. Sabot. 1976. *Migration and Urban Surplus Labour: The Case of Tanzania.* Paris: Development Centre of the Organization for Economic Co-operation and Development.

Barongo, Longin R, Martien W. Borgdorff, Frank F. Mosha, Angus Nicoll, Heiner Groskurth, Kesheni P. Senkoro, James N. Newell, John Changalucha, Arnoud H. Klokke, Japhet Z. Killewo, Johan P. Velema, Richard J. Hayes, David T. Dunn, Lex A. S. Muller, and Joas B. Rugemalila. 1992. "The Epidemiology of HIV-1 Infection in Urban Areas, Roadside Settlements and Rural Villages in Mwanza Region, Tanzania." *AIDS* 6: 1521–28.

Barton, Thomas G. 1991. *Sexuality and Health in Sub-Saharan Africa. An Annotated Bibliography.* Nairobi: African Medical and Research Foundation.

Bassett, Mary T., and Marvelous Mhloyi. 1991. "Women and AIDS in Zimbabwe: The Making of an Epidemic." *International Journal of Health Services* 21 (1): 143–56.

Bauni, Evasius. 1992. "The Changing Sexual Patterns of the Meru People of the Chogoria Region of Kenya." In *Sexual Behaviour and Networking: Anthropological and Socio-Cultural Studies on the Transmission of HIV,* T. Dyson, ed., pp. 335–51. Liège: Editions Derouaux Ordina.

Becker, Charles and Rene Collignon. 1999. "A History of STDs and AIDS in Senegal: Difficulties in Accounting for 'Social Logics' in Health Policy." In *Histories of Sexually Transmitted Diseases and HIV/AIDS in Sub-Saharan Africa,* Philip Setel, Milton Lewis and Maryinez Lyons, eds., pp. 65–98. Westport, CT: Greenwood Press.

Beidelman, Thomas O. 1982. *Colonial Evangelism: A Socio-Historical Study of an East African Mission.* Bloomington: Indiana University Press.

———. 1987 [1980]. "Women and Men in Two East African Societies." In *Explorations in African Systems of Thought,* I. Karp and C. S. Bird, eds. pp. 141–64. Washington, DC: Smithsonian Institution Press.

Benenson, Abram S. 1990. *Control of Communicable Diseases in Man.* Washington, DC: American Public Health Association.

Bernard, H. Russell. 1988. *Research Methods in Cultural Anthropology.* Newbury Park, CA: Sage.

Bierman, Werner, and John Campbell. 1989. "The Chronology of Crisis in Tanzania, 1974–1986." In *The IMF, the World Bank, and the African Debt.* Vol. I: *The Economic Impact,* B. Onimode, ed., pp. 66–88. London: Zed Books.

Bledsoe, Caroline. 1980. *Women and Marriage in Kpelle Society.* Stanford: Stanford University Press.

———. 1990. "The Politics of AIDS, Condoms, and Heterosexual Relations in Africa: Recent Evidence from the Local Print Media." In *Births and Power: Social Change and the Politics of Reproduction,* W. P. Handwerker, ed., pp. 197–223. Boulder, CO: Westview Press.

Boerma, J. Ties, Andrew J. Nunn, and James A. G. Whitworth. 1998. "Mortality Impact of the AIDS Epidemic: Evidence from Community Studies in Less Developed Countries." *AIDS* 12 (supp. 1): 3–14.

Borgdorff, Martien, Longin Barongo, Ellen van Jaarsveld, Arnoud Klokke, Kesheni Senkoro, James Newell, Angus Nicoll, Frank Mosha, Heiner Grosskurth, Ronald Swai, Henri van Asten, Johan Velema, Richard Hayes, Lex Muller, and Joas Rugemalila. 1993. "Sentinel Surveillance for HIV-1 Infection: How Representative Are Blood Donors, Outpatients with Fever, Anaemia, or Sexually Transmitted Diseases, and Antenatal Clinic Attenders in Mwanza Region, Tanzania?" *AIDS* 7:567–72.

Bourdieu, Pierre. 1977. *Outline of a Theory of Practice.* Trans. Richard Nice. Cambridge: Cambridge University Press.

Brandt, Allan M. 1987. *No Magic Bullet: A Social History of Venereal Disease in the United States since 1880.* New York: Oxford University Press.

Bureau of Statistics, United Republic of Tanzania. 1973. *National Demographic Survey of Tanzania, 1973.* Vol. 1: *Regional and National Data.* Dar es Salaam: Bureau of Statistics, President's Office.

———. 1990. *Population Census Regional Profile: Kilimanjaro, 1988 Census.* Dar es Salaam: Bureau of Statistics, President's Office.

Bureau of Statistics, United Republic of Tanzania, and Macro International. 1993. *Tanzania Demographic and Health Survey, 1991/1992.* Calverton, MD: Macro International Inc / Dar es Salaam: Bureau of Statistics, President's Office.

Caldwell, John C., Pat Caldwell, and Pat Quiggin. 1989. "The Social Context of AIDS in Sub-Saharan Africa." *Population and Development Review* 15 (2): 185–235.

———. 1991. "The African Sexual System: Reply to Le Blanc et al." *Population and Development Review* 17 (3): 506–15.

Caldwell, John C., I. O. Orubuloye, and Pat Caldwell. 1991. "The Destabilization of the Traditional Yoruba Sexual System." *Population and Development Review* 17 (2): 229–62.

———. 1992. "Underreaction to AIDS in Sub-Saharan Africa." *Social Science and Medicine* 34 (11): 1169–82.

Campbell, Horace, and Howard Stein, eds. 1992. *Tanzania and the IMF: The Dynamics of Liberalization.* Boulder, CO: Westview Press.

Caplan, Pat, ed. 1987. *The Cultural Construction of Sexuality.* London: Tavistock.

Caprara, Andrea, Dedy Seri, Giulio C. De Gregorio, Alessandro Parenzi, Carlos M. Salazar, and Tapé Gozé. 1993. "The Perception of AIDS in the Bete and Baoule of the Ivory Coast." *Social Science and Medicine* 36 (9): 1229–35.

Caraël, Michel. 1996. "Women, AIDS and STDs in Sub-Saharan Africa: The Impact of Marriage Change." In *AIDS and the Grassroots. Problems, Challenges, and Opportunities,* C. Cabrera, D. Pitt, and F. Staugård, eds., pp. 53–82. Gaborone: Ipelegeng Publishers.

Caraël, Michel, John Cleland, and Roger Ingham. 1994. "Extramarital Sex: Implications of Survey Results for STD / HIV Transmission." *Health Transition Review* 4 (supp.): 153–72.

Cheru, Fantu. 1989. "The Role of the IMF and World Bank in the Agrarian Crisis of Sudan and Tanzania: Sovereignty vs Control." In *The IMF, The World Bank and the African Debt.* Vol. 2: *The Social and Political Impact,* B. Onimode, ed., pp. 77–94. London: Institute for African Alternatives.

Chin, James. 1991. "The Epidemiology and Projected Mortality of AIDS." In *Disease and Mortality in Sub-Saharan Africa,* R. G. Feacham and D. T. Jamison, eds., pp. 203–13. Oxford: Oxford University Press.

Chirimuuta, Richard, and Rosalind Chirimuuta. 1989. *AIDS, Africa, and Racism.* London: Free Association Books.

Chirwa, Wiseman Chijere. 1999. "Sexually Transmitted Diseases in Colonial Malawi." In *Histories of Sexually Transmitted Diseases and HIV/AIDS in Sub-Saharan Africa,* Philip Setel, Milton Lewis and Maryinez Lyons, eds., pp. 143–66. Westport, CT: Greenwood.

Claeson, Claes-Fredrik, and Bertil Egero. 1972. *Migration and the Urban Population: A Demographic Analysis of Population Census Data for Tanzania.* Dar es Salaam: BRALUP.

Cleland, John, and Benoît Ferry. 1995. *Sexual Behaviour and AIDS in the Developing World.* Social Aspects of AIDS, P. Aggleton, series ed. London: Taylor and Francis.

Clifford, James. 1988. *The Predicament of Culture: Twentieth Century Ethnography, Literature, and Art.* Cambridge: Harvard University Press.

Clyde, David F. 1962. *History of the Medical Services of Tanganyika.* Dar es Salaam: Government Printers.

Cohen, Barney, and James Trussell. 1996. *Preventing and Mitigating AIDS in Sub-Saharan Africa.* Washington, DC: National Research Council.

Comaroff, Jean. 1985. *Body of Power, Spirit of Resistance: The Culture and History of a South African People.* Chicago: University of Chicago Press.

———. 1993. "The Diseased Heart of Africa: Medicine, Colonialism and the Black Body." In *Knowledge, Power, and Practice: The Anthropology of Medicine and Everyday Life,* S. Lindenbaum and M. Lock, eds., pp. 305–29. Berkeley: University of California Press.

Conant, Francis P. 1988a. "The Social Consequences of AIDS: Implications for East Africa and the Eastern United States." In *AIDS 1988: AAAS Symposia Papers,* R. Kulstad, ed., pp. 147–56. Washington, DC: American Association for the Advancement of Science.

———. 1988b. "Using and Rating Cultural Data on HIV Transmission in Africa." In *AIDS 1988: AAAS Symposia Papers,* R. Kulstad, ed., pp. 201–74. Washington, DC: American Association for the Advancement of Science.

Cooper, Frederick. 1983. "Urban Space, Industrial Time, and Wage Labor in Africa." In *Struggle for the City: Migrant Labor, Capital, and the State in Urban Africa,.* F. Cooper, ed., pp. 7–50. Vol. 8 of Series on African Modernization and Development. Beverly Hills: Sage.

Cordell, Dennis D, Joel Gregory, and Victor Piché. 1992. "The Demographic Reproduction of Health and Disease: Colonial Central African Republic and Contemporary Burkina Faso." In *The Social Basis of Health and Healing in Africa,* S. Feierman and J. M. Janzen, eds. pp. 39–70. Berkeley: University of California Press.

Csordas, Thomas. 1988. "Embodiment as a Paradigm for Anthropology." *Ethos* 18:5–47.

Curtin, Philip. 1985. "Medical Knowledge and Urban Planning in Colonial Tropical Africa." *American Historical Review* 90 (3): 594–613.

*Daily News* (Dar es Salaam). 1988a. [Letter to the editor]. *Daily News,* June 1.

———. 1988b. "The Social Side of AIDS . . . "*Daily News,* May 21.

Daniel, E. Valentine. 1984. *Fluid Signs: Being a Person the Tamil Way.* Berkeley: University of California Press.

———. 1994. "The Individual in Terror." In *Embodiment and Experience: The Existential Ground of Culture and Self,* T. J. Csordas, ed., pp. 229–47. Cambridge: Cambridge University Press.

Dare, O. O., and J. G. Cleland. 1994. "Reliability and Validity of Survey Data on Sexual Behaviour." *Health Transition Review* 4 (supp.): 93–110.

Dawson, Marc H. 1992. "Socioeconomic Change and Disease: Smallpox in Colonial Kenya, 1820–1920." In *The Social Basis of Health and Healing in Africa,* S. Feierman and J. M. Janzen, eds. pp. 90–103. Berkeley: University of California Press.

de Zalduondo, Barbara O. 1990. "Prostitution Viewed Cross-Culturally: Toward Recontextualising Commercial Sex Work for Improved AIDS Intervention Research." Paper prepared for the seminar "Anthropologists at Work on AIDS," American Anthropological Association Task Force on AIDS, Washington, DC.

de Zalduondo, Barbara O., Gernard I. Msamanga, and Lincoln Chen. 1989. "AIDS in Africa: Diversity in the Global Pandemic." *Daedalus* 118 (3): 165–204.

Derrida, Jacques. 1973. *Speech and Phenomena and Other Essays on Husserl's Theory of Signs.* Trans. David B. Allison. Evanston, IL: Northwestern University Press.

Dixon-Mueller, Ruth. 1993. "The Sexuality Connection in Reproductive Health." *Studies in Family Planning* 20 (6): 297–307.

Dundas, Charles. 1924. *Kilimanjaro and Its People.* London: H.F. & G. Witherby.

Enel, Catherine, and Gilles Pison. 1992. "Sexual Relations in the Rural Area of Mlomp (Casamance, Senegal)." In *Sexual Behavior and Networking: Anthropological and Socio-Cultural Studies on the Transmission of HIV,* T. Dyson, ed., pp. 249–67. Liège: Editions Derouaux Ordina.

Epstein, A. L. 1981. *Urbanization and Kinship: The Domestic Domain on the Copperbelt of Zambia.* London: Academic Press.

Evans, Barry G. 1991. "Estimating Underreporting of AIDS: Straightforward in Theory, Difficult in Practice." [Editorial comment.] *AIDS* 5:1261–62.

Fapohunda, Eleanor R., and Michael Todaro. 1988. "Family Structure, Implicit Contracts, and the Demand for Children in Southern Nigeria." *Population and Development Review* 14 (4): 571–94.

Farmer, Paul. 1988. "Bad Blood, Spoiled Milk: Bodily Fluids as Moral Barometers in Rural Haiti." *American Ethnologist* 15 (1): 62–83.

———. 1992. *AIDS and Accusation: Haiti and the Geography of Blame.* Berkeley: University of California Press.

———. 1995. "Culture, Poverty, and the Dynamics of HIV Transmission in Rural Haiti." In *Culture and Sexual Risk: Anthropological Perspectives on AIDS,* Han ten Brummelhuis and Gilbert Herdt, eds., pp. 3–28. Luxembourg: Gordon and Breach.

Feierman, Steven. 1985. "Struggles for Control: The Social Roots of Health and Healing in Modern Africa." *African Studies Review* 28 (2/3): 73–147.

———. 1993. "Defending the Promise of Subsistence: Population Growth and Agriculture in the West Usambara Mountains, 1920–1980." In *Population Growth and Agricultural Change in Africa,* B. L. Turner, G. Hyden, and R. Kates, eds., pp. 114–44. Gainesville: University of Florida Press.

Fleming, Bruce E. 1990. "African Perceptions of AIDS: Another Way of Dying." *The Nation* (April 2): 446–50.

Fortes, Meyer. 1987. *Religion, Morality and the Person: Essays on Tallensi Religion.* Ed. Jack Goody. Cambridge: Cambridge University Press.

Forthal, D. N., F. S. Mhalu, A. Dahoma, K. M. Nyamuryekunge, J. Kidenya, C. A. Schable, J. W. Curran, and J. B. McCormick. 1986. "AIDS in Tanzania." Paper presented at Third International Conference on AIDS, Washington, DC.

Fosbrooke, Henry A. 1952. [Letter]. *Tanganyika Notes and Records* 32:100–102.

Foucault, Michel. 1980a. *The History of Sexuality.* Vol. 1: *An Introduction.* Trans. Robert Hurley. New York: Vintage.

———. 1980b. *Power/Knowledge: Selected Interviews and Other Writings, 1972–1977.* Trans. Colin Gordon. Brighton: Harvester Press.

Frankenberg, Ronald. 1992. "The Other Who Is Also the Same: The Relevance of Epidemics in Space and Time for Prevention of HIV Infection." *International Journal of Health Services* 22 (1): 73–88.

Freyhold, M., K. Sawaki, and M. Zalla. 1973. "Moshi District." In *The Young Child in Tanzania,* pp. 166–240. Dar es Salaam: UNICEF.

Gallagher, Catherine, and Thomas Laqueur, eds. 1987. *The Making of the Modern Body: Sexuality and Society in the Nineteenth Century.* Berkeley: University of California Press.

Garenne, Michel, Charles Becker, and Rosario Cardenas. 1992. "Heterogeneity, Life Cycle, and the Potential Demographic Impact of AIDS in a Rural Area of Africa." In

*Sexual Behaviour and Networking: Anthropological and Socio- Cultural Studies on the Transmission of HIV,* T. Dyson, ed., pp. 269–82. Liège: Editions Derouaux Ordina.

Gay, Peter. 1984. *Education of the Senses: The Bourgeois Experience, Victoria to Freud.* New York: Oxford University Press.

Gilman, Sander L. 1985. *Difference and Pathology: Stereotypes of Sexuality, Race and Madness.* Ithaca, NY: Cornell University Press.

Gogarty, H. A. 1927. *Kilima-njaro: An East-African Vicariate.* New York: Society for the Propagation of the Faith.

Goldsmith, Marsha F. 1988. "AIDS around the World: Analyzing Complex Patterns." *Journal of the American Medical Association* 259 (13): 1917–19.

Good, Byron J. 1994. *Medicine, Rationality, and Experience: An Anthropological Perspective.* Cambridge: Cambridge University Press.

Good, Charles M. 1991. "AIDS, STDs and Urbanization in Africa." *African Urban Quarterly* 6 (1/2): 1–7.

Gould, Peter. 1993. *The Slow Plague: A Geography of the AIDS Pandemic.* Oxford: Blackwell.

Graeber, David. 1996. "Beads and Money: Notes toward a Theory of Wealth and Power." *American Ethnologist* 23 (1): 4–24.

Green, Allen J. 1986. "A Political Economy of Moshi Town, 1920–1960." Ph.D. diss., Department of History, UCLA.

Greenhalgh, Susan. 1995. "Anthropology Theorizes Reproduction: Integrating Practice, Political Economic, and Feminist Perspectives." In *Situating Fertility: Anthropology and Demographic Inquiry,* Susan Greenhalgh, ed., pp. 1–28. Cambridge: Cambridge University Press.

Grmek, Mirko D. 1990. *History of AIDS: Emergence and Origin of a Modern Epidemic.* Princeton, NJ: Princeton University Press.

Grosskurth, Heiner, Frank Mosha, James Todd, Ezra Mwijaribu, Arnoud Klokke, Kesheni Senkoro, Philippe Mayaud, John Changalucha, Angus Nicoll, Gina ka-Gina, James Newell, Kokugonza Mugeye, David Mabey, and Richard Hayes. 1995. "Impact of Improved Treatment of Sexually Transmitted Diseases on HIV Infection in Rural Tanzania: Randomised Controlled Trial." *Lancet* 346:530–36.

Grosz, Elizabeth. 1994. *Volatile Bodies: Toward a Corporeal Feminism.* St. Leonards: Allen & Unwin.

Gutmann, Bruno. 1926. *Das Recht der Dschagga.* Trans. A. M. Nagler. Human Relations Area Files (HRAF), Yale University Library.

———. 1932. *Die Stammeslehren der Dschagga.* Trans. Ward Goodenough and Dorothy Crawford [1958]. HRAF, Yale University Library.

Guyer, Jane I. 1981. "Household and Community in African Studies." *African Studies Review* 24 (2/3): 87–137.

———. 1996. "Traditions of Invention in Equatorial Africa." *African Studies Review* 39 (3): 1–28.

Håkansson, N. Thomas. 1990. "The Appropriation of Fertility: Descent and Sex Among the Gusii." In *The Creative Communion: African Folk Models of Fertility and the Regeneration of Life,* A. Jacobson-Widding and W. van Beek, eds., pp. 187–99. Vol. 15 of Uppsala Studies in Cultural Anthropology. Stockholm: Almqvist & Wiksell.

Haley, Bruce. 1978. *The Healthy Body and Victorian Culture.* Cambridge, MA: Harvard University Press.

Hammar, Lawrence. 1993. "Reflections on Sex and Ethnographer Shame." *Synergia* 3: 73–87.

———. 1996. "Bad Canoes and *Bafalo:* The Political Economy of Sex on Daru Island, Western Province, Papua New Guinea." *Genders* 23:212–43.

Hammel, Eugene A. 1990. "A Theory of Culture for Demography." *Population and Development Review* 16 (3): 455–85.

Haram, Liv. 1995. "Negotiating Sexuality in Times of Economic Want: The Young and Modern Meru Women." In *Young People at Risk: Fighting AIDS in Northern Tanzania,*

K.-I. Klepp, P. M. Biswalo, and A. Talle, eds., pp. 31–48. Oslo: Scandinavian University Press.

Haraway, Donna J. 1987. *It's 8:30. Do You Know Where Your Brains Are? Donna Haraway Reads the National Geographics of Primates.* New York: Paper Tiger Television.

———. 1991. *Simians, Cyborgs, and Women: The Reinvention of Nature.* New York: Routledge.

Harries, Patrick. 1990. "La Symbolique du sexe: L'identité culturelle au début de l'exploitation des mines d'or du Witwatersrand." *Cahiers d'études Africaines* 120: 451–74.

Harris, Judith Rich. 1998. *The Nurture Assumption: Why Children Turn Out the Way They Do.* New York: Free Press.

Higgins, Donna L., Christine Galavotti, Kevin R. O'Reilly, Daniel J. Schnell, Melinda Moore, Deborah L. Rugg, and Robert Johnson. 1991. "Evidence for the Effects of HIV Antibody Counseling and Testing on Risk Behaviors." *Journal of the American Medical Association* 266 (17): 2419–29.

Hooper, Ed. 1990. *Slim: A Reporter's Own Story of AIDS in East Africa.* London: Bodley Head.

Howard, Mary Theresa. 1980. "Kwashiorkor on Kilimanjaro: The Social Handling of Malnutrition." Ph.D. diss., Michigan State University.

Howlett, William, and Watoki M. M. M. Nkya. 1987. "AIDS Control Programme." KCMC, Tanzania. Ms.

———. [n.d.]. "Tuberculosis in HIV Disease in Northern Tanzania." Ms.

Howlett, W. P., W. M. M. M. Nkya, and K. Mmuni. 1987. "AIDS in Kilimanjaro Christian Medical Center." Ms.

Howlett, William P., Watoki M. M. M. Nkya, Konrad A. Mmuni, and Werner R. Missalek. 1988. "Clinical Features of AIDS in the Northern Zone of Tanzania." Ms.

Hrdy, Daniel B. 1987. "Cultural Practices Contributing to the Transmission of Human Immunodeficiency Virus in Africa." *Review of Infectious Diseases* 9 (6): 1109–19.

Hunt, C. W. 1989. "Migrant Labour and Sexually Transmitted Disease: AIDS in Africa." *Journal of Health and Social Behaviour* 30:353–73.

Hunt, Nancy Rose. 1992. "Negotiated Colonialism: Domesticity, Hygiene, and Birth Work in the Belgian Congo." Ph.D. diss., University of Wisconsin, Madison.

Hunter, David J. 1993. "AIDS in Sub-Saharan Africa: The Epidemiology of Heterosexual Transmission and the Prospects for Prevention." *Epidemiology* 4 (1): 63–72.

Huygens, Pierre, Ellen Kajura, Janet Seeley, and Tom Barton. 1996. "Rethinking Methods for the Study of Sexual Behaviour." *Social Science and Medicine* 42 (2): 221–31.

Iliffe, John. 1979. *A Modern History of Tanganyika.* Cambridge: Cambridge University Press.

International Labour Organisation. 1992. "The State and the Informal Sector in Tanzania: Report of a Study on the Development Policies and Institutional Environment and Informal Sector in Tanzania." Addis Ababa: International Labour Organisation, Jobs and Skills Programme for Africa.

Irwin, Kathleen, Jane Bertrand, Ndili Mibandumba, Kashama Mbuyi, Chirezi Muremeri, Makolo Mukoka, Kamenga Munkolenkole, Nzila Nzilambi, Ngaly Bosenge, Robert Ryder, Herbert Peterson, Nancy C. Lee, Phyllis Wingo, Kevin O'Reilly, and Kathy Rufo. 1991. "Knowledge, Attitudes and Beliefs about HIV Infection and AIDS among Healthy Factory Workers and Their Wives, Kinshasa, Zaire." *Social Science and Medicine* 32 (8): 917–30.

Jackson, Michael. 1989. *Paths toward a Clearing: Radical Empiricism and Ethnographic Inquiry.* Bloomington: Indiana University Press.

Jackson, Michael, and Ivan Karp. 1990. *Personhood and Agency: The Experience of Self and Other in African Culture.* Stockholm: Almqvist & Wiksell.

Jeater, Diana. 1993. *Marriage, Perversion, and Power: The Construction of Moral Discourse in Southern Rhodesia, 1894–1930.* Oxford: Clarendon Press.

Jochelson, Karen. 1991. "HIV and Syphilis in the Republic of South Africa: The Creation of an Epidemic." *African Urban Quarterly* 6 (1/2): 20–34.

Jochelson, Karen, Monyaola Mothibeli, and Jean-Patrick Leger. 1991. "Human Immuno-deficiency Virus and Migrant Labor in South Africa." *International Journal of Health Services* 21 (1): 157–73.

Johnson, Frederick. 1939. *A Standard Swahili–English Dictionary.* Oxford: Oxford University Press.

Johnston, H. H. 1886. *The Kilima-Njaro Expedition.* London: Kegan Paul, Trench.

Kaijage, Fred J. 1989. "The AIDS Crisis in Kagera Region, Tanzania, in Historical Perspective." In *Behavioral and Epidemiological Aspects of AIDS Research in Tanzania: Proceedings from a Workshop in Dar es Salaam,* J. Z. Killewo and G. K. Lwihula, eds., pp. 52–61. Dar es Salaam: SAREC.

———. 1993. "AIDS Control and the Burden of History in Northwestern Tanzania." *Population and Environment* 14 (3): 279–300.

Kapiga, Saidi H., G. Nachtigal, and D. J. Hunter. 1991. "Knowledge of AIDS among Secondary School Pupils in Bagamoyo and Dar-es-Salaam, Tanzania." *AIDS* 5 (3): 325–28.

Kapiga, Saidi H., John F. Shao, George K. Lwihula, and David J. Hunter. 1994. "Risk Factors for HIV Infection among Women in Dar-es-Salaam, Tanzania." *Journal of Acquired Immune Deficiency Syndromes* 7:301–9.

Kasfir, Nelson. 1993. "Agricultural Transformation in the Robusta Coffee/Banana Zone of Bushenyi, Uganda." In *Population Growth and Agricultural Change in Africa,* B. L. Turner, G. Hyden, and R. Kates, eds., pp. 41–79. Gainesville: University of Florida Press.

Katz, J. 1976. *Gay American History.* Crowell: New York.

Kerner, Donna O. 1988. "'Hard Work' and Informal Sector Trade in Tanzania." In *Traders versus the State: Anthropological Approaches to Unofficial Economies,* G. Clark, ed., pp. 41–56. Boulder, CO: Westview Press.

Kertzer, David I., and Tom Fricke, eds. 1997a. *Anthropological Demography: Toward a New Synthesis.* Chicago: University of Chicago Press.

———. 1997b. "Toward an Anthropological Demography." In *Anthropological Demography. Toward a New Synthesis,* D. I. Kertzer and T. Fricke, eds., pp. 1–35. Chicago: University of Chicago Press.

Kessy, Anna Tengia. 1995. "Risk Factors and Prevalence of Sexually Transmitted Diseases among Youths in Moshi Rural District, Kilimanjaro Region, 1995." Paper presented at the conference "Youth and Related Problems," Dar es Salaam, Oct. 19–21.

Killewo, J., J. Comoro, J. Lugalla, and G. Kwesigabo. 1993. "Systemic Interventions and Their Evaluation against HIV/AIDS in Kagera Region, Tanzania: Proceedings of a Workshop Held in Bukoba, Tanzania, 10–11 May." Dar es Salaam: Muhibili University College of Health Sciences, Department of Epidemiology and Biostatistics.

Killewo, J., L. Dahlgren, and A. Sandström. 1994. "Socio-Geographic Patterns of HIV-1 Transmission in Kagera Region, Tanzania." *Social Science and Medicine* 38 (1): 129–34.

Killewo, Japhet, Klinton Nyamuryekunge, Anita Sandström, Ulla Bredberg-Rådén, Stig Wall, Fred Mhalu, and Gunnel Biberfeld. 1990. "Prevalence of HIV-1 Infection in the Kagera Region of Tanzania: A Population-based Study." *AIDS:* 1081–85.

Kimambo, Isaria N. 1996. "Environmental Control and Hunger in the Mountains and Plains of Nineteenth-Century Northeastern Tanzania." In *Custodians of the Land: Ecology and Culture in the History of Tanzania,* G. Maddox, J. Giblin, and I. N. Kimambo, eds., pp. 71–95. London: James Currey.

Klepp, Knut-Inge, Paul M. Biswalo, and Aud Talle, eds. 1995. *Young People at Risk: Fighting AIDS in Northern Tanzania.* Oslo: Scandinavian University Press.

Klepp, K. I., S. S. Ndeki, and G. R. Z. Mliga. 1994. "Knowledge, Perceived Risk of AIDS

and Sexual Behavior among Primary School Children in Two Areas of Tanzania."
*Health Education Research* 9 (1): 133–38.

Klepp, Knut-Inge, S. J. Ngaliwa, and N. L. Ole-Kingʊri. 1993. "The Joint Tanzanian-Norwegian AIDS Project." In "Status Report No. 3." Tanzania-Norway AIDS Project. Moshi: MUTAN.

Klouman, Elise, Elisante J. Masenga, Noel E. Sam, and Zebedia Lauwo. 1995. "Control of Sexually Transmitted Diseases: Experiences from a Rural and an Urban Community." In *Young People at Risk: Fighting AIDS in Northern Tanzania,* K.-I. Klepp, P. M. Biswalo, and A. Talle, eds., pp. 204–21. Oslo: Scandinavian University Press.

Konde-Lule, Joseph K. 1995. "The Declining HIV Seroprevalence in Uganda: What Evidence?" *Health Transition Review* 5 (supp.): 27–34.

Konde-Lule, Joseph K., M. Musagara, and S. Musgrave. 1993. "Focus Group Interviews about AIDS in Rakai District of Uganda." *Social Science and Medicine* 37 (5): 679–84.

Konoky-Ahulu, F. I. D. 1989. *What Is AIDS?* Watford: Tetteh-A'Domeno.

Koponen, Juhani. 1988. *People and Production in Late Precolonial Tanzania: History and Structures.* Helsinki: Finnish Anthropological Society.

———. 1994. *Development for Exploitation: German Colonial Policies in Mainland Tanzania, 1884–1914.* Uppsala: Nordic Africa Institute.

———. 1996. "Population: A Dependent Variable." In *Custodians of the Land: Ecology and Culture in the History of Tanzania,* Gregory Maddox, James Giblin, and Isaria N. Kimambo, eds., pp. 19–42. London: James Curry.

Krapf, J. Lewis. 1860. *Travels, Researches and Missionary Labors.* Boston: Ticknor & Fields.

Kreiss, Joan K., Davy Koech, Francis A. Plummer, King K. Holmes, Marilyn Lightfoote, Peter Piot, Allan R. Ronald, J. O. Ndinya-Achola, Lourdes J. D'Costa, Pacita Roberts, Elizabeth N. Ngugi, and Thomas Quinn. 1986. "AIDS Virus Infection in Nairobi Prostitutes: Spread of the Epidemic to East Africa." *New England Journal of Medicine* 314 (7): 414–18.

Kunitz, Stephen. 1994. *Disease and Social Diversity: The European Impact on the Health of Non-Europeans.* New York: Oxford University Press.

Laga, Maria. 1995. "Commentary: STD Control for HIV Prevention—It Works!" *Lancet* 346:518.

Laquer, Thomas. 1990. *Making Sex: Body and Gender from the Greeks to Freud.* Cambridge, MA: Harvard University Press.

Larson, Ann. 1989. "Social Context of Human Immunodeficiency Virus Transmission in Africa: Historical and Cultural Bases of East and Central African Sexual Relations." *Reviews of Infectious Diseases* 11 (5): 716–31.

Last, Murray. 1992. "The Importance of Knowing about Not Knowing: Observations from Hausaland." In *The Social Basis of Health and Healing in Africa,* S. Feierman and J. M. Janzen, eds., pp. 393–406. Berkeley: University of California Press.

Lawuo, Z. E. 1980. *Education and Social Change in a Rural Community: A Study of Colonial Education and Local Response among the Chagga between 1920 and 1945.* Dar es Salaam: University of Dar es Salaam Press.

Le Blanc, Marie-Nathalie, Dierdre Meintel, and Victor Piché. 1991. "The African Sexual System: Comment on Caldwell et al." *Population and Development Review* 17 (3): 497–505.

Legge, Kate. 1997. "Life Sucks, Timmy." *Australian Magazine* (Mar. 8–9): 10–18.

Le Roy, A. 1889. *Au Kilima-Ndjaro: Afrique Orientale.* Paris: L. de Soye et fils.

Lehmann, Rudolf. 1941. "Some Field-notes on the Chaga of Kilimanjaro." *Bantu Studies* 15 (4): 379–96.

Lemenye, Justin. 1953. *Maisha ya Sameni Ole Kivasis yaani Justin Lemenye.* Kampala: Eagle Press.

———. 1955. "The Life of Justin: An African Autobiography." *Tanganyika Notes and Records* 41:30–56.

Leshabari, M. T., and S. F. Kaaya. 1995. "Youth in Jeopardy: Failure of Success in Tanzania." Paper presented at the conference "Youth and Related Problems," Dar es Salaam, Oct. 19–21.

Lesthaeghe, Ron J. 1989. "Production and Reproduction in Sub-Saharan Africa: An Overview of Organizing Principles." In *Reproduction and Social Organization in Sub-Saharan Africa*, R. J. Lesthaeghe, ed., pp. 13–59. Berkeley: University of California Press.

Lesthaeghe, Ron J., Georgia Kaufmann, and Dominique Meekers. 1989. "The Nuptiality Regimes in Sub-Saharan Africa." In *Reproduction and Social Organization in Sub-Saharan Africa*, R. J. Lesthaeghe, ed., pp. 238–337. Berkeley: University of California Press.

Lie, Gro Therese, and Paul M. Biswalo. 1993. "Perceptions of the Good HIV / AIDS Counsellor in Arusha and Kilimanjaro Regions of Tanzania: Implications for Hospital Counseling in Tanzanian Norwegian AIDS Project." In "Status Report No. 3." Tanzania-Norway AIDS Project. Moshi: MUTAN.

———. 1995. "Community Counselling: Experiences from a Village in the Arusha Region." In *Young People at Risk: Fighting AIDS in Northern Tanzania*, K.-I. Klepp, P. M. Biswalo, and A. Talle, eds., pp. 165–83. Oslo: Scandinavian University Press.

Lock, Margaret. 1993. "Cultivating the Body: Anthropology and Epistemologies of Bodily Practice and Knowledge." *Annual Review of Anthropology* 22:133–55.

Lockwood, Matthew. 1995. "Structure and Behavior in the Social Demography of Africa." *Population and Development Review* 21 (1): 1–32.

Lugala, Joseph. 1994. "Structural Adjustment Programs and Health Care in Tanzania." Paper presented at the conference "Social Change and Health in Africa," Harvard Medical School, Boston, MA.

Lurie, Peter, Percy Hintzen, and Robert A. Lowe. 1995. "Socioeconomic Obstacles to HIV Prevention and Treatment in Developing Countries: The Roles of the International Monetary Fund and the World Bank." *AIDS* 9 (6): 539–46.

Luvanga, N. E. 1996. "Towards the Development of Informal Sector Policy in Tanzania: Some Policy Issues." Dar es Salaam: University of Dar es Salaam, Economic Research Bureau.

Lwihula, George. 1988. "Social Cultural Factors Associated with the Transmission of HIV Virus in Tanzania: The Kagera Experience." Paper presented at the workshop "Counseling AIDS Patients," Sokoine University of Agriculture, Morogoro.

———. 1990. "Sexual Practices and Patterns of Interaction in the Kagera Area with Reference to the Spread of HIV." Paper presented at the seminar "Anthropological Studies Relevant to Sexual Transmission of HIV," International Union for the Scientific Study of Population, Committee on Anthropology and Demography, Sønderborg, Denmark.

Lyons, Maryinez. 1992. *The Colonial Disease: A Social History of Sleeping Sickness in Northern Zaire, 1900–1940.* Cambridge: Cambridge University Press.

Lyttleton, Chris. 1996. "Health and Development: Knowledge Systems and Local Practice in Rural Thailand." *Health Transition Review* 6 (1): 25–48.

McGrath, Janet, Charles B. Rwabukwali, Debra A. Schumann, Jonnie-Pearson Marks, Sylvia Nakayiwa, Barbara Namande, Lucy Nakyobe, and Rebecca Mukasa. 1993. "Anthropology and AIDS: The Cultural Context of Sexual Risk Behavior among Urban Women in Kampala, Uganda." *Social Science and Medicine* 36 (4): 429–439.

Makundi, J. E. S. 1969. "Pre-Colonial Forces against the Creation of One Chagga Nation." Ms., University of Dar es Salaam.

Manderson, Lenore. 1996. *Sickness and the State: Health and Illness in Colonial Malaya, 1870–1940.* Cambridge: Cambridge University Press.

Mann, Jonathan M. 1987. "The Epidemiology of LAV / HTLV-III in Africa." *Annales Institute Pasteur/Virology* 138:113–18.

Mann, Jonathan M., Henry Francis, Thomas Quinn, Pangu Kaza Asila, Ngaly Bosenge, Nzila Nzilambi, Kapita Bila, Muyembe Tamfum, Kalisi Ruti, Peter Piot, Joseph McCormick, and James W. Curran. 1986. "Surveillance for AIDS in a Central African City." *Journal of the American Medical Association* 255 (23): 3255–59.

Mann, Jonathan M, Thomas C. Quinn, Peter Piot, Ngaly Bosenge, Nzila Nzilambi, Mpunga Kalala, Henry Francis, Robert L. Colebunders, Robert Byers, Pangu Kasa Azila, and James W. Curran. 1987. "Condom Use and HIV Infections among Prostitutes in Zaire." [Letter]. *New England Journal of Medicine* 316 (6): 345.

Mann, Jonathan M., Daniel J. M. Tarantola, and Thomas W. Netter. 1992. *AIDS in the World: A Global Report.* Cambridge, MA: Harvard University Press.

Marcus, George, and Michael M. J. Fischer. 1986. *Anthropology as Cultural Critique: An Experimental Moment in the Human Sciences.* Chicago: University of Chicago Press.

Marealle, Thomas L. M. 1952. "The Wachagga of Kilimanjaro." *Tanganyika Notes and Records* 32:57–64.

Maro, Paul S. 1975. *Population Growth and Agricultural Change in Kilimanjaro, 1920–1970.* Dar es Salaam: BRALUP.

Martin, Emily. 1992. *The Woman in the Body: A Cultural Analysis of Reproduction.* Boston: Beacon Press.

Maruma, Oliver J. 1969. *Chagga Politics, 1930–1952.* Ms., University of Dar es Salaam.

Mauss, Marcel. 1967. *The Gift: Forms and Functions of Exchange in Archaic Societies.* New York: W. W. Norton.

———. 1979. *Sociology and Psychology: Essays.* Trans. Ben Brewster. London: Routledge & Kegan Paul.

Mbaga, J. M., K. J. Pallangyo, M. Bakari, and E. A. Aris. 1990. "Survival Time of Patients with Acquired Immune Deficiency Syndrome: Experience with 274 Patients in Dar-es-Salaam." *East African Medical Journal* 67 (2): 95–99.

Meghji, Zakia Mohammed. 1977. *The Development of Women Wage Labor: The Case of Industries in Moshi District.* M.A. thesis, University of Dar es Salaam.

Merinyo, Clement. 1988. *Kifo cha AIDS.* Dar es Salaam: Grand Arts Promotions.

Merlin, M., R. Josse, J. P. Gonzales, E. Delaporte, A. Dupont, D. Salaun, M. C. Georeges-Courbot, H. Fluery, R. Josserand, D. Kouka Bemba, J. B. McCormick, J. Limbassa, F. Barré-Sinoussi, J. C. Chermann, and A. J. Georges. 1987. "Epidemiology of HIV-1 Infection among Randomized Representative Central African Populations." *Annales Institute Pasteur/Virology* 138:503–10.

Merton, Robert K. 1949. *Social Theory and Social Structure.* Glencoe: Free Press.

Mhalu, Fred S., Abdalla Dahoma, Ephraim Mbena, Samuel Maselle, Ulla Bredberg-Råden, and Gunnel Biberfeld. 1988. "Some Aspects of the Epidemiology of AIDS and Infections with the Human Immunodeficiency Virus in the United Republic of Tanzania." In *AIDS and Associated Cancers in Africa,* G. Giraldo, E. Beth-Giraldo, N. Clumeck, M.-R. Gharbi, S. K. Kyalwazi, and G. D. Thé eds., pp. 50–60. Basel: Karger.

Mhalu, Fred, Karim Hirji, Petrida Ijumba, John Shao, Ephraim Mbena, Davis Mwakagile, Caroline Akim, Paul Senge, Hussein Mponezya, Ulla Bredberg Raden, and Gunnel Biberfeld. 1991. "A Cross-Sectional Study of a Program for HIV Infection Control among Public House Workers." *Journal of Acquired Immune Deficiency Syndromes* 4 (3): 290–96.

Ministry of Health and AMMP Team. 1997. "The Policy Implications of Adult Morbidity and Mortality: End of Phase 1 Report." Dar es Salaam: United Republic of Tanzania.

Mnyika, Kagoma Selemani. 1996. "Epidemiology of HIV-1 Infection in Northern Tanzania." Ph.D. diss., University of Bergen and Muhimbili University College of Health Sciences, University of Dar es Salaam.

Mnyika, Kagoma S., Knut-Inge Klepp, Gunnar Kvåle, Steinar Nilssen, Peter E. Kissila, and Naphthal Ole-King'ori. 1994. "Prevalence of HIV-1 Infection in Urban, Semi-Urban and Rural Areas in Arusha Region, Tanzania." *AIDS* 8:1477–81.

Mogensen, Hanne Overgaard. 1997. "The Narrative of AIDS among the Tonga of Zambia." *Social Science and Medicine* 44 (4): 431–39.

Moore, Henrietta L. 1996 [1986]. *Space, Text, and Gender: An Anthropological Study of the Marakwet in Kenya.* New York: Guilford Press.

Moore, J. E. 1971. *Rural Population Carrying Capacities of the Districts of Tanzania.* BRALUP Research Paper No. 18. Dar es Salaam: BRALUP.

Moore, Sally Falk. 1976. "The Secret of the Men: A Fiction of Chagga Initiation and Its Relation to the Logic of Chagga Symbolism." *Africa* 46 (4): 357–70.

———. 1977. "The Chagga." In *The Chagga and Meru of Tanzania,* S. F. Moore and P. Pruritt, eds., pp. 1–85. London: International African Institute.

———. 1981. "Chagga 'Customary' Law and the Property of the Dead." In *Mortality and Immortality: The Anthropology and Archaeology of Death,* S. C. Humphreys and Helen King, eds., pp. 225–48. London: Academic Press.

———. 1986. *Social Facts and Fabrications: "Customary" Law on Kilimanjaro, 1880–1980.* Cambridge: Cambridge University Press.

Moshi Diocese. 1990. *The Catholic Church in Moshi: A Centenary Memorial, 1890–1990.* Ndanda: Ndanda Mission Press.

Mpangile, Gottlieb S., M. T. Leshabari, and David Kihwele. 1993. "Factors Associated with Induced Abortion in Public Hospitals in Dar es Salaam, Tanzania." *Reproductive Health Matters* (Nov.): 21–31.

Mpensela, Henry S. 1990. *Magonjwa ya Maendeleo.* Ndanda: Benedictine Publications.

Muhondwa, Eustace P. Y. 1991. "Contending with Unbelief and Fatalism among the Youth concerning HIV/AIDS Control in Tanzania." Ms.

Mukiza-Gapere, Jackson, and James P. M. Ntozi. [n.d.]. "Impact of AIDS on Marriage Patterns, Customs, and Practices in Uganda." Ms.

Munn, Nancy. 1986. *The Fame of Gawa: A Symbolic Transformation in a Massim (Papua New Guinea) Society.* Cambridge: Cambridge University Press.

MUTAN. 1993. "Status Report No. 3." Tanzania-Norway AIDS Project. Moshi: MUTAN.

Mwale, Genevieve, and Philip Burnard. 1992. *Women and AIDS in Rural Africa. Rural Women's Views of AIDS in Zambia.* Hampshire: Avebury.

Nabaitu, Januario, Cissy Bachengana, and Janet Seeley. 1994. "Marital Instability in a Rural Population in South-West Uganda: Implications for the Spread of HIV-1 Infection." *Africa* 64 (2): 243–51.

NACP. 1991. "National AIDS Control Programme AIDS Surveillance Report No. 5." Dar es Salaam: United Republic of Tanzania, Ministry of Health.

———. 1992. "National AIDS Control Programme AIDS Surveillance Report No. 6." Dar es Salaam: United Republic of Tanzania, Ministry of Health.

———. 1994. "National AIDS Control Programme HIV/AIDS/STD Surveillance Report No. 8." Dar es Salaam: United Republic of Tanzania, Ministry of Health.

———. 1997. "National AIDS Control Programme HIV/AIDS/STD Surveillance Report No. 12." Dar es Salaam: United Republic of Tanzania, Ministry of Health.

Ndeki, S. S., K. I. Klepp, A. M. Seha, and M. T. Leshabari. 1994. "Exposure to HIV/AIDS Information, AIDS Knowledge, Perceived Risk and Attitudes toward People with AIDS among Primary-School Children in Northern Tanzania." *AIDS Care* 6 (2): 183–91.

New, Charles. 1873. *Life, Wanderings, and Labours in Eastern Africa.* London: Hodder & Stoughton.

Nguma, Justin, M. T. Leshabari, and G. S. Mpangile. 1991. "Perceived Risk and Adoption of Protective Behavior against HIV Infection among Truck Drivers, Casual Laborers, and Post-Secondary School Pupils in Dar es Salaam." Paper presented at the workshop "The Development of the Second Medium Term Plan for AIDS Control in Tanzania," Kibaha.

Nkrumah, F. K., R. G. Choto, J. Emmanuel, and R. Kumar. 1990. "Clinical Presentation of Symptomatic Human Immuno-Deficiency Virus in Children." *Central African Journal of Medicine* 36 (5): 116–20.

Nkya, W. M., S. H. Gillespie, W. Howlett, J. Elford, C. Nyamuryekunge, C. Assenga, and B. Nyombi. 1991. "Sexually Transmitted Diseases in Prostitutes in Moshi and Arusha, N. Tanzania." *International Journal of STD & AIDS* 2 (6): 432–35.

Nkya, W. M. M. M., William P. Howlett, C. Assenga, and B. Nyombi. 1988a. "AIDS in Northern Tanzania: An Urban Disease Model." Paper presented at the Fourth International Conference on AIDS, Stockholm, Jun. 12–16.

———. 1988b. "Seroepidemiology of HIV-1 Infection in the Kilimanjaro Region." In *AIDS and Associated Cancers in Africa*, G. Giraldo, E. Beth-Giraldo, N. Clumeck, M.-R. Gharbi, S. K. Kyalwazi, and G. d. Thé, eds. pp. 61–65. Basel: Karger.

Nkya, W. M. M. M., W. Howlett, B. Nyombi, and C. Assenga. 1987. "AIDS Situation in the Northern Zone of Tanzania." Ms.

Nnko, Soori, and Robert Pool. 1995. "Love, Lust, Deceit and Money: Tanzanian School Pupils and the Discourses of Sex." Paper presented at Ninth International Conference on AIDS and STD in Africa, Kampala.

———. 1997. "Sexual Discourse in the Context of AIDS: Dominant Themes on Sexual Relations among School Children in Mwanza, Tanzania." Paper presented at the workshop "Multi-Partnered Sexuality and Sexual Networking in Eastern and Southern Africa," University of Natal, Durban.

Obbo, Christine. 1988. "Is AIDS Just Another Disease?" In *AIDS 1988: Symposia Papers*, R. Kulstad, ed., pp. 191–98. Washington, DC: American Association for the Advancement of Science.

———. 1991. "The Language of AIDS in Rural and Urban Uganda." *African Urban Quarterly* 6 (1/2): 83–92.

1993. "HIV Transmission through Social and Geographical Networks in Uganda." *Social Science and Medicine* 36 (7): 949–55.

———. 1995. "Gender, Age and Class: Discourses on HIV Transmission and Control in Uganda." In *Culture and Sexual Risk: Anthropological Perspectives on AIDS*, H. ten Brummelhuis and G. Herdt, eds., pp. 79–95. Luxembourg: Gordon & Breach.

O'Connor, Patricia, M. T. Leshabari, and George Lwihula. 1992. "Ethnographic Study of the Truck Stop Environment in Tanzania." Dar es Salaam: Family Health International/AIDSTECH/Muhimbili Medical Center.

Odner, Knut. 1971. "Report on an Archeology Survey on the Slopes of Kilimanjaro." *Azania* 6:131–49.

Orubuloye, I. O., John C. Caldwell, and Pat Caldwell. 1992. "Sexual Networking and the Risk of AIDS in Southwest Nigeria." In *Sexual Behaviour and Networking: Anthropological and Socio Cultural Studies on the Transmission of HIV*, T. Dyson, ed., pp. 283–301. Liège: Editions Derouaux Ordina.

Orubuloye, I. O., Pat Caldwell, and John C. Caldwell. 1993. "The Role of High-Risk Occupations in the Spread of AIDS: Truck Drivers and Itinerant Market Women in Nigeria." *International Family Planning Perspectives* 19 (2): 43–48 and 71.

Packard, Randall M. 1989. *White Plague, Black Labor*. Berkeley: University of California Press.

Packard, Randall M., and Paul Epstein. 1991. "Epidemiologists, Social Scientists, and the Structure of Medical Research on AIDS in Africa." *Social Science and Medicine* 33 (7): 771–94.

Palca, J. 1990. "African AIDS: Whose Research Rules?" *Science* 250:199–201.

Patton, Cindy. 1990. *Inventing AIDS*. New York: Routledge.

Pela, A. Ona, and Jerome Platt. 1989. "AIDS in Africa: Emerging Trends." *Social Science and Medicine* 28 (1): 1–8.

Pellow, Deborah. 1990. "Sexuality in Africa." *Trends in History* 4 (4): 71–96.

Phillips, Andrew, Caroline A. Sabin, Jonathan Elford, Margarita Bofill, George Janossy, and Christine A. Lee. 1994. "Use of CD4 Lymphocyte Count to Predict Long Term Survival Free of AIDS after HIV Infection." *British Medical Journal* 309 (6950): 309–13.

Pickering, H, and H. A. Wilkins. 1993. "Do Unmarried Women in African Towns Have to Sell Sex, or Is it a Matter of Choice?" *Health Transition Review* 3 (supp.): 17–27.

Piot, Peter, Francis A. Plummer, Fred S. Mhalu, Jean-Louis Lamboray, James Chin, and Jonathan M. Mann. 1988. "AIDS: An International Perspective." *Science* 239 (Feb. 5): 573–79.

Piot, Peter, Francis A Plummer, Marie-Ann Rey, Elisabeth N. Ngugi, Christine Rouzioux, Josiah O Ndinya-Achola, Gaby Veracaurteren, Lourdes J. D'Costa, Marie Laga, Herbert Nsanze, Lieve Fransen, David Haase, Guido van der Groen, Robert C. Brunham, Allan R. Ronald, and Françoise Brun-Vézinet. 1987. "Retrospective Seroepidemiology of AIDS Virus Infection in Nairobi Populations." *Journal of Infectious Diseases* 155 (6): 1108–12.

Pollock, Donald. 1996. "Personhood and Illness among the Kulina." *Medical Anthropology Quarterly* 10 (3): 319–41.

Pool, Robert, Mary Masawe, J. Ties Boerma, and Soori Nnko. 1996. "The Price of Promiscuity: Why Urban Males in Tanzania Are Changing Their Sexual Behavior." *Health Transition Review* 6 (2): 203–22.

Preston-Whyte, Eleanor M. 1995. "'Bring Us the Female Condom': HIV Intervention, Gender, and Political Empowerment in Two South African Communities." *Health Transition Review* 5 (supp.): 209–22.

Quinn, Thomas C. 1994. "Population Migration and the Spread of Types 1 and 2 Human Immunodeficiency Viruses." *Proceedings of the National Academy of Sciences* 91 (Mar.): 2407–14.

Ranger, Terence O. 1981. "Godly Medicine: The Ambiguities of the Medical Mission in Southeast Tanzania, 1900–1945." *Social Science and Medicine* 15B:261–77.

Ratliffe, Eric A. 1996. "Self and Society through the Red Light: Changing Identities in the Go-Go Bar and Their Importance in STD/AIDS Control." Paper presented at American Anthropological Association Meetings, San Francisco, Nov. 19–24.

Raum, Otto F. 1939. "Female Initiation among the Chagga." *American Anthropologist* 41: 554–65.

———. 1940. *Chaga Childhood: A Description of Indigenous Education in an East African Tribe.* Oxford: Oxford University Press.

Renne, Elisha P. 1993. "Changes in Adolescent Sexuality and the Perception of Virginity in a Southwestern Nigerian Village." *Health Transition Review* 3 (supp.): 121–33.

Richards, Audrey I. 1956. *Chisungu: A Girls' Initiation Ceremony among the Bemba of Northern Rhodesia.* London: Faber.

Riesman, Paul. 1986. "The Person and the Life Cycle in African Social Life and Thought." *African Studies Review* 29 (2): 71–138.

Rochberg-Halton, Eugene. 1986. *Meaning and Modernity: Social Theory in the Pragmatic Attitude.* Chicago: University of Chicago Press.

Romero-Daza, Nancy. 1993. "Migrant Labor, Multiple Sexual Partners, and Sexually Transmitted Diseases: The Makings for an AIDS Epidemic in Rural Lesotho." Ph.D. diss., State University of New York, Buffalo.

Rosaldo, Michelle. 1980. *Knowledge and Passion: Ilongot Notions of Self and Social Life.* Cambridge: Cambridge University Press.

Rushing, William A. 1995. *The AIDS Epidemic: Social Dimensions of an Infectious Disease.* Boulder, CO: Westview Press.

Rushton, J. Philippe, and Anthony F. Bogaert. 1989. "Population Differences in Susceptibility to AIDS: An Evolutionary Analysis." *Social Science and Medicine* 28 (12): 1211–20.

Rutenberg, Naomi, Ann K. Blanc, and Saidi Kapiga. 1994. "Sexual Behaviour, Social Change, and Family Planning among Men and Women in Tanzania." *Health Transition Review* 4 (supp.): 173–96.

Sabatier, Renee. 1988. *Blaming Others: Prejudice, Race, and Worldwide AIDS.* Philadelphia: New Society Publishers.

Samoff, Joel. 1974. *Tanzania: Local Politics and the Structure of Power.* Madison: University of Wisconsin Press.

Sanders, David, and Abdulrahman Sambo. 1991. "AIDS in Africa: The Implications of Economic Recession and Structural Adjustment." *Health Policy and Planning* 6 (2): 157–65.

Schanz, Johannes. 1913. *"Mitteilungen über die Besiedlung des Kilimandscharo durch die Dschagga und deren Geschichte."* Baessler-Archiv, Supp. 4.

Scheper-Hughes, Nancy, and Margaret Lock. 1987. "The Mindful Body: A Prolegomenon to Future Work in Medical Anthropology." *Medical Anthropology Quarterly* 1 (1): 6–41.

Schoepf, Brooke G. 1988. "Women, AIDS, and Economic Crisis in Central Africa." *Canadian Journal of African Studies* 22 (3): 625–44.

———. 1991a. "Ethical, Methodological and Political Issues of AIDS Research in Central Africa." *Social Science and Medicine* 33 (7): 749–63.

———. 1991b. "Political Economy, Sex and Cultural Logics: A View From Zaire." *African Urban Quarterly* 6 (1/2): 94–106.

———. 1992. "Sex, Gender and Society in Zaire." In *Sexual Behavior and Networking. Anthropological and Socio-Cultural Studies on the Transmission of HIV,* T. Dyson, ed., pp. 353–75. Liège: Editions Derouaux Ordina.

———. 1993a. "Gender, Development and AIDS: A Political Economy and Cultural Framework." *Women and International Development Annual* 3:53–85.

———. 1993b. "The Social Epidemiology of Women and AIDS in Africa." In *Women and HIV/AIDS: An International Resource Book,* M. Berer and S. Ra, eds., pp. 51–54. London: Pandora.

———. 1995. "Culture, Sex Research and AIDS Prevention in Africa." In *Culture and Sexual Risk: Anthropological Perspectives on AIDS,* H. ten Brummelhuis and G. Herdt, eds., pp. 29–52. Luxembourg: Gordon & Breach.

Schoepf, B. G., R. wa Nkera, C. Shoepf, W. Engundu, and P. Ntsomo. 1988. "AIDS and Society in Central Africa: A View from Zaire." In *AIDS in Africa: The Social and Policy Impact,* N. Miller and R. C. Rockwell, eds., pp. 211–29. Lewiston: Edwin Mellen Press.

Seeley, Janet. 1993. "Searching for Indicators of Vulnerability: A Study of Household Coping Strategies in Rural South West Uganda." Entebbe: MRC/ODA Research Programme on AIDS in Uganda.

Seidel, Gill. 1993. "The Competing Discourses of HIV/AIDS in Sub-Saharan Africa: Discourses of Rights and Empowerment vs. Discourses of Control and Exclusion." *Social Science and Medicine* 36 (3): 175–94.

Serwadda, David, Maria J. Wawer, Stanley Musgrave, Nelson K. Sewankambo, Jonathan E. Kaplan, and Ronald H. Gray. 1992. "HIV Risk Factors in Three Geographic Strata of Rural Rakai District, Uganda." *AIDS* (9): 983–89.

Setel, Philip. 1989. "Symbols of a New Disease: AIDS in the Tanzanian Press." Ms.

———. 1991a. "'A Good Moral Tone': Victorian Ideals of Health and the Judgement of Persons in Nineteenth Century Travel and Mission Accounts from East Africa." Working Papers in African Studies No. 150, Boston University African Studies Center.

———. 1991b. "Upside-down and Backwards: Epistemologies of AIDS in the West as Applied to Africa." Ms.

———. 1994. "Power, 'Text,' and the Representation of Historical Consciousness in the Autobiography of Assefa Woldegebriel." *Journal of Narrative and Life History* 4 (3): 193–213.

———. 1995a. "Bo'n Town Life: Youth, AIDS, and the Changing Character of Adulthood in Kilimanjaro, Tanzania." Ph.D. diss., Department of Anthropology, Boston University.

———. 1995b. "The Effect of HIV and AIDS on Fertility in East and Central Africa." *Health Transition Review* 5 (supp.): 179–90.

———. 1995c. "The Social Context of AIDS Education among Young Men in Northern

Kilimanjaro." In *Young People at Risk: Fighting AIDS in Northern Tanzania,* K.-I. Klepp, P. M. Biswalo, and A. Talle, eds., pp. 49–68. Oslo: Scandinavian University Press.

———. 1995d. "The Social Life of My Social Life: Fieldwork and Personal Experience in Northern Tanzania." Ms.

———. 1996. "AIDS as a Paradox of Manhood and Development in Kilimanjaro, Tanzania." *Social Science and Medicine* 43 (8): 1169–78.

———. 1997. "Overcoming Structural Obstacles among Local Implementors Is Key to AIDS Prevention." *World Health Forum* 18 (2): 215–17.

———. 1999a. "The History of Sexually Transmitted Diseases and HIV / AIDS in Africa." In *Histories of Sexually Transmitted Diseases and HIV/AIDS,* P. Setel, M. Lewis, and M. Lyons, eds. Westport, CT: Greenwood.

———. 1999b. "'Someone to Take my Place': Fertility and the Male Life Course among Coastal Boiken, East Sepik Province, Papua New Guinea." In *Fertility and the Male Life Cycle in an Era of Fertility Decline,* C. Bledsoe, S. Lerner, and J. Guyer, eds. Oxford / Liege: Oxford University Press and the International Union for the Scientific Study of Population.

Setel, Philip, and Gertrude Kessy. 1992. "Preliminary Results of a Household Survey on Youth and AIDS in Moshi, Tanzania." Paper presented at the Sixth International Conference on Women and AIDS in Africa, Arusha, Tanzania.

Setel, Philip, Remy Lyimo, Elizabeth Urio, and Frank Mndasha. 1996. "Male Perspectives on Fertility and Fatherhood in Urban Kilimanjaro." Paper presented at annual meeting of the American Anthropological Association, San Francisco, November 20–24.

Setel, Philip, and Sabine Mtweve. 1995. "KIWAKKUKI: A Brief History and Analysis of a Community-Based Response to AIDS." In *Young People at Risk: Fighting AIDS in Northern Tanzania,* K.-I. Klepp, P. M. Biswalo, and A. Talle, eds., pp. 149–64. Oslo: Scandinavian University Press.

Shann, G. N. 1956. "The Early Development of Education among the Chagga." *Tanganyika Notes and Records* 45:21–32.

Shivji, Issa G. 1992. "The Politics of Liberalization in Tanzania: The Crisis of Ideological Hegemony." In *Tanzania and the IMF: The Dynamics of Liberalization,* H. Campbell and H. Stein, eds., pp. 41–58. Boulder, CO: Westview Press.

Silberschmidt, Margarethe. 1992. "Have Men Become the Weaker Sex? Changing Life Situations in Kisii District, Kenya." *Journal of Modern African Studies* 30 (2): 237–53.

Sontag, Susan. 1989. *AIDS and Its Metaphors.* New York: Farrar, Straus & Giroux.

Stahl, Kathleen. 1964. *History of the Chagga People of Kilimanjaro.* London: Mouton.

Stambach, Amy. 1996a. "Kutoa Mimba: Debates about Schoolgirl Abortion in Northern Tanzania." Paper presented at IUSSP seminar "Socio-Cultural and Political Aspects of Abortion from an Anthropological Perspective," Trivandrum.

———. 1996b. "'The Secret Is, There Is No Secret': Thoughts on Chagga Initiation and Ritual Knowledge." Paper presented at American Anthropological Association Meetings, San Francisco, November 19–24.

———. 1998. "'Education is My Husband': Marriage, Gender and Reproduction in Northern Tanzania." In *Women and Education in Sub-Saharan Africa,* M. Bloch, R. Tabachnik, and J. Beoku-Betts, eds., pp. 185–200. Boulder, CO: Lynne Rienner.

Swantz, Marja-Liisa, Ulla-Stina Henricson, and Mary Zalla. 1975. "Socio-Economic Causes of Malnutrition in Moshi District." Dar es Salaam: Bureau of Resource Assessment and Land Use Planning.

Sweat, Michael D., and Julie A. Denison. 1995. "Reducing HIV Incidence in Developing Countries with Structural and Environmental Interventions." *AIDS* 9 (supp.): S251–S257.

Talle, Aud. 1995. "Bar Workers at the Border." In *Young People at Risk. Fighting AIDS in Northern Tanzania,* K.-I. Klepp, P. M. Biswalo, and A. Talle, eds., pp. 18–30. Oslo: Scandinavian University Press.

Tanganyika Health Division. 1963. "Annual Report."

Tanganyika Territory. 1957. Census Part 2. *General African Census, August 1957: Tribal Analysis, Part 1—Territorial, Provincial, District.* Dar es Salaam: Government Printer.

Tanganyika Territory Medical Department. 1950–57. "Annual Report." Dar es Salaam: Government Printer.

Taussig, Michael. 1993. *Mimesis and Alterity: A Particular History of the Senses.* New York: Routledge.

Taylor, Christopher. 1990. "Condoms and Cosmology: The 'Fractal' Person and Sexual Risk in Rwanda." *Social Science and Medicine* 31 (9): 1023–28.

Thomas, Ian D. 1967. "Population Density in Tanzania, 1967." Research Paper No. 5b. Dar es Salaam: BRALUP.

Timaeus, Ian, and Wendy Graham. 1989. "Labor Circulation, Marriage, and Fertility in Southern Africa." In *Reproduction and Social Organization in Sub-Saharan Africa,* R. J. Lesthaeghe, ed., pp. 365–400. Berkeley: University of California Press.

Treichler, Paula. 1987. "AIDS, Homophobia, and Biomedical Discourse: An Epidemic of Signification." In *AIDS: Cultural Analysis and Cultural Activism,* D. Crimp, ed., pp. 31–70. Cambridge: MIT Press.

———. 1989. "AIDS and HIV Infection in the Third World: A First World Chronicle." In *Remaking History: Discussions in Contemporary Culture,* vol. 4, B. K. Kruger and P. Mariani, eds., pp. 31–86. Seattle: DIA Arts Council.

Tripp, Aili Mari. 1989. "Women and the Changing Urban Household Economy in Tanzania." *Journal of Modern African Studies* 27 (4): 601–23.

Trostle, James. 1992. "Introduction: Research Capacity Building in International Health—Definitions, Evaluations and Strategies for Success." *Social Science and Medicine* 35 (11): 1321–24.

Tumbo-Masabo, Zubeida, and Rita Liljeström. 1994. *Chelewa, Chelewa: The Dilemma of Teenage Girls.* Uppsala: Scandinavian Institute of African Studies.

Turner, Bryan S. 1984. *The Body and Society.* Oxford: Basil Blackwell.

Turshen, Meredith. 1984. *The Political Ecology of Disease in Tanzania.* New Brunswick, NJ: Rutgers University Press.

UNAIDS. 1997. "Report on the Global HIV/AIDS Epidemic." Geneva: World Health Organization.

———. 1998. "Report on the Global HIV/AIDS Epidemic." Geneva: World Health Organization.

United Nations. 1994. *AIDS and the Demography of Africa.* New York: United Nations Department for Economic and Policy Analysis.

United Republic of Tanzania. 1992. "1988 Population Census Preliminary Report." Dar es Salaam: Bureau of Statistics, Ministry of Finance, Economic Affairs, and Planning.

———. 1994. "1988 Population Census National Profile: The Population of Tanzania— The Analytical Report." Dar es Salaam: Bureau of Statistics, President's Office, Planning Commission.

van Etten, G. M. 1976. *Rural Health Development in Tanzania.* Assen: Van Gorcum.

van der Straten, A., R. King, O. Grinstead, A. Serufilira, and S. Allen. 1995. "Couple Communication, Sexual Coercion and HIV Risk Reduction in Kigali, Rwanda." *AIDS* 9 (8): 935–44.

van Onselen, Charles. 1982a. *Studies in the Social and Economic History of Witwatersrand, 1886–1914.* Vol 1: *New Babylon.* Harlow: Longman.

———. 1982b. *Studies in the Social and Economic History of Witwatersrand, 1886–1914.* Vol. 2: *New Nineveh.* Harlow: Longman.

Vance, Carole S. 1991. "Anthropology Rediscovers Sexuality: A Theoretical Comment." *Social Science and Medicine* 33 (8): 875–84.

Vasseleu, Cathryn. 1991. "Life Itself." In *Cartographies: Poststructuralism and the Mapping of Bodies and Spaces*, R. Diprose and R. Ferrell, eds., pp. 55–64. St. Leonard: Allen & Unwin.

Vaughan, Megan. 1991. *Curing Their Ills: Colonial Power and African Illness.* Stanford, CA: Stanford University Press.

Volderbing, Paul, and P. T. Cohen. 1990. "Clinical Spectrum of HIV Infection." In *The AIDS Knowledge Base*, P. T. Cohen, M. Sande, and P. Volderbing, eds., sect. 4.1.1. Waltham, MA: Medical Publishing Group.

von Troil, Margaretha. 1992. "Looking for a Better Life in Town: The Case of Tanzania." In *The Urban-Rural Interface in Africa: Expansion and Adaptation*, J. Baker and P. O. Pedersen, eds., pp. 1223–37. Uppsala: Scandinavian Institute of African Studies.

Wallace, Roderick. 1991. "Traveling Waves of HIV Infection on a Low Dimensional 'Socio-Geographic' Network." *Social Science and Medicine* 32 (7): 847–52.

Watney, Simon. 1989. "AIDS, Language and the Third World." In *Taking Liberties. AIDS and Cultural Politics*, E. C. Carter and S. Watney, eds., pp. 183–192. London: Serpent's Tail.

Wawer, M. J., D. Serwadda, S. Musgrave, J. K. Konde-Lule, M. Musagara, and N. K. Sewankambo. 1991. "Dynamics of Spread of HIV-1 Infection in a Rural District of Uganda." *British Medical Journal* 303 (23): 1303–6.

Weinstein, Kia I., Sylvester Ngallaba, Anne R. Cross, and F. M. Mburu. 1995. "Tanzania Knowledge, Attitudes and Practices Survey 1994." Dar es Salaam: United Republic of Tanzania, Bureau of Statistics, Planning Commission.

Weiss, Brad. 1993. "'Buying Her Grave': Money, Movement, and AIDS in North-West Tanzania." *Africa* 63 (1): 19–35.

———. 1996. *The Making and Unmaking of the Haya Lived World: Consumption, Commoditization, and Everyday Practice.* Durham, NC: Duke University Press.

White, Luise. 1990. *The Comforts of Home: Prostitution in Colonial Nairobi.* Chicago: University of Chicago Press.

Wilhelm, J., G. Möhlig, and J. C. Winter. 1982. "Language and Dialect Atlas of Kilimanjaro." In *Recent German Research on Africa: Language and Culture*, Deutsche Forschungsgemeinschaft and the Institute for Scientific Co-operation, ed., pp. 62–68. Tübingen: Institute for Scientific Co-operation.

Wilson, David, Shiela Msimanga, and Ruth Greenspan. 1988. "Knowledge about AIDS and Self-Reported Sexual Behaviour among Adults in Bulawayo, Zimbabwe." *Central African Journal of Medicine* 34 (5): 95–97.

Winter, J. C. 1979. *Bruno Gutmann, 1876–1966: A German Approach to Social Anthropology.* Oxford: Clarendon Press.

Working Group on Demographic Effects of Economic and Social Reversals. 1993. *Demographic Effects of Economic Reversals in Sub-Saharan Africa.* Washington, DC: National Academy Press.

World Bank. 1993. *World Development Report, 1993: Investing in Health.* New York: World Bank/Oxford University Press.

World Health Organization. 1992. "A Study of the Sexual Experience of Young People in Eleven African Countries: The Narrative Research Method." Geneva: World Health Organization, Adolescent Health Programme.

———. 1995. "Acquired Immunodeficiency Syndrome (AIDS): Data as at 15 December 1995." *Weekly Epidemiological Record* 70 (50): 353–54.

Yelvington, Kevin A. 1996. "Flirting in the Factory." *Journal of the Royal Anthropological Institute* 2:313–33.

Zaba, Basia, Ties Boerma, and Tanya Marchant. 1998. "Family Planning in the Era of AIDS: A Social Science Research Agenda." Liège: International Union for the Scientific Study of Population.

Zaba, Basia, and Simon Gregson. 1998. "Measuring the Impact of HIV on Fertility in Africa." *AIDS* 12 (supp. 1): S41–S50.

# Index

abduction. *See* bride capture

abortion: for extramarital pregnancy, 77; as illegal in Tanzania, 177, 267n.31, 271n.45; increase in, 112; as morally forbidden, 123; precolonial, 45; for premarital pregnancy, 115–16; techniques of, 258n.35

adolescence: moral character developing in, 97–100; puberty, 97, 109. *See also* young adults

adultery. *See* marital infidelity

adulthood: circumcision conferring adult status, 37; and the economic collapse of the 1980s, 144–49; the elderly, 97, 265n.8; marriage and *kihamba* ownership, 142; the "whole person," 93–94. *See also* young adults; men; women

affines, 32

Africa: culture blamed for AIDS in, 198–99; incidence of AIDS in, 1, 2; as proving ground for science and technology, 241; sexual intercourse as commonest mode of HIV transmission in, 4; sexuality in, 16–17, 27–28, 237; sexuality responding to sociopolitical changes in, 259n.44; transactional nature of sexual encounters and relationships in, 141–42. *See also* Kenya; Tanzania; Uganda; Zambia; *and other countries and peoples by name*

African District Sanitary Inspectors (ADSIs), 192

age-grade system *(rika):* banana leaves as symbolic of, 255n.14; clan allegiance crosscut by, 33, 253n.4; each grade relinquishing reproduction when a new grade is initiated, 45, 257n.26; and initiation rituals, 37, 39, 256n.18

agnates, 32

Ahlberg, Beth Maina: on AIDS education, 180; on moral regimes in public discourse about sexuality, 122–23; on openness in sexual relationships, 18, 101; on religion and premarital pregnancy, 113; on sexual pleasure, 92; on sexual relationships in Africa, 17, 28

AIDS: age and sex structure in Tanzania, 18–20, *19*; ambiguity and uncertainty in, 218, 220–23; bad moral character associated with, 3, 29, 147; bodies and discourse in study of, 10–14; bodies as icons of disordered desire in, 100; and business, 165–71, 172, 176, 204; characteristics of AIDS patients at Kilimanjaro Christian Medical Centre, *210;* children orphaned by, 82; commercial sex work in transmission of, 120; competing discourses of, 172; confidentiality of patients violated, 219; confusion regarding, 232–35; conspiracy theories of, 239–40; cultural loss associated with, 173; cultural rhetorics of, 234; demographic variables in study of, 5, 251n.4; and desire, 3, 65, 90; development linked with, 146, 234, 237; dislocation linked with, 59–60, 64, 73, 75, 204–5, 211, 222, 233, 234; early cases in Kilimanjaro Region, 84; early epidemiology in Tanzania, 18–22; early cultural experience of, 219–32; and economic conditions, 144–82, 237; emphasizing as matter of reproductive

AIDS (*continued*)
health, 246; as epidemic of signification, 144; euphemisms for, 162–63; and
fertility, 53; gallows humor about, 179;
gender relations eroded by, 77–78;
HIV as precondition for, 4, 251n.2;
imagined sexual mores in discourse
about, 28; incidence in Africa, 1, 2; incidence globally, 2; as "Juliana," 204,
240; knowledge and expectation in
early responses to, 210–19; marriage affected by, 131; mean latency period of,
19; medico-moral discourse on, 172–75;
mobility associated with, 60, 148, 198,
208; and moral character, 3, 29, 90–
91, 93, 172–73; moral demographies
and, 55–59; and oral demography of
Chagga, 50; the "othering" of, 149, 215,
233; as paradox of gender and development, 87; people's responses to in
Kilimanjaro, 178–80; and personhood,
14–18, 90; and poverty, 237, 275n.1;
projections of epidemic's effects, 21–
22; promiscuity associated with, 174,
184, 212; recognition as a new illness,
260n.4; reporting problems in Tanzania, 18–19, 273n.17; research on associated with development sector, 24; and
secrecy in sexual relationships, 103;
self-testing for, 179, 271n.49; sentinel
surveillance programs, 19–20, 206,
252n.19, 274n.21; and sexuality, 14–18,
145; shunning people with, 221–22; significations of and the bodies of young
adults, 183–87; signs of, 185, 211; slang
names for, 145, 204, 240; and social reproduction, 2, 21, 233, 236; sociogeographic networks in spreading, 203,
208, 273n.16; stories and rumors about,
20, 186; towns and markets associated
with, 153–63; and sexual culture, 140–
43; urban disease model of, 197–204;
and wasting syndromes, 218; women's
response to, 86–88; and work, 163–65;
young people and, 87–88. *See also*
AIDS education; HIV; risk
AIDS education: AIDS patients in, 219–
20; criticisms of, 176–77; on desire and
character and AIDS, 90, 93; expatriate
women in, 175, 219; at Kilimanjaro
Christian Medical Centre, 208, 274n.20;
as limited by circumstance, 22; Lu-

theran Health Education Department
workshops, 77; Moshi drop-in center,
14; pragmatics of, 180–82; signifying
risk in AIDS control messages, 171–82;
skepticism about messages of, 212
Ainsworth, Martha, 19, 22, 202
*akili*, 94, 164
alcohol, 98
anal intercourse, 122, 174, 257n.28
anal plug. See *ngoso*
Arusha (Tanzania): Chagga men employed in, 67, 68, 71; HIV risk and
relationship status in, 84, 265n.43;
and urban disease model of AIDS,
200; young people migrating to,
153

bad moral character (*tabia mbaya*): in adolescents, 97–98; AIDS associated with,
3, 29, 147; business associated with,
153; in children, 95; excessive desire
associated with, 59; as individual response to social forces, 58
Bailey, B. T., 189, 192
banana plant, symbolism of, 255n.14
bank tellers, 166, 167, 168
barmaids, 120–22; as core transmitter
group, 208; HIV seroprevalence
among, 206, *207*; low status of, 165; in
male-female relationship matrix, *104*
Barnett, Tony, 21, 163, 186, 203, 212
Barongo, Longin R., 20, 83, 85, 86, 200,
203
beer belly (*kitambi*), 170–71, 174, 196
Bété, 218
betrothal, 47–48, 259n.42
biomedicine: as an African healing practice, 242, 245; contested place of, 240–
46; and culture, 102, 246–47; and development, 196; power and appeal in the
colonial era, 187–97; in social experience of AIDS epidemic, 21
birth control, 45
birth spacing, 45, 46, 258n.34
black market (*magendo*), 147, 148, 156
Blaikie, Piers, 21, 163, 186, 203, 212
Bledsoe, Caroline, 10, 130
blood, 36, 48
blood donors: HIV seroprevalence
among, 206, *207*; as sentinel group,
19–20, 206, 252n.20, 274n.21
blood transfusion, 251n.3

bodies: AIDS transforming into icons of disordered desire, 100; the Body in anthropological theory, 11, 252n.13; Chagga conceiving as social, 36; Chagga ritual focusing on, 41; Chagga using in cultural interpretation, 35; cultural dimension of, 246–47; homologies between *vihamba* and, 256n.24; ideology in definition of, 16; moral demographies relating personhood and, 56–57; and personhood, 11, 56–57, 90; as qualisigns, 57; sexuality as the cultivation of embodiment, 140–43; significations of AIDS and the bodies of young adults, 183–87; in study of AIDS, 10–14

bride capture, 47, 48, 92, *106*, 128, 260nn. 49, 50

bridewealth *(ngosa)*: affines and, 32; bar transactions as parody of, 122; commercial aspect of, 141; example of, 140; group nature of, 259n.41; and *ngoso,* 258n.40; as obstacle to marriage, 175–76, 271n.42; patrikin providing, 33, 47; payment of, 47, 259n.42

Bukoba (Tanzania), 86, 211

Burundi, incidence of AIDS in, 2

business: AIDS associated with, 165–71, 172, 176, 204; as antithesis of work, 165; bad *tabia* and *tamaa* associated with, 153; in local accounts of AIDS transmission, 147–48; *mitumba* trade, 132, 160; in Moshi Rural and Urban Districts, *151*; as most common occupation in Moshi, 268n.6; *wahuni* associated with, 165–71; women in, 75, 99, 134, 154. *See also* informal sector; markets

Caldwell, John C., 5, 17, 28, 54, 91, 92

Caldwell, Pat, 5, 17, 28, 54, 91, 92

Caraël, Michel, 52, 84, 86, 201

cash (money), 61, 62, 98–99, 166, 211, 261n.15, 274n.22

casual labor, 122, 264n.30

Chagga: and biomedicine, 187–97, 242; the body conceived as social by, 36; the body used in cultural interpretation by, 35; chiefdoms of, 44, 253n.2; coffee cultivation, 263n.24; as conventional term, 253n.2; on cultural loss, 50, 58; demographic tradition of, 27; descent among, 253n.6; on disease, 188;

employment in health care, 194–95; individualism among, 255n.16; initiation rituals, 37–41; interdependence of dominant and subordinate elements in, 34, 254n.10; inward-looking censure emerging in, 148; *mangis,* 59, 66, 195; modernity as contradictory for, 3; nostalgia over decline of culture and tradition, 50; origins of, 44; precolonial population dynamics and growth, 41–46; prostitution among, 148; recession of the 1980s, 75–76, 144–49; returning home to die, 206; slave trading among, 45, 258n.36; therapeutic knowledge among, 255n.13; wide distribution of, 68. *See also* children; *kihamba* regime; Kilimanjaro Region; men; women; young adults

Chagga Medical Executive Committee, 196, 272n.10

children: AIDS leaving orphaned, 82; colonial imagery in play of, 62; cursing of, 271n.3; grandparents in socializing of, 35, 41; imitation in development of, 35–36, 41, 254n.11; development of moral character in, 94–97; rituals for, 95; of "the market," 158–59, 269n.15

Christianity, 57–58, 61, 113, 127, 130, 261n.8

church, the, as AIDS education source, 178

church weddings, *108,* 130

circumcision, female, 36, 40, 92, 256n.19, 267n.53

circumcision, male 38–39; adult status and sexual rights conferred by, 37; symbolism of, 36

cities. *See* towns

civil weddings, *108,* 130

Cleland, John, 83, 103, 201

clitoridectomy, 36, 40, 92, 256n.19, 267n.53

Clyde, David F., 189–90, 194, 258n.38

coffee cultivation, 49, 51, 61, 66, 149, 262n.24

cohabiting relationships, 85, *108,* 129, 132, 265n.44, 266n.19

colonialism: African disease ecology shifting due to, 51–52; demographic pressures as due to, 41–42; scientific colonialism, 241; *tamaa* and, 60–61, 261n.15

Comaroff, Jean, 16, 189, 242